A Practical Approach to Regional Anesthesiology and Acute Pain Medicine

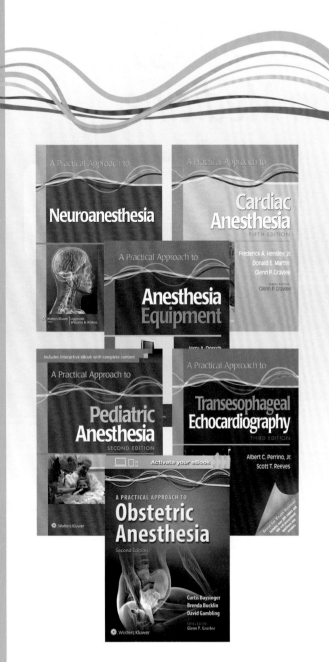

A Practical Approach to Regional Anesthesiology and Acute Pain Medicine

Fifth Edition

Editors

JOSEPH M. NEAL, MD
Anesthesiology Faculty
Department of Anesthesiology
Virginia Mason Medical Center
Seattle, Washington

DE Q.H. TRAN, MD, FRCPC
Professor
Department of Anesthesiology
Montreal General Hospital
McGill University
Montreal, Québec, Canada

FRANCIS V. SALINAS, MD
US Anesthesia Partners-Washington
Department of Anesthesiology
Staff Anesthesiologist
Swedish Medical Center
Swedish Orthopedic Institute
Seattle, Washington

Editor of the Previous Editions

MICHAEL F. MULROY, MD
Emeritus Faculty Anesthesiologist
Department of Anesthesiology
Virginia Mason Medical Center
Seattle, Washington

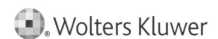

Wolters Kluwer

Philadelphia · Baltimore · New York · London
Buenos Aires · Hong Kong · Sydney · Tokyo

Acquisitions Editor: Keith Donnellan
Development Editor: Kristina Oberle
Editorial Coordinator: Emily Buccieri
Marketing Manager: Dan Dressler
Production Project Manager: David Orzechowski
Design Coordinator: Holly McLaughlin
Manufacturing Coordinator: Beth Welsh
Prepress Vendor: S4Carlisle Publishing Services

Fifth Edition

9 8 7 6 5 4 3 2 1

Printed in China

Library of Congress Cataloging-in-Publication Data

Names: Neal, Joseph M., editor. | Tran, De Q.H. editor. | Salinas, Francis
V., editor.
Title: A practical approach to regional anesthesiology and acute pain
medicine / editors, Joseph M. Neal, De Q.H. Tran, Francis V. Salinas.
Other titles: Practical approach to regional anesthesia.
Description: 5th edition. | Philadelphia: Wolters Kluwer Health, [2018] |
Preceded by Practical approach to regional anesthesia / Michael F. Mulroy
... [et al.]. 4th ed. 2009. | Includes bibliographical references and index.
Identifiers: LCCN 2017024590| ISBN 9781469896830 (pbk.) | ISBN 1469896834 (pbk.)
Subjects: | MESH: Anesthesia, Conduction | Pain, Postoperative—drug therapy
| Acute Pain—drug therapy | Anesthetics—therapeutic use |
Analgesics—therapeutic use | Handbooks
Classification: LCC RD84 | NLM WO 231 | DDC 617.9/64–dc23 LC record available at
https://lccn.loc.gov/2017024590

CCS0817

Dedication

To my wife Kay and children Erin and Pete for their love and patience, to my friends throughout the regional anesthesia community, and to my Virginia Mason colleagues, residents, and fellows—each of you have taught me more than you can ever imagine.
Joe Neal

For Drs. Quang Hieu Tran, Le Thu Dinh, Silvia Duong, and Mr. Tadao Ando
De Tran

I would like to thank my wife Joanne and my children Alex, Brandon, and Cameryn for their love, support, and inspiration. I would also like to express my heartfelt gratitude to both Dr. Mulroy and Dr. Neal, who have been my teachers, mentors, role-models, colleagues, and most of all great friends.
Francis Salinas

In memory of our departed colleagues
Christopher M. Bernards, MD and Daniel C. Moore, MD

Contributors

Julian Aliste, MD
Clinical Instructor
Department of Anesthesiology
Hospital Clinico Universidad de Chile
University of Chile
Santiago, Chile

Ki J. Chin, MBBS (Hons), FRCPC
Associate Professor
Department of Anesthesia and Pain
Management
University Health Network
Toronto Western Hospital
Toronto, Ontario, Canada

Roderick J. Finlayson, MD, FRCPC
Professor
Department of Anesthesia
Montreal General Hospital
Montreal, Quebec, Canada

Andrew T. Gray, MD, PhD
Professor
Department of Anesthesia and
Perioperative Care
Zuckerberg San Francisco General
Hospital
University of California, San Francisco
San Francisco, California

Michael D. Herrick, MD
Assistant Professor of Anesthesiology
Department of Anesthesiology
Dartmouth-Hitchcock Medical Center
Geisel School of Medicine at Dartmouth
Lebanon, New Hampshire

Rebecca L. Johnson, MD
Assistant Professor of Anesthesiology
Department of Anesthesiology
Mayo Clinic College of Medicine
Rochester, Minnesota

Monica Liu, MBChB, FRCA
Fellow
Department of Anesthesia and Pain
Management
Toronto Western Hospital
University Health Network
Toronto, Ontario, Canada

Edward R. Mariano, MD, MAS (Clinical
Research)
Professor of Anesthesiology, Perioperative
and Pain Medicine
Department of Anesthesiology
Stanford University School of Medicine
Chief, Anesthesiology and Perioperative
Care Service
Veterans Affairs Palo Alto Health Care
System
Palo Alto, California

Susan B. McDonald, MD
Vice President for Medical Affairs
Sentara RMH Medical Center
Harrisonburg, Virginia

Kathleen L. McGinn, MD
Clinical Instructor
Department of Anesthesiology,
Perioperative
and Pain Medicine
Lucile Packard Children's Hospital
Stanford University
Stanford, California

Michael F. Mulroy, MD
Emeritus, Anesthesiology Faculty
Department of Anesthesiology
Virginia Mason Medical Center
Seattle, Washington

Joseph M. Neal, MD
Anesthesiology Faculty
Department of Anesthesiology
Virginia Mason Medical Center
Seattle, Washington

Christine L. Oryhan, MD
Anesthesiology Faculty
Associate Director, Pain Medicine
Fellowship
Department of Anesthesiology and Pain
Medicine
Virginia Mason Medical Center
Seattle, Washington

Francis V. Salinas, MD
US Anesthesia Partners-Washington
Department of Anesthesiology
Staff Anesthesiologist
Swedish Medical Center
Swedish Orthopedic Institute
Seattle, Washington

Brian D. Sites, MD, MS
Professor of Anesthesiology and
Orthopedic Surgery
Department of Anesthesiology
Dartmouth-Hitchcock Medical Center
Geisel School of Medicine at Dartmouth
Lebanon, New Hampshire

De Q.H. Tran, MD, FRCPC
Professor
Department of Anesthesiology
Montreal General Hospital
McGill University
Montreal, Québec, Canada

Kevin E. Vorenkamp, MD
Anesthesiology Faculty
Director, Pain Medicine Fellowship
Department of Anesthesiology and Pain
Medicine
Virginia Mason Medical Center
Seattle, Washington

Preface to the Fifth Edition

The fifth edition of **A Practical Approach to Regional Anesthesiology and Acute Pain Medicine** commemorates and celebrates many milestones apropos to a textbook that has been in continuous publication for nearly 30 years. Our friend, colleague, and mentor Michael F. Mulroy, MD was the sole author for the first (1989) and second (1996) editions of *Regional Anesthesia: An Illustrated Procedural Guide*. For the third edition, Dr. Mulroy remained the primary author and editor, but brought on contributors for pediatric regional anesthesia and chronic pain medicine. The fourth edition (2009) became part of Wolters Kluwers' *Practical Approach* series and introduced three coeditors, all Virginia Mason Medical Center colleagues and former trainees of Dr. Mulroy—Christopher M. Bernards, MD, Susan B. McDonald, MD, and Francis V. Salinas, MD.

The interval between the fourth and fifth editions marked notable passages. From the book's beginnings, Dr. Mulroy's inspiration was his colleague Daniel C. Moore, MD, the founding member of the Virginia Mason Clinic Department of Anesthesiology and the author of several textbooks including *Regional Block*, which was considered by many during the 1950s through the early 1980s as the quintessential regional anesthesia textbook. Few anesthesiologists of any generation matched the influence of Dan Moore on his department, the practice of regional anesthesia, and anesthesiology worldwide. Dr. Moore died in 2015, just three days shy of his 97th birthday. Our friend and colleague Chris Bernards died in January 2012 at the age of 53. His contributions to pharmacology and pharmacokinetics have shaped regional anesthesia and pain medicine and will continue to do so for many years. With our greatest respect and admiration, we dedicate this fifth edition to our departed and sorely missed colleagues Chris Bernards and Dan Moore.

The eight years between the fourth and fifth edition also witnessed remarkable changes in regional anesthesia and acute pain medicine, so much so that we have changed the book's title to **A Practical Approach to Regional Anesthesiology and Acute Pain Medicine** to reflect this evolution. As this book was being prepared, the Accreditation Council for Graduate Medical Education approved Regional Anesthesiology and Acute Pain Medicine as the newest anesthesiology fellowship. Other major developments include ultrasound guidance as the preferred nerve localization tool for peripheral nerve blocks, and health care delivery changes that endorse the concept of the perioperative surgical home and the regional anesthesiologist/acute pain medicine physician's opportunity to assume a leadership role in these changes. The evolution of other anesthesiology specialties prompted us to retire topics that have surpassed their traditional regional anesthesia roots, such as obstetrical anesthesia, chronic pain medicine, and their related blocks. In their place, we have expanded our discussions of truncal blocks, systems-based practice, and acute pain medicine. Concurrent with the focus on ultrasound-guided techniques we have expanded and updated illustrations relevant to these procedures. Throughout the book we have strived to maintain a balanced approach to indications, complications, and techniques, while maintaining a focused, outlined template to enhance readability and consistency across chapters. As it has always been, this book does not intend to be a comprehensive treatise on regional anesthesia. Many books and atlases written by colleagues that we admire and respect serve that purpose. To paraphrase the preface to the fourth edition, ". . .the book aspires to be a concise and practical manual for both beginning learners of the subspecialty and those more experienced, such that all will find it a resource to expand their understanding, dexterity, and comfort with regional anesthesia and all of its postoperative benefits."

Dr. Mulroy retired from clinical practice in 2014, but his inspiration and involvement are omnipresent. Our colleague Susan McDonald has taken on new challenges in medical administration. Thus, Drs. Neal and Salinas are delighted to welcome De Q.H. Tran, MD, FRCPC as coeditor. We have known Dr. Tran since his fellowship at Virginia Mason, and are extremely proud of his significant contributions to academic regional anesthesiology. As past and current coeditors, we gratefully acknowledge the significant contributions of the Wolters Kluwer/Lippincott Williams & Wilkins team of Acquisitions Editor Keith Donnellan, Development Editor Kristina Oberle, Editorial Coordinator Emily Buccieri, and Senior Project Manager Jeethu Abraham. Likewise, we are most grateful for the previous edition artwork of Jennifer Smith, along with new illustrations that the American Society of Regional Anesthesia and Pain Medicine commissioned from Jennifer Gentry.

Joseph M. Neal, MD
De Q.H. Tran, MD, FRCPC
Francis V. Salinas, MD

Contents

1

Regional Anesthesia Systems

Edward R. Mariano

KEY POINTS

1. Health-care is about value, not volume. Every new program or service will be evaluated based on its value contribution.

2. The American Society of Anesthesiologists (ASA) has proposed a physician anesthesiologist–led, patient-centered model known as the Perioperative Surgical Home (PSH) that coordinates this process. Regional anesthesiology and acute pain medicine (RAAPM) is an essential component of this model.

3. There are two compelling reasons for starting a RAAPM system: curbing perioperative opioid use and improving the patient experience.

4. Despite start-up costs, RAAPM may be the catalyst that promotes cost-saving processes within a hospital.

5. Clinical pathways, sometimes referred to as enhanced recovery protocols, can be nested within the PSH model and can decrease costs for joint replacement surgery by streamlining the surgical process and minimizing variability.

(continued)

6. A RAAPM program should promote fall prevention education for patients who receive a lower extremity peripheral nerve block, with special emphasis on the joint replacement population. These blocks facilitate early mobility after surgery, which decreases the incidence of other hospital-acquired conditions (e.g., pressure ulcers, deep venous thrombosis).

7. When feasible, the use of a block room to allow parallel processing of surgical patients eligible for regional anesthesia decreases anesthesia-controlled turnover time and thereby increases patient access to regional anesthesia procedures.

8. Proper documentation and coding are essential for capturing eligible charges and quantifying work, and should be developed in collaboration with the billing service.

9. Home management of patients with perineural catheter requires special consideration and proper patient selection but does not have to be overly burdensome.

10. The role of acute pain medicine has evolved beyond a catheter management service; prevention and treatment of acute pain requires a multidisciplinary, team-based, multimodal approach.

THE CLINICAL PRACTICE OF REGIONAL ANESTHESIA has evolved into modern-day regional anesthesiology and acute pain medicine (RAAPM). This medical subspecialty continues to change based on new health-care initiatives, technological advances, and scientific breakthroughs in understanding pain mechanisms and the human body's responses to pain and pain relief. The use of regional analgesia techniques for pain management is typically combined with systemic nonopioid analgesics in a multimodal approach (1). When setting up a RAAPM system, one must first understand the context in which a new system will be developed, the practical aspects of initiating a new service line, and trends that may direct the system's future goals.

I. **Value, not volume.** Health-care systems stress value and not volume—every new program or service will be evaluated based on its value contribution. **According to the Triple Aim for health, the three primary goals of any health-care program should be to improve the patient experience, reduce costs of care, and advance population health** (2). Anesthesiology practice itself is evolving with the emergence of large anesthesia groups and multispecialty national health-care companies. Competition for contracts creates demand for innovation and value. "Value-based purchasing" (3) is a program designed by the Centers for Medicare and Medicaid Services (CMS) to encourage "better outcomes, patient outcomes, and innovations (4)." Value, according to CMS, is composed of three domains—clinical processes, patient experience, and outcomes (mortality rates)—which align well with the Triple Aim (4). Data related to these domains are publicly available and comparable across health-care institutions consistent with the Institute of Medicine's recommendation to make health-care performance data more transparent for consumers (5).

II. **The Perioperative Surgical Home.** From the perspective of a patient or family member, the process of undergoing surgery, from the decision to schedule until full recovery, can be an incredibly disjointed and intimidating one. **The American Society of Anesthesiologists (ASA) has proposed a physician anesthesiologist-led, patient-centered model, known as the Perioperative Surgical Home (PSH) that coordinates this process** (6). To date, there are few practical models of PSH to follow but most depend on the existence of a RAAPM program (7,8). For a PSH model to be accepted within a health-care system, the example set by a functioning RAAPM program is essential. **The patient's experience of pain is woven throughout the perioperative period** (9). RAAPM encompasses preoperative preparation of the anticipated difficult pain patient (e.g., high-dose opioids or chronic pain at baseline), the coordination of intraoperative anesthesia care and postoperative pain management through clinical pathways (10), and the transition of analgesic regimens from inpatient to outpatient.

III. **Rationale for a RAAPM system.** Using value as a starting point and considering the societal issues affecting health-care priorities, **there are two compelling reasons for starting a RAAPM system: curbing perioperative opioid use and improving the patient experience**.

    A. **Opioid crisis.** The crisis of prescription opioid overuse and abuse has affected countries around the world; anesthesiologists are ideally positioned to make positive changes toward reversing this trend (11). **Even minor outpatient surgical procedures, and their associated anesthesia and analgesia techniques, can lead to long-term opioid use** (12). It is impossible to predict which opioid-naïve patients are predisposed to developing chronic opioid use postoperatively. Patients who present for surgery with an active opioid prescription are very likely to still be on opioids after a year (13). A RAAPM program that coordinates inpatient and outpatient pain management can make a difference in patient outcomes. **Regional analgesia, especially continuous peripheral nerve block techniques, has been shown to reduce the need for opioid analgesia in the acute postoperative period** (14).

    B. **Patient experience.** Effective expectation management is a primary determinant of patient satisfaction. Patients wish to avoid nausea, vomiting, and most importantly pain (15), which has a particularly strong influence on overall patient experience. Indeed, seven of the CMS survey questions relate to pain (3), and this theme of effective pain management is expected to persist into the future. Opioid-sparing regional analgesic techniques that provide targeted pain control with minimal side effects will play a crucial role in creating a more positive patient experience. **The optimal duration of regional analgesia continues to be studied, but current evidence demonstrates advantages of continuous over single-injection techniques in terms of overall pain control, opioid requirements, and patient-reported satisfaction** (16).

IV. **Hospital cost considerations.** Nearly half the costs of providing care for the hospitalized surgical patient are fixed (17); the remaining variable costs may be influenced by care models. **Despite associated start-up costs, RAAPM may be the catalyst that promotes cost-saving processes within a hospital.**

    A. **Clinical pathways.** Clinical pathways, such as those for joint replacement surgery, decrease hospitalization costs. **Coordinated perioperative pain management that includes regional analgesic techniques is a key component of these protocols** (18). Also called **enhanced recovery protocols, clinical pathways can be nested within the PSH model and decrease costs by streamlining the surgical process and minimizing variability** (19). The advantage of a PSH is that it provides stable oversight and leadership for clinical pathway development and continuous improvement (10).

    B. **Postoperative complications.** Postoperative complications also influence hospitalization costs. Certain postoperative "hospital-acquired conditions" (HACs) are ineligible for payment by CMS. **Examples of HACs include catheter-associated urinary tract infection, surgical-site infection after orthopedic surgery, inpatient falls and trauma, hospital-acquired pressure ulcers, and deep venous thrombosis or pulmonary embolism** (20). The incidence of HACs after joint replacement is estimated to be 1.3% and may cost hospitals a collective 70 million dollars annually (20). HACs are also considered within the clinical processes domain of value-based purchasing (4). Although use of regional anesthesia and analgesia may not directly prevent HACs, evidence suggests that certain techniques such as neuraxial anesthesia may be associated with a lower rate of inpatient falls (21) and postoperative infection (22), and the use of peripheral nerve blocks has not been shown conclusively to increase fall risk (21). **Moreover, a comprehensive RAAPM program should incorporate fall prevention for patients undergoing lower extremity peripheral nerve blocks, especially the joint replacement population** (23). Regional analgesia-facilitated early mobility after surgery may indirectly decrease the incidence of pressure ulcers, blood clots, and the need for continuous urinary bladder catheterization. Joint replacement surgery represents an important target for health-care cost reduction programs given the increasing number of new joint replacements per year (24).

> **CLINICAL PEARL**   Fall prevention takes a multipronged approach: increasing patient and family education and awareness regarding fall risk; instituting a standard fall risk assessment tool (e.g., Morse fall scale); and improving communication among team members through alert systems (e.g., colored wrist bands, signs, bed alarms; Fig. 1.1) (23).

   C. Hospital length of stay. A RAAPM program may influence length of hospitalization in joint replacement patients who depend on achievement of physical therapy goals to meet discharge criteria (25). **Shorter length of stay may offer cost savings but may also risk increasing readmission rates after joint replacement** (26). The target hospital length of stay is institution-specific and should take into account the patient population served, post-discharge resources available to patients, availability of on-call physicians, and timeline for serious complications based on type of surgery.

How *high* is your risk for *falling*?

- ⬤ High risk for falls
- ◯ Moderate risk for falls
- ◯ Low risk for falls

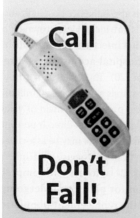

Call

Don't Fall!

- **Call for help** if you need to use the bathroom
- Wear **non-skid socks** at all times
- Use your **cane** or **walker**
- Ask to have your bedside table **within your reach**
- **Call for help** if you need to get out of bed
- If you are moderate to high risk, your **bed alarm** will be turned on to let us know that you need help

If you want more information on Fall Prevention, educational pamphlets are available at the nurses' station and upon request.

FIGURE 1.1   Example of a communication tool to help promote fall risk awareness and prevent falls.

D. **Outpatient length of stay.** For ambulatory surgery patients, postoperative nausea and vomiting and poorly controlled pain can prolong postanesthesia care unit (PACU) discharge time (27). **Regional anesthesia techniques can decrease the incidence of these adverse events and, thus, the time to meet discharge criteria.** If a step-down or phase II recovery unit is available, patients who receive regional anesthesia may be able to bypass PACU and go directly to phase II, which can also result in cost savings by reducing nursing costs (28).

E. **Operating room efficiency.** One of the great concerns when starting a RAAPM program is the potential negative effect on operating room efficiency. **Surgeons raise concerns regarding the potential for failed blocks, complications, and case delays** (29). Certain aspects of patient preparation (e.g., education, consent) may be performed before the day of surgery to decrease delays (30,31). The model of regional anesthesia delivery may influence efficiency on the day of surgery. **For example, parallel processing of surgical patients eligible for regional anesthesia (i.e., performing blocks before surgery in a separate area while the previously scheduled case is underway in the operating room) has the potential to decrease anesthesia-controlled turnover time and increase patient access to regional anesthesia procedures** (32).

V. **Practical tips for regional anesthesia**

A. **Block room.** For certain practices, setting up a dedicated induction area for regional anesthesia procedures outside the operating room may make sense. A block room need not be dedicated fully to RAAPM but rather may be shared with the preoperative patient holding area or PACU (Fig. 1.2) (31). The space enhances parallel processing by allowing performance of regional anesthesia procedures before surgery. Having a dedicated block room staff for all RAAPM procedures and consults is one staffing paradigm (7,8), but may not be feasible for all settings depending on case volume, staffing, and availability of other resources. The block room model may be ideal when the same anesthesiologist performs both the block and the intraoperative anesthetic, thereby facilitating block placement while the operating room is being turned over. **The block room represents a**

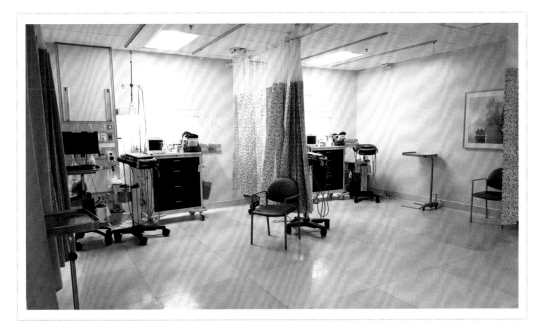

FIGURE 1.2   A regional anesthesia induction area or block room with standard monitoring, oxygen source, resuscitation equipment, and regional anesthesia supplies.

common area to store regional anesthesia supplies (see Chapter 2) and equipment (e.g., ultrasound machines, nerve stimulators, and positioning devices). If this space is regularly used for RAAPM procedures, common supplies (e.g., needles, catheter kits, gowns, gloves, hats, and masks) may be stored on shelves or in cabinets in the block room. Medications may be stored in a lockable mobile "block cart" that can be shared between more than one procedural space. The number of ultrasound machines needed for a block room depends entirely on the expected number and frequency of procedures to be performed; high-volume centers with multiple simultaneous procedures may require one ultrasound machine per bay ideally. Each procedural space should also have a dedicated computer terminal loaded with the institution's anesthesia record keeping system and electronic medical record (EMR), when applicable.

   B. Logistics. An efficient system requires advance planning and good communication. For teaching hospitals, greater efficiency equates to more time for training residents and fellows in RAAPM procedures. **To save time on the day of surgery, a RAAPM team member (e.g., physician, advanced practice provider, or nurse) can counsel eligible patients by phone the night before.** Patients for RAAPM procedures should be identified in advance on the operating room schedule, with explicit notification of the clerical staff members who check patients in and perioperative nursing staff. In academic programs, performing RAAPM procedures outside the operating room while the previous surgery is still underway allows the most time for teaching without negatively affecting efficiency but does require a block room model with either a resident or fellow outside the operating room dedicated only to RAAPM or a facilitator to relieve the trainee temporarily from operating room duties.

CLINICAL PEARL   Dedicated nursing staff for RAAPM or a resource nurse assigned daily to prepare RAAPM patients will help facilitate the process of preoperative patient preparation on the day of surgery by regularly communicating with the front desk during the day and getting patients for RAAPM procedures ready as soon as they arrive.

   C. Set-up. A nurse or advanced practice provider may set up a tray of supplies and medications before the procedure, apply monitors, insert the peripheral intravenous catheter, participate in the preprocedural time-out, and administer intravenous sedation when appropriate. In terms of ergonomics, the ultrasound machine should be placed directly across from the performing physician (Fig. 1.3). The tray of supplies and medications is best located on the performer's dominant side to avoid contaminating the sterile field. The patient should be optimally positioned for the block to be performed, and the bed height should be adjusted so the performing physician's elbows are bent at approximately 90 degrees.

   D. Safety systems. Regional anesthesia procedures need to be performed in a safe environment, either in the operating room or in a dedicated procedural area. All patients should be monitored according to ASA standards: pulse oximetry, electrocardiogram, and noninvasive blood pressure. **If intravenous sedation is administered, a second clinician (e.g., physician, advanced practice provider, or nurse) must be present to monitor the patient.** A continuous oxygen supply and variety of delivery systems must be available as well as suction, resuscitation, and advanced airway management equipment in case of emergency. **Before performing each regional anesthesia procedure, the anesthesiologist must conduct a preprocedural time-out that entails confirmation (with the patient himself/herself as well as a second clinician) of the patient's identity, allergies, planned surgical procedure as verified by a consent form, planned block procedure with laterality and site marking, and availability of medications and equipment; the time-out process is facilitated by the bedside posting of a cognitive aid (e.g., time-out checklist** (33)**; Fig. 1.4).** One special rescue medication that must be available wherever regional anesthesia procedures are performed is lipid emulsion for local anesthetic systemic toxicity (34).

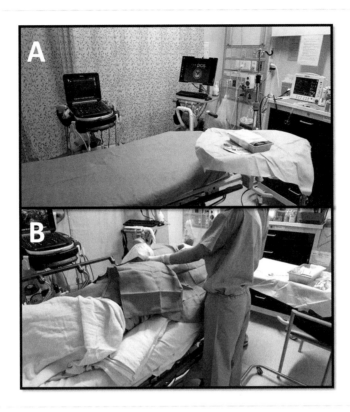

FIGURE 1.3   Equipment set-up demonstrating optimal ergonomics: **(A)** before the procedure and **(B)** during the procedure.

E. **Training and implementation.** Despite evidence supporting the efficacy of regional anesthesia techniques in perioperative pain management, the penetrance continues to be low. Even for common procedures like total knee replacement, only one in four patients receives a nerve block (35). The advent of ultrasound guidance in regional anesthesia has led to standardized training guidelines (36) that have been incorporated into residencies and/or simulation-based training programs for practicing anesthesiologists (37). A successful system requires more than just well-trained clinical staff. It takes physician leadership and a culture open to continuous improvement (10).

F. **Documentation. Proper documentation and coding are essential for capturing eligible charges and quantifying work**. The former influences practice income, whereas the latter may be used to justify the hiring of additional personnel. For regional anesthesia procedures performed for acute pain management, a standardized procedure note separate from the anesthesia record is recommended (31), either in paper form or as a template in the EMR. A standardized EMR template or procedure note may also facilitate proper coding of procedures and application of modifiers. Current Procedural Terminology (CPT) codes are changed and/or added every year, so forms must be regularly reviewed and updated as necessary.

CLINICAL PEARL   The practice's billing manager or external billing company should be involved in the development of standardized documentation for regional anesthesia procedures and acute pain medicine consults (31).

VA Palo Alto Health Care System
Regional Anesthesia Procedure Checklist

Pre-Procedure Patient Safety Briefing:
(Conducted by Anesthesiology Attending, Fellow, or Resident M.D.)

☐ Identify patient by confirming full name and SSN.
☐ Verify that a valid IMED Consent is in the chart.
* If the patient is scheduled for surgery, a separate informed consent for the regional anesthesia procedure is not necessary.
* If the patient is NOT having surgery but a regional anesthesia procedure is indicated, a separate informed consent for the regional anesthesia procedure needs to be completed.
☐ Confirm regional anesthesia procedure site is marked by M.D.

TIME OUT STOP (Performed immediately prior to procedure by Anesthesiology Attending, Fellow, or Resident M.D.)

☐ ALL Activity Stopped for Time Out.

☐ Patient Name: _____ SSN:_____
☐ Procedure: _____
☐ Site/Side:_____
☐ Allergies: _____
☐ Confirm Pre-Procedure Patient Safety Briefing is Complete.

FIGURE 1.4   Sample cognitive aid for performing a time-out before regional anesthesia procedures.

9   G. **Outpatient perineural catheter management.** The management of perineural catheter in patients at home requires special considerations. First, not all patients are good candidates for outpatient catheters, so proper patient selection is a key. Phone calls may be made by a physician, advanced practice provider, or nurse with referral back to a RAAPM physician in the event of any issues or concerns. Patients should have a caretaker (e.g., friend or family member) immediately available. The caretaker may be able to see the catheter site better than the patient in certain anatomical locations (e.g., interscalene) and can report pertinent information to the regional

anesthesiologist. Outpatient with perineural catheter should receive written instructions for the portable infusion device, catheter removal, and information about common and uncommon issues associated with perineural catheter maintenance. Many of these common issues can be addressed by preemptively calling patients later in the evening on the day of surgery; patients can easily become overwhelmed with the quantity of information received. Finally, patients should have the direct contact number of a regional anesthesiologist who will be available 24 hours a day. Currently, there is no evidence in the published literature to support limiting patient selection for ambulatory perineural infusion based on distance from the hospital alone; however, individual practices may have their own criteria.

CLINICAL PEARL The ambulatory perineural catheter patient needs to have a reliable phone number for daily follow up from a regional anesthesiology team member until catheter removal (nearly all patients are comfortable removing their own perineural catheters) (38).

VI. **Emergence of acute pain medicine.** There is a clear need for acute pain medicine specialists. The most recent guidelines for fellowship training combine regional anesthesiology with acute pain medicine. **The role of acute pain medicine has evolved beyond merely a catheter management service, and the prevention and treatment of acute pain often take a multidisciplinary, team-based, multimodal approach.** Acute pain medicine consultation may involve the treatment of an acutely ill patient on the medical service suffering from a sickle cell crisis or pancreatitis. Another growing role for acute pain physicians is the coordination of care for hospitalized patients on high doses of opioids, chronic pain syndromes, and complex analgesic regimens including buprenorphine–naloxone, which is growing in popularity as a substance abuse deterrent. Initial and follow-up consultations for acute pain are categorized as evaluation and management services with dedicated CPT codes. Proper coding and billing for consults and procedures may help justify the development of an acute pain medicine program. Physician specialists in RAAPM can take the lead in developing enhanced recovery protocols for surgical patients as well as other clinical pathways that provide better coordination of the perioperative process and improve patient outcomes.

CONFLICTS OF INTEREST

Dr. Mariano has received unrestricted funding for educational programs paid to his institution from Halyard Health (Alpharetta, GA) and B. Braun (Bethlehem, PA). These companies had no input in any aspect of the present book chapter.

REFERENCES

1. Chou R, Gordon DB, de Leon-Casasola OA, et al. Management of Postoperative Pain: A Clinical Practice Guideline From the American Pain Society, the American Society of Regional Anesthesia and Pain Medicine, and the American Society of Anesthesiologists' Committee on Regional Anesthesia, Executive Committee, and Administrative Council. *J Pain* 2016;17(2):131–157.
2. Berwick DM, Nolan TW, Whittington J. The triple aim: care, health, and cost. *Health Aff (Millwood)* 2008;27(3):759–769.
3. Mariano ER, Miller B, Salinas FV. The expanding role of multimodal analgesia in acute perioperative pain management. *Adv Anesth* 2013;31(1):119–136.
4. Center for Medicare and Medicaid Services. *Hospital Value-Based Purchasing.* Washington, DC: Department of Health and Human Services; 2012.
5. Institute of Medicine. *Best Care at Lower Cost: The Path to Continuously Learning Health Care in America.* Washington, DC: National Academies Press; 2012.

6. Kain ZN, Vakharia S, Garson L, et al. The perioperative surgical home as a future perioperative practice model. *Anesth Analg* 2014;118(5):1126–1130.
7. Walters TL, Howard SK, Kou A, et al. Design and implementation of a perioperative surgical home at a veterans affairs hospital. *Semin Cardiothorac Vasc Anesth* 2016;20(2):133–140.
8. Garson L, Schwarzkopf R, Vakharia S, et al. Implementation of a total joint replacement-focused perioperative surgical home: a management case report. *Anesth Analg* 2014;118(5):1081–1089.
9. Walters TL, Mariano ER, Clark JD. Perioperative surgical home and the integral role of pain medicine. *Pain Med* 2015;16(9):1666–1672.
10. Mudumbai SC, Walters TL, Howard SK, et al. The Perioperative Surgical Home model facilitates change implementation in anesthetic technique within a clinical pathway for total knee arthroplasty. *Healthc (Amst)* 2016;4(4):334–339.
11. Alam A, Juurlink DN. The prescription opioid epidemic: an overview for anesthesiologists. *Can J Anaesth* 2016;63(1):61–68.
12. Sun EC, Darnall BD, Baker LC, et al. Incidence of and risk factors for chronic opioid use among opioid-naive patients in the postoperative period. *JAMA Intern Med* 2016;176(9):1286–1293.
13. Mudumbai SC, Oliva EM, Lewis ET, et al. Time-to-cessation of postoperative opioids: a population-level analysis of the veterans affairs health care system. *Pain Med* 2016;17(9):1732–1743.
14. Richman JM, Liu SS, Courpas G, et al. Does continuous peripheral nerve block provide superior pain control to opioids? A meta-analysis. *Anesth Analg* 2006;102(1):248–257.
15. Macario A, Weinger M, Carney S, et al. Which clinical anesthesia outcomes are important to avoid? The perspective of patients. *Anesth Analg* 1999;89(3):652–658.
16. Bingham AE, Fu R, Horn JL, et al. Continuous peripheral nerve block compared with single-injection peripheral nerve block: a systematic review and meta-analysis of randomized controlled trials. *Reg Anesth Pain Med* 2012;37(6):583–594.
17. Macario A, Vitez TS, Dunn B, et al. Where are the costs in perioperative care? Analysis of hospital costs and charges for inpatient surgical care. *Anesthesiology* 1995;83(6):1138–1144.
18. Webb CA, Mariano ER. Best multimodal analgesic protocol for total knee arthroplasty. *Pain Manag* 2015;5(3):185–196.
19. Raphael DR, Cannesson M, Schwarzkopf R, et al. Total joint Perioperative Surgical Home: an observational financial review. *Perioper Med (Lond)* 2014;3:6.
20. Duchman KR, Pugely AJ, Martin CT, et al. Medicare's hospital-acquired conditions policy: a problem of nonpayment after total joint arthroplasty. *J Arthroplasty* 2016;31(9 Suppl):31–36.
21. Memtsoudis SG, Danninger T, Rasul R, et al. Inpatient falls after total knee arthroplasty: the role of anesthesia type and peripheral nerve blocks. *Anesthesiology* 2014;120(3):551–563.
22. Liu J, Ma C, Elkassabany N, et al. Neuraxial anesthesia decreases postoperative systemic infection risk compared with general anesthesia in knee arthroplasty. *Anesth Analg* 2013;117(4):1010–1016.
23. Kim TE, Mariano ER. Developing a multidisciplinary fall reduction program for lower-extremity joint arthroplasty patients. *Anesthesiol Clin* 2014;32(4):853–864.
24. Laucis NC, Chowdhury M, Dasgupta A, et al. Trend toward high-volume hospitals and the influence on complications in knee and hip arthroplasty. *J Bone Joint Surg Am* 2016;98(9):707–712.
25. Capdevila X, Barthelet Y, Biboulet P, et al. Effects of perioperative analgesic technique on the surgical outcome and duration of rehabilitation after major knee surgery. *Anesthesiology* 1999;91(1):8–15.
26. Cram P, Lu X, Kates SL, et al. Total knee arthroplasty volume, utilization, and outcomes among Medicare beneficiaries, 1991–2010. *JAMA* 2012;308(12):1227–1236.
27. Chung F, Mezei G. Factors contributing to a prolonged stay after ambulatory surgery. *Anesth Analg* 1999;89(6):1352–1359.
28. Williams BA, Kentor ML, Vogt MT, et al. Economics of nerve block pain management after anterior cruciate ligament reconstruction: potential hospital cost savings via associated postanesthesia care unit bypass and same-day discharge. *Anesthesiology* 2004;100(3):697–706.
29. Oldman M, McCartney CJ, Leung A, et al. A survey of orthopedic surgeons' attitudes and knowledge regarding regional anesthesia. *Anesth Analg* 2004;98(5):1486–1490.
30. Brooks BS, Barman J, Ponce BA, et al. An electronic surgical order, undertaking patient education, and obtaining informed consent for regional analgesia before the day of surgery reduce block-related delays. *Local Reg Anesth* 2016;9:59–64.

31. Mariano ER. Making it work: setting up a regional anesthesia program that provides value. *Anesthesiol Clin* 2008;26(4):681–692, vi.

32. Chazapis M, Kaur N, Kamming D. Improving the Peri-operative care of Patients by instituting a 'Block Room' for regional anaesthesia. *BMJ Qual Improv Rep* 2014;3(1).

33. Mulroy MF, Weller RS, Liguori GA. A checklist for performing regional nerve blocks. *Reg Anesth Pain Med* 2014;39(3):195–199.

34. Neal JM, Mulroy MF, Weinberg GL. American Society of Regional Anesthesia and Pain Medicine checklist for managing local anesthetic systemic toxicity: 2012 version. *Reg Anesth Pain Med* 2012;37(1):16–18.

35. Gabriel RA, Kaye AD, Nagrebetsky A, et al. Utilization of femoral nerve blocks for total knee arthroplasty. *J Arthroplasty* 2016;31(8):1680–1685.

36. Sites BD, Chan VW, Neal JM, et al. The American Society of Regional Anesthesia and Pain Medicine and the European Society Of Regional Anaesthesia and Pain Therapy Joint Committee recommendations for education and training in ultrasound-guided regional anesthesia. *Reg Anesth Pain Med* 2009;34(1):40–46.

37. Mariano ER, Harrison TK, Kim TE, et al. Evaluation of a standardized program for training practicing anesthesiologists in ultrasound-guided regional anesthesia skills. *J Ultrasound Med* 2015;34(10):1883–1893.

38. Ilfeld BM, Esener DE, Morey TE, et al. Ambulatory perineural infusion: the patients' perspective. *Reg Anesth Pain Med* 2003;28(5):418–423.

2 Equipment

Andrew T. Gray

KEY POINTS

1. Nerve stimulation can be used to locate peripheral nerves for regional blocks. Short-duration impulses (0.1 ms) are effective in stimulating motor fibers, whereas long-duration impulses (0.3 ms) will also stimulate sensory fibers.

2. Electrically insulated needles have a high current density at the tip. This allows more precise identification of peripheral nerves.

3. Needle tip visibility on ultrasound scans depends on a number of factors, including needle diameter and the angle of insertion.

4. Small volumes of injected saline or local anesthetic (e.g., 1 mL) can be used to help identify the needle or catheter tip with ultrasound imaging.

5. A smooth piece of metal (a test tool) can be used to detect functional lines of insonation from an ultrasound transducer when the scan head is covered with a thin layer of gel.

I. General principles

A. Regional anesthesia techniques can be performed with almost any syringe and needle. Success depends more on knowledge of anatomy and the operator's skill set than the quality of the instruments. Nevertheless, selection of proper equipment can optimize the performance of regional anesthesia techniques.

II. Block trays

A. Equipment for regional blocks is usually stocked in prepared sterile trays. The latter usually contain skin-preparation swabs, drapes, needles, syringes, solution cups, and a sterility indicator. The choice of equipment will be dictated by the specific blocks attempted and by personal preference. However, some general comments are warranted. Concern about infectious diseases, especially newer ones that are resistant to conventional sterilization techniques, has created a greater reliance on **disposable equipment**. The quality of disposable trays has improved, and the willingness of the manufacturers to *"customize"* trays to the needs of individual institutions is widespread. They remove the burden of sterilization from the local department or hospital (but not the responsibility of checking for sterility).

III. Peripheral nerve stimulators

A. Peripheral nerve stimulators deliver a pulsed electric current to a needle. As the latter approaches a nerve, depolarization is produced. Efferent motor nerves (A-α fibers) are most easily depolarized, so these devices confer the distinct benefit of identifying mixed peripheral nerves by producing muscular contraction rather than eliciting uncomfortable sensory paresthesiae.

B. **The degree of stimulation depends on the total current (amperage) and (presumably) the distance between the current source and the nerve.** This principle led to the development of nerve stimulators with variable outputs. A high current (approximately 1 to 2 mA) can be used to confirm that the needle is approaching a nerve. A progressively lower current may document increasing proximity between the needle and a nerve. In practice, 2 mA will produce depolarization of a motor nerve at a distance. As the needle is moved closer to the nerve, a smaller current suggests adequate proximity to the latter. However, recent reports have challenged the relationship between the current and neural proximity, bringing into question whether any correlation can be assumed. Specifically, needles in direct contact with nerves (based on paresthesiae) may require currents from 0.1 mA to greater than 1 mA in order to produce an evoked motor response, so the relevance of the final stimulating current remains unclear (1). Current practice suggests that a current of 0.5 mA is ideal, but adequate anesthesia can be produced with greater and lesser stimulating currents.

C. The characteristics of the stimulating current can also be modified to produce a sensory response. **The short-duration impulse commonly used (0.1 ms) is effective in stimulating motor fibers, but a longer duration pulse (0.3 ms) will also stimulate sensory fibers, a useful feature if a pure sensory nerve (e.g., lateral femoral cutaneous or saphenous nerve) is being sought.**

D. The ideal nerve stimulator possesses a variable linear output with a clear display of current delivered. The positive (red, anode) lead of the stimulator is connected to a skin electrode (the anatomic location of the anode does not influence stimulation). The negative (black, cathode) lead is attached to the exploring needle. The connection can be secured with an "alligator"-type clamp, but commercial needles with electrical connectors incorporated into their design are more commonly used. **Cathodal stimulation via the needle is approximately twice as efficient as anodal stimulation, so lead polarity is important.**

E. **Electrically insulated (sheathed, Teflon-coated) needles concentrate more current at the needle tip, thus causing neural depolarization to decrease after the needle tip passes the nerve.** In contrast, noninsulated needles can continue to stimulate the target nerve with their shafts even when the needle tips have moved beyond the neural target. Therefore, although more expensive, insulated needles constitute the criterion standard for neurostimulation-guided nerve blocks. Injection of a small volume of local anesthetic (1 mL, the Raj test) will eliminate the evoked response when the needle tip is adjacent to the nerve target. This is because of dissipation of the current density at the needle tip and depends on the ionic strength of the injectate (2).

F. Nerve stimulators do not provide a substitute for knowledge of anatomy and proper initial needle placement. They will only help document the proximity of the needle to the nerve. Although it is speculated that their use may reduce the potential for nerve damage, no study has shown an increased safety margin with nerve stimulators, because nerve injuries can still occur despite their use. Thus neurostimulators do not eliminate the risk of nerve injury when blocks are performed on unconscious adults.

CLINICAL PEARL   A basic understanding of peripheral nerve stimulator functions and limitations optimizes their usefulness to the regional anesthesiologist.

IV. Ultrasound machines (Fig. 2.1)

A. Ultrasound imaging allows direct visualization of peripheral nerves. Ultrasound machines have been critically evaluated for their ability to meet the needs of regional anesthesiologists (3). Several features have been identified as important to ergonomics and overall ease of use.

B. The start-up time (from power on to readiness for scanning) is important in a busy practice, particularly if the machine requires an uninterrupted power source rather than battery life. Screen size, positioning (swivel, articulating arm, etc.), and angle can influence image viewing. **Basic image quality controls (adjustment of depth, receiver gain, and probe selection)** are critical to assessment of a machine. Expectedly, novices prefer a relatively straightforward user interface (3).

C. Many commercial ultrasound machines are now marketed with nerve imaging presets so that fewer adjustments of imaging quality control are necessary in clinical practice. Most important is the identification of nerve fascicles. Machines and transducers can be evaluated on live models for their ability to resolve the fine layers of collagen that divide peripheral nerves into neural fascicles (i.e., the fascicle count). When evaluating ultrasound equipment, it is important to control for factors that influence image interpretation (e.g., the model, the anatomic region and peripheral nerve, room lighting, etc.). The portability of ultrasound machines is paramount for settings where blocks are performed in the induction room, operating room, and recovery room.

V. Transducers (Fig. 2.2A and B)

A. **Ultrasound transducers have an array of piezoelectric crystals that emit and receive sound waves that travel through soft tissues**. A wide variety of transducers are available for clinical imaging purposes. Transducer selection is critical for optimal regional anesthesia imaging.

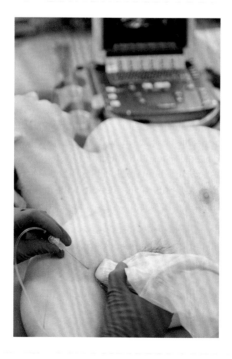

FIGURE 2.1 Ultrasound machine for regional anesthesia. In this figure, a laptop platform has been positioned for an axillary block.

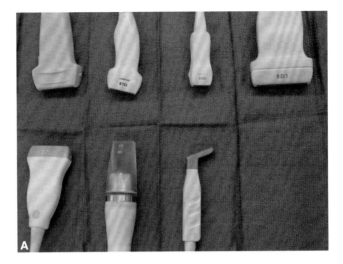

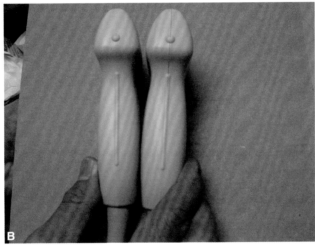

FIGURE 2.2   **A:** Ultrasound transducers for nerve blocks. A wide variety of transducers are available with different sizes in footprint (i.e., the length of the active face of the transducer). **B:** Transducer damage. A crack in the seam of an ultrasound transducer is shown (*right*). For comparison, an intact transducer is shown (*left*).

B. Most practitioners use **linear arrays** with a large footprint for regional blocks. These transducers contain a large number of crystals (elements) for high-resolution imaging of peripheral nerves and a broad field of view. For deeper blocks or blocks that require a larger viewing field (such as neuraxial, lumbar plexus, and parasacral/subgluteal/anterior sciatic blocks), **curved arrays** are often used.

C. Higher insonation **frequencies** allow better imaging quality (smaller wavelength). However, **attenuation** of sound waves is frequency dependent. It is particularly important to select the highest frequency that will allow sound waves to travel to the target and back to the transducer. Increasing the receiver gain remains a poor remedy when the insonation frequency is too high, because it results in amplification of the background noise. There exists considerable variation in attenuation among patients and anatomic regions. As an approximate guide, the penetration depth (cm) is 60/center frequency (MHz) (4). For example, a transducer with a center frequency of 10 MHz has a penetration depth of 6 cm.

VI. Doppler (Fig. 2.3)

A. Most ultrasound machines possess a **variety of Doppler imaging modalities** that allow detection of blood flow. Power Doppler (integration of the power spectrum of the Doppler shift) is particularly useful for the detection of small arteries that accompany peripheral nerves. Power Doppler displays significant advantages over traditional color Doppler (5). It is more sensitive (by a factor of 3 to 5 in some cases), exhibits less angle dependence, and there has no aliasing of the signals. Aliasing arises when the signal is off scale because of undersampling from too low pulse repetition frequency. The potential disadvantages of power Doppler stem from the absence of directional information and the high sensitivity to motion (resulting in flash artifact). Power Doppler appears to be the best current Doppler modality to detect intraneural blood flow (6). Many practitioners prescan (scout imaging) with power Doppler to detect adjacent blood vessels prior to the performance of regional blocks.

VII. Spatial compound imaging (Fig. 2.4)

A. With conventional sonography, tissue is insonated from a single direction. With spatial compound sonography, images are obtained from several different imaging angles and combined into a single image at real-time frame rates (7). Only a portion of the field of imaging receives all the different lines of sight (this region is triangular in shape for linear arrays).

B. Spatial compound images are formed when the ultrasound beam is directed at a set of angles from each element in the transducer. This technology reduces angle-dependent artifacts (such as acoustic shadowing and enhancement) and can improve needle tip visibility over a limited range of insertion angles (8). **A test tool (a smooth paper clip or solid metal stylet work well) can be used to detect the lines of insonation from a transducer when the scan head is covered with a thin layer of gel** (9).

C. **Spatial compound imaging confers significant advantages for regional anesthesia and musculoskeletal imaging** (10). This imaging technology allows trapezoidal formatting of the displayed image, thereby providing a wider view for a given transducer footprint. Although commonly applied to linear arrays, spatial compound imaging is currently being developed for curved arrays as well.

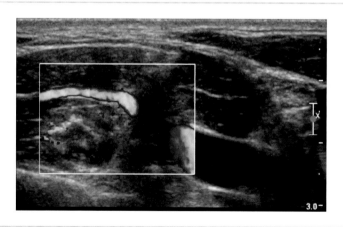

FIGURE 2.3   Power Doppler imaging. In this figure, duplex power Doppler imaging is shown during interscalene block. A large dorsal scapular artery crosses the brachial plexus in the interscalene groove.

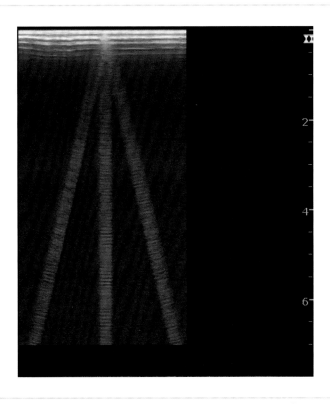

FIGURE 2.4 Spatial compound imaging. In this figure, a linear array test tool image is used to reveal three lines of sight for spatial compound imaging.

VIII. Acoustic coupling and transducer covers (Fig. 2.5)

A. Air must be excluded from the transducer–skin interface for adequate sound transmission to soft tissues (acoustic coupling). The author recommends sterile, single-use gel packs to minimize the risk of infection and cross-contamination, although extremely low rates of block-related infection have been reported (11,12).

B. A number of studies have examined whether gel contamination can promote nerve injury in animal models (13). Although it is unclear if functional deficits can occur, our practice is to remove excess gel from the needle entry site using sterile dry gauzes. Gel removal is particularly important when ultrasound is used for neuraxial blocks to avoid gel entrainment into the epidural or subarchnoid space. When peripheral nerve catheters are placed using ultrasound guidance, one must remove all gel from the field prior to securing the catheter. A number of gel substitutes have been studied: for instance, dextrose (D5W) appears to have favorable acoustic properties (14). Sterile transducer cover substitutes include gloves or adhesive dressings (15).

CLINICAL PEARL   A thorough appreciation of ultrasound physics, machine adjustments, and limitations allows the practitioner to maximize his or her ability to effectively localize nerves and accurately inject drugs around them.

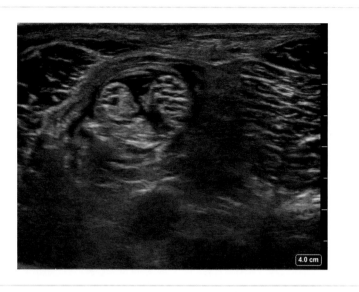

FIGURE 2.5   Neural imaging with ultrasound (acoustic coupling with sterile gel and transducer cover). The two major branches of the sciatic nerve in the popliteal fossa (the tibial and common peroneal nerves) are shown. The fascicular architecture of the nerves can be easily appreciated after a subparaneural popliteal sciatic nerve block.

IX. **Echogenic needles** (Fig. 2.6A and B)

A. Conventional needles are composed of smooth stainless steel. **Because of the marked acoustic impedance mismatch with soft tissue, these needles will strongly reflect ultrasound waves if the latter strike the shaft perpendicularly (i.e., when the needles are placed parallel to the skin surface and the active face of the transducer).** However, when the needles are inserted at an angle with the ultrasound beam, the returning echoes from the needle tip diminish (16). Thus, a number of important technologies have been developed to improve needle tip echoes from block needles.

B. Echogenic needles display textured surfaces. Patterns include diffuse roughness (sandblast), dimple, sawtooth, "X" etchings, cubic corners, and so on. Some of these patterns are believed to specifically promote reflection back to the transducer wave source regardless of angle (retroreflection technology). Other needles are coated with polymers that trap air on their surface, thereby enhancing sound wave reflection.

C. The best assessment of echogenic needles is carried out under clinical conditions rather than with tissue equivalent phantoms (which often optimize imaging). Use of echogenic needles may decrease procedural time. However, given the low incidence of adverse events, a reduction in the latter can be been difficult to demonstrate.

D. Several **additional strategies can be used to improve needle tip visibility**. Small volume test injections (0.5 to 1 mL) can help identify the needle tip. The transducer can be rocked back to improve the angle of insonation with the needle. Larger diameter needles can be easier to visualize, especially for deeper blocks. Rotating the needle so that its bevel faces the transducer can help identify the cut on the bevel. Gentle movement of the needle (slight to-and-fro movement) also improves visibility of its tip.

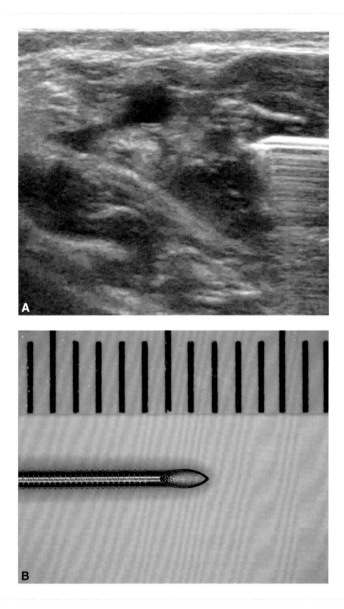

FIGURE 2.6 A: Needle imaging during in-plane approach to axillary block. In this figure, a conventional stainless steel needle approaches near parallel to the active face of the transducer. The cut on the bevel is clearly identified. Reverberation artifact from the shaft walls is observed but does not extend to the bevel opening at the tip. **B:** Close-up photograph of an echogenically modified needle. The surface of the needle shaft has been textured to enhance received echoes near the tip.

   X. **Echogenic catheters** (Fig. 2.7)

       A. For perineural catheter placement, more homogenous procedural times have been reported with ultrasound guidance compared to neurostimulation. A number of perineural catheters kits are currently marketed, including catheter through needle and catheter over needle designs. There exists a wide range of echogenicity among commercial catheters (17,18).

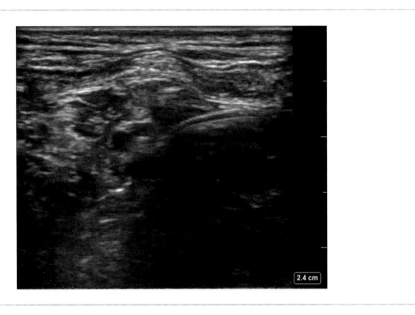

FIGURE 2.7 Catheter imaging for continuous interscalene block. The dark lumen and echogenic walls of the catheter are identified. The catheter tip is not evident in the field of imaging.

B. Catheter tips can be difficult to identify with ultrasound imaging. Visualization of the dark lumen between the echogenic walls of the catheter constitutes the best method for lumen identification (parallel white lines) (19). Catheter coils often display a serpentine appearance on ultrasound scans.

C. Injection of small volumes of saline or air (0.5 to 1 mL) can help identify the catheter tip (20,21). The priming volume of the catheter is often sufficient for the air test. Injecting saline or local anesthetic through an unprimed catheter is an excellent way to perform a catheter air test. Some practitioners also administer agitated dextrose (D5W) while imaging with color Doppler to identify the catheter tip (22,23). Manually moving an inner guide wire back and forth can also enhance catheter visibility on color Doppler or M-mode sonography (24).

D. A number of new echogenic designs for perineural catheters are under development. Metallic reinforcement of the catheter walls or metallic inner stylet can improve catheter visibility on ultrasound scans. The clinical impact of these new designs and the predictive value of the aforementioned test injections are currently being studied. Three-dimensional ultrasound has been used as a tool to guide and evaluate peripheral nerve catheter placement.

CLINICAL PEARL No localization technique (nerve stimulation or ultrasound) has been shown to reduce the chance of nerve injury after regional block.

XI. Infusion devices

A. Anesthesiologists have become actively involved in the prolongation of regional techniques for pain relief in the postoperative period. There exist several continuous infusion devices available for local anesthetic delivery.

B. For inpatients, small electrically driven pumps can provide a continuous infusion of local anesthetic as well as a patient-controlled option that allows supplemental doses at times of increased need. These devices are individually programmable and demonstrate a high degree of flexibility. They also possess a lockout interval to prevent excessive intake by the patients. Because mechanical failure is rare, these pumps are highly effective for inpatient postoperative analgesia.

C. Several modalities are available for outpatient local anesthetic infusion.

1. The simplest devices are **elastomeric bulbs** that contain a fixed amount of local anesthetic under a constant pressure, which is then delivered at a fixed rate through a flow valve connected to the catheter. These pumps can provide continuous perineural infusions for 24 to 60 hours for both upper and lower extremity analgesia. The main limitation associated with elastomeric pumps stems from the fixed delivery rate. However, newer devices can provide on-demand boluses for breakthrough pain.

2. There exist **spring-loaded mechanical pumps** that are similar to elastomeric pumps in their simplicity. They also rely on a constant tension to deliver the solution, and have been equipped with bolus capability.

3. Alternatively, **small battery-operated, programmable, mechanical pumps** are available. They provide the same options as the inpatient devices: in addition to a continuous infusion, they can also deliver on-demand boluses. Again, mechanical problems with these pumps are rare and they appear to provide a useful option for prolonging postoperative analgesia in outpatients.

CONFLICTS OF INTEREST

Dr. Gray discloses involvement with Smiths Medical (consulting) and Elsevier-Saunders (royalties).

ACKNOWLEDGMENTS

The author wishes to acknowledge the contribution of Michael F. Mulroy, MD, who authored the chapter on equipment in the previous edition.

REFERENCES

1. Perlas A, Niazi A, McCartney C, et al. The sensitivity of motor response to nerve stimulation and paresthesia for nerve localization as evaluated by ultrasound. *Reg Anesth Pain Med* 2006;31(5):445–450.
2. Tsui BC, Wagner A, Finucane B. Electrophysiologic effect of injectates on peripheral nerve stimulation. *Reg Anesth Pain Med* 2004;29(3):189–193.
3. Wynd KP, Smith HM, Jacob AK, et al. Ultrasound machine comparison: an evaluation of ergonomic design, data management, ease of use, and image quality. *Reg Anesth Pain Med* 2009;34(4):349–356.
4. Szabo TL, Lewin PA. Ultrasound transducer selection in clinical imaging practice. *J Ultrasound Med.* 2013;32(4):573–582.
5. Rubin JM, Bude RO, Carson PL, et al. Power Doppler US: a potentially useful alternative to mean frequency-based color Doppler US. *Radiology* 1994;190(3):853–856.
6. Vanderschueren GA, Meys VE, Beekman R. Doppler sonography for the diagnosis of carpal tunnel syndrome: a critical review. *Muscle Nerve* 2014;50(2):159–163.
7. Wilhjelm JE, Jensen MS, Jespersen SK, et al. Visual and quantitative evaluation of selected image combination schemes in ultrasound spatial compound scanning. *IEEE Trans Med Imaging* 2004;23(2):181–190.
8. Wiesmann T, Borntröger A, Zoremba M, et al. Compound imaging technology and echogenic needle design: effects on needle visibility and tissue imaging. *Reg Anesth Pain Med* 2013;38(5):452–455.
9. Goldstein A, Ranney D, McLeary RD. Linear array test tool. *J Ultrasound Med* 1989;8:385–397.
10. Lin DC, Nazarian LN, O'Kane PL, et al. Advantages of real-time spatial compound sonography of the musculoskeletal system versus conventional sonography. *AJR Am J Roentgenol* 2002;179(6):1629–1631.

11. Provenzano DA, Liebert MA, Steen B, et al. Investigation of current infection-control practices for ultrasound coupling gel: a survey, microbiological analysis, and examination of practice patterns. *Reg Anesth Pain Med* 2013;38(5):415–424.
12. Alakkad H, Naeeni A, Chan VW, et al. Infection related to ultrasound-guided single-injection peripheral nerve blockade: a decade of experience at Toronto Western hospital. *Reg Anesth Pain Med* 2015;40(1):82–84.
13. Pintaric TS, Cvetko E, Strbenc M, et al. Intraneural and perineural inflammatory changes in piglets after inject of ultrasound gel, endotoxin, 0.9% NaCl, or needle insertion without injection. *Anesth Analg* 2014;118(4):869–873.
14. Tsui BC. Dextrose 5% in water as an alternative medium to gel for performing ultrasound-guided peripheral nerve blocks. *Reg Anesth Pain Med* 2009;34(5):525–527.
15. Tsui BC, Twomey C, Finucane BT. Visualization of the brachial plexus in the supraclavicular region using a curved ultrasound probe with a sterile transparent dressing. *Reg Anesth Pain Med* 2006;31(2):182–184.
16. Schafhalter-Zoppoth I, McCulloch CE, Gray AT. Ultrasound visibility of needles used for regional nerve block: an in vitro study. *Reg Anesth Pain Med* 2004;29(5):480–488.
17. McGahan JP. Laboratory assessment of ultrasonic needle and catheter visualization. *J Ultrasound Med* 1986;5:373–377.
18. Mariano ER, Yun RD, Kim TE, et al. Application of echogenic technology for catheters used in ultrasound-guided continuous peripheral nerve blocks. *J Ultrasound Med* 2014;33(5):905–911.
19. Takatani J, Takeshima N, Okuda K, et al. Ultrasound visibility of regional anesthesia catheters: an in vitro study. *Korean J Anesthesiol* 2012;63(1):59–64.
20. Swenson JD, Davis JJ, DeCou JA. A novel approach for assessing catheter position after ultrasound-guided placement of continuous interscalene block. *Anesth Analg* 2008;106(3):1015–1016.
21. Kan JM, Harrison TK, Kim TE, et al. An in vitro study to evaluate the utility of the "air test" to infer perineural catheter tip location. *J Ultrasound Med* 2013;32(3):529–533.
22. Dhir S, Ganapathy S. Use of ultrasound guidance and contrast enhancement: a study of continuous infraclavicular brachial plexus approach. *Acta Anaesthesiol Scand* 2008;52(3):338–342.
23. Brookes J, Sondekoppam R, Armstrong K, et al. Comparative evaluation of the visibility and block characteristics of a stimulating needle and catheter vs an echogenic needle and catheter for sciatic nerve block with a low-frequency ultrasound probe. *Br J Anaesth* 2015;115(6):912–919.
24. Elsharkawy H, Salmasi V, Abd-Elsayed A, et al. Identification of location of nerve catheters using pumping maneuver and M-Mode – a novel technique. *J Clin Anesth* 2015;27(4):325–330.

3. Ultrasound-Guided Regional Anesthesiology

Michael D. Herrick and Brian D. Sites

KEY POINTS

1. Ultrasound technology allows the intimate imaging of nerves, needle, and surrounding structures.

2. Ultrasound images are generated when ultrasound waves reflect off of structures and return to the transducer. The degree to which ultrasound is reflected determines how bright and white the image appears on the display screen.

3. In order to optimize image quality and distinguish neural from non-neural structures, the anesthesiologist should understand machine controls and the underlying basic principles of ultrasound physics.

4. Ultrasound artifacts are common and their recognition is important for maximizing quality and safety of ultrasound-guided regional anesthesia.

THE USE OF ULTRASOUND TO FACILITATE NERVE LOCALIZATION has revolutionized the practice of regional anesthesia. To optimize the benefits of ultrasonography and minimize potential harm, the anesthesiologist should understand several important physical principles of sound energy. Such an understanding should translate into optimization of image quality as well as the appreciation of artifacts and technical limitations.

I. Terminology

It is crucial to understand several ultrasound terms and techniques to appreciate why ultrasound physics is important for generating optimal images in the performance of ultrasound-guided regional anesthesiology.

A. Glossary

1. **Hyperechoic.** Structures that strongly reflect sound waves back to the transducer and appear white on the ultrasound screen.

2. **Hypoechoic.** Structures that weakly reflect sound waves and appear less white on the ultrasound screen.

3. **Anechoic.** Structures that do not reflect sound waves and appear dark on the ultrasound screen.

4. **Attenuation.** The weakening of ultrasound waves as they are transmitted to greater depth.

B. Technique

1. **In-plane.** Insertion of the needle in relation to transducer so that the entire needle can be imaged in its long axis as it enters the body and approaches the target structure (Fig. 3.1). The advantage of this approach is that the entire needle and tip can be visualized and directed away from various non-neural structures such as blood vessels and pleura.

2. **Out-of-plane.** Insertion of the needle in relation to the transducer so that a short-axis (cross-sectional) view of the needle is generated (Fig. 3.1). Only a portion of the needle is visualized with this technique. The out-of-plane technique has the advantage that it mimics

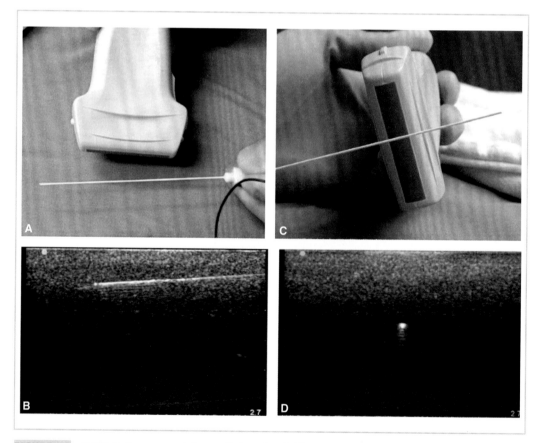

FIGURE 3.1 **A:** The *in-plane approach* for needle insertion. **B:** The corresponding ultrasound needle image for the in-plane approach. **C:** The out-of-plane approach for needle insertion. **D:** The corresponding ultrasound needle image for the out-of-plane approach. (Adapted from Sites BD, Brull R, Chan VW, et al. Artifacts and pitfall errors associated with ultrasound-guided regional anesthesia. Part I: understanding the basic principles of ultrasound physics and machine operations. *Reg Anesth Pain Med* 2007;32:415. Copyright 2007 by Lippincott Williams & Wilkins.)

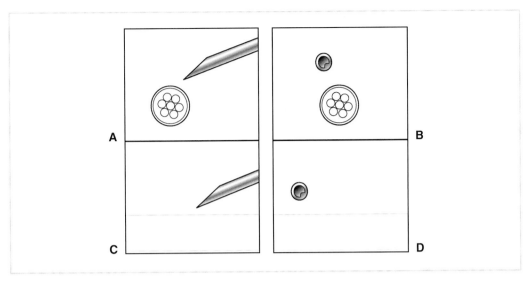

FIGURE 3.2   Various approaches to visualizing the nerve and the needle. **A:** Nerve in cross-section (short-axis) and needle in-plane. **B:** Nerve in short-axis, needle "out-of-plane." **C:** Nerve in longitudinal axis (long-axis) view, needle in-plane. **D:** Nerve in long-axis, needle out-of-plane. (Adapted from Mulroy MF, Bernards CM, McDonald SB, et al. *A Practical Approach to Regional Anesthesia.* 4th ed. Baltimore, MD: Lippincott Williams & Wilkins; 2009. Copyright 2009 by Lippincott Williams & Wilkins.)

conventional approaches to performing nerve blocks and minimizes the amount of tissue that the needle must transgress prior to reaching the target structures.

3. **Short-axis nerve imaging.** In this approach, the nerve is visualized in cross-section (Fig. 3.2). This is the most common approach used to visualize nerves.

4. **Long-axis nerve imaging.** In this approach, the nerve is visualized longitudinally (Fig. 3.2).

CLINICAL PEARL   Axis refers to how the nerve is imaged with the transducer, while the plane technique refers to how the needle is inserted in relation to the image.

II. Ultrasound physics

Prior to adjusting the ultrasound machine interface to optimize image quality, it is helpful to understand how ultrasound waves are generated, how they interact with different tissues in the body, and how an image is generated from the return of ultrasound waves to the transducer.

A. Ultrasound wave generation

An ultrasound wave is generated when an electrical voltage is applied to piezoelectric crystals that are located inside the transducer. When this current is applied to the crystals, it causes them to vibrate and create sound waves that are longitudinally transmitted from the transducer to the patient through a conductive gel (1,2). Each longitudinal sound wave is characterized by compressions (high pressure) and rarefactions (low pressure). **Wavelength** is simply the distance between pressure peaks and **frequency** is the number of pressure peaks per second (Fig. 3.3). **Period** is the time it takes to complete a single cycle of a peak and a trough. The speed of sound in soft tissue is believed to be the constant value of 1,540 m/s (v). Frequency and wavelength are inversely related and together are proportionally related to the speed of sound:

$$1{,}540 \text{ m/s} \sim \text{frequency} \times \text{wavelength}$$

Ultrasound frequencies used in regional anesthesiology typically range from 1 to 15 MHz (1,2).

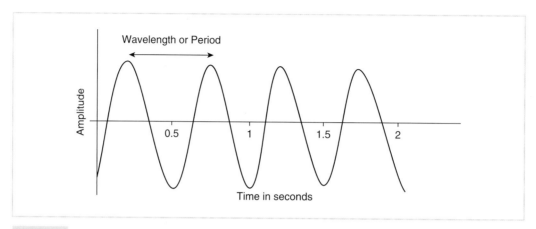

FIGURE 3.3 Depiction of an ultrasound wave. Wavelength is the distance between pressure peaks, and period is the time between pressure peaks. Frequency is the number of pressure peaks per second. In this figure, there are two pressures peaks per second so the frequency would be 2 Hz.

    B. **Interaction with tissues.** The ultrasound waves enter the body and are either transmitted, reflected, scattered, or refracted as they encounter body tissues (Fig. 3.4) (3).

        1. **Transmission.** When ultrasound waves encounter a boundary between two different types of tissue, part of that energy is transmitted through the boundary to interact with deeper

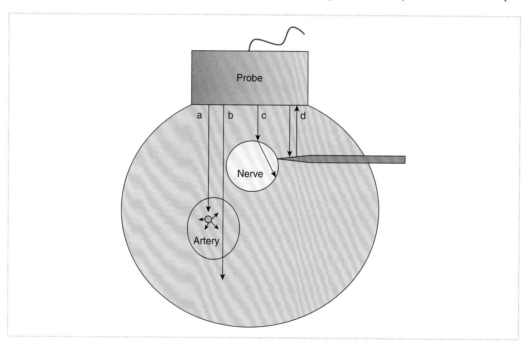

FIGURE 3.4 The many responses that an ultrasound wave produces when traveling through tissue. *(A)* Scatter reflection: the ultrasound wave is deflected in several random directions both to and away from the probe. Scattering occurs with small or irregular objects. *(B)* Transmission: the ultrasound wave continues through the tissue away from the probe. *(C)* Refraction: when an ultrasound wave contacts the interface between two media with different propagation velocities, the ultrasound wave is refracted (bent) depending upon the differences in velocities. *(D)* Specular reflection: reflection from a large, smooth object (such as the needle) which returns the ultrasound wave toward the probe when it is perpendicular to the ultrasound beam. (Adapted from Sites BD, Brull R, Chan VW, et al. Artifacts and pitfall errors associated with ultrasound-guided regional anesthesia. Part I: understanding the basic principles of ultrasound physics and machine operations. *Reg Anesth Pain Med* 2007;32:413. Copyright 2007 by Lippincott Williams & Wilkins.)

tissues. **Attenuation** at deeper depths is caused by reflection, scatter, and absorption. This concept is important to understand when a transducer or transducer setting is selected for different types of blocks. High-frequency transducers are ideal for imaging superficial structures (e.g., interscalene brachial plexus) because they facilitate the best detail and tissue distinction. In ultrasound terminology, high-frequency ultrasound provides better axial and lateral resolution. However, as a result of attenuation, high-frequency ultrasound is limited in its ability to reach deeper structures (e.g., lumbar plexus; Fig. 3.5) (1,2).

CLINICAL PEARL   Most ultrasound machines allow the operator to adjust the emitting ultrasound frequency. Try different settings to see which frequency optimizes your image.

2. **Reflection.** Reflection is the key event that results in the generation of an ultrasound image. Reflection occurs when sound waves encounter a boundary between two tissues that have different acoustic impedances. **Acoustic impedance** is the tendency of a tissue to resist the passage of ultrasound. Interfaces that have large differences in their acoustic impedances (e.g., fluid–soft tissue interfaces) reflect most of the ultrasound wave back to the transducer. For a given interface, reflection is maximized when the ultrasound beam is perpendicular to the target. A **spectral reflector** is a large smooth structure (e.g., a block needle) that acts like a mirror and causes organized sound to be reflected back to the transducer and produces a hyperechoic structure.

3. **Scatter.** Most tissues have a rough service and are called **diffuse reflectors**. They cause the ultrasound beam to scatter in different directions including some that travel back to the transducer and contribute to image generation. Higher frequency transducers cause more scatter compared to their lower frequency counterparts (1,2).

4. **Refraction.** Refraction occurs when an ultrasound wave passes through an interface between two tissues that have slightly different acoustic impedances and changes its trajectory. More refraction occurs when the angle of the ultrasound beam is not perpendicular to the target structures (2).

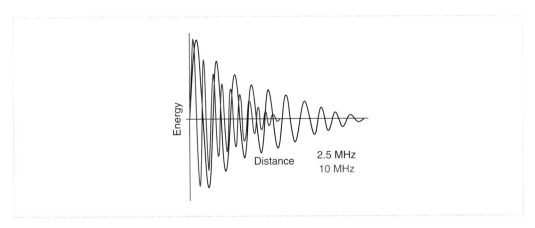

FIGURE 3.5   Attenuation is estimated as the attenuation coefficient × frequency × path length. Notice the lower frequency wave (2.5 MHz) has less attenuation at a given distance when compared with the 10 MHz wave. Thus, the 2.5 MHz wave is able to penetrate the tissue more effectively than the 10 MHz wave. (Adapted from Sites BD, Brull R, Chan VW, et al. Artifacts and pitfall errors associated with ultrasound-guided regional anesthesia. Part I: understanding the basic principles of ultrasound physics and machine operations. *Reg Anesth Pain Med* 2007;32:416. Copyright 2007 by Lippincott Williams & Wilkins.)

CLINICAL PEARL   Try to image structures using angles of insonation that approach the perpendicular in order to maximize reflection and minimize refraction.

2   **C. Image generation**

After serving as ultrasound wave generators, the piezoelectric crystals switch modes and become image receivers that capture sound waves that reflect off structures and return to the transducer. The sound waves cause the crystals to vibrate and generate electrical energy that is transmitted to a receiver that processes and cleans the image. The image that is generated is a two-dimensional image that displays structure on a grayscale continuum. Structures that strongly reflect the sound waves back to the transducer appear **hyperechoic**, structures that weakly reflect the sound waves appear **hypoechoic**, and structures that do not reflect sound waves appear **anechoic**. The receiver performs numerous functions that sharpen the image.

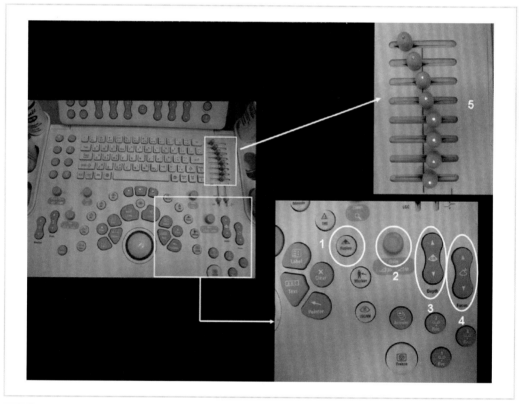

3   **FIGURE 3.6**   An image of a typical ultrasound interface. (1) Probe frequency control. In the depicted system and probe, the frequency can be adjusted from 3 to 12 MHz. The wavelength cannot be adjusted independently; however, manual adjustments to frequency result in corresponding changes in wavelength. (2) Overall gain button. This dial changes how bright or dark the entire image appears. (3) Depth control. The objective is to set the depth to just below the target of interest, thereby optimizing temporal resolution. (4) Focus button. It is important to position the focus of the ultrasound beam at the same level as the target of interest. This will optimize both lateral and axial resolution. (5) Time gain compensation (TGC). These toggle dials control the gain at consecutive depth intervals. The top dials control superficial gain and the bottom dials control deeper gain. Because attenuation occurs more with deeper imaging, the typical pattern of the TGC dials is a progressive increase in gain as indicated in the figure. (Reprinted from Sites BD, Brull R, Chan VW, et al. Artifacts and pitfall errors associated with ultrasound-guided regional anesthesia. Part I: understanding the basic principles of ultrasound physics and machine operations. *Reg Anesth Pain Med* 2007;32:416. Copyright 2007 by Lippincott Williams & Wilkins.)

Amplification is the ability of the receiver to brighten the entire image by amplifying the signals equally. Gain is adjusted by turning the gain control dial up or down. Another function of the receiver that can be adjusted is the **time gain compensation (TGC) dials**. As discussed above, images attenuate at greater depth. TGC adjustment allows deeper structures to be brightened more than more superficial structures, so similar tissues can appear the same color even when situated at different depths (Fig. 3.6).

D. **Color Doppler.** The interaction between ultrasound waves and red blood cells is discussed in the "Blood flow artifact" section.

III. **Limits of ultrasound.** Ultrasound has provided the regional anesthesiologist the ability to visualize the target structure, the needle trajectory, and the spread of local anesthetic. Despite all these advantages, there are some limitations of ultrasound.

A. **Image resolution and quality vary inversely with depth of penetration (3). In particular, deep blocks in obese patients may be pose distinct challenges based on poor image quality**.

B. **Ultrasound waves are not transmitted in air, and as a result, any structure deep to an air-filled pocket will not be seen. Ultrasound waves are highly attenuated by certain structures, such as bone, which can make it challenging to image deeper structures (see dropout (acoustic) shadowing).**

C. **Numerous artifacts can be created (see section IV: ultrasound-related artifacts) that may result in erroneous diagnosis, patient injuries, or failed blocks.**

D. **Ultrasound imaging and needle insertion techniques are additional skills that require education and training to master.**

IV. **Ultrasound-related artifacts**
An ultrasound artifact is a structure in an ultrasound image that does not have a corresponding anatomic tissue structure. Artifacts are frequent findings on the screen display because they usually result from the physical properties of ultrasound itself. **Ultrasound artifacts are important to recognize because they may alter the size, location, and shape of the target, as well as reference structures or even show structures that are not present (4,5).**

A. **Gain artifact.** The gain settings on an ultrasound machine can be thought as similar to the volume control on any device that is playing music (audible sound). The gain is adjusted either by an overall gain dial or by TGC dials. When the gain is turned up, the returning echo signals are amplified and will appear brighter and whiter. The existing structures may appear dark or absent on ultrasound if the overall gain is set too low (Fig. 3.7). If the overall gain is set too high, the existing structures can be very bright and even obscured. To "compensate" for attenuation, TGC dials are set to alter the gain at different depths on the ultrasound image. Based on attenuation principles, the dials are usually set in a diagonal configuration so that echoes returning from deeper aspects of the patient are amplified more than those from more superficial areas. Similar to overall gain, if the dials are not positioned properly, they can cause an existing object to appear as absent or obscured (Fig. 3.8) (5).

B. **Lateral resolution artifact.** Lateral resolution is the ability of the imaging system to distinguish between two objects that are at the same depth (side by side) in an ultrasound image. In order to maximize resolution, it is important to select the correct frequency transducer for imaging the targeted structures. Higher frequencies are better for shallower structures, and lower frequencies provide better penetration and lateral resolution for deeper structures (Fig. 3.9). Additionally, in order to maximize lateral resolution, the ultrasound beam should be focused onto the structures

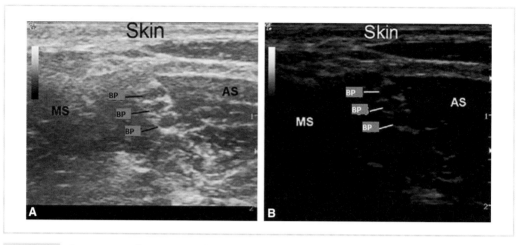

FIGURE 3.7 Incorrect overall gain setting. This is a short-axis view of the brachial plexus at the interscalene level. **A:** Overall gain is set too high. **B:** Overall gain is set to low. AS, anterior scalene muscle; MS, middle scalene muscle; BP, brachial plexus roots/trunks. (Adapted from Sites BD, Brull R, Chan VW, et al. Artifacts and pitfall errors associated with ultrasound-guided regional anesthesia. Part II: a pictorial approach to understanding and avoidance. *Reg Anesth Pain Med* 2007;32:420. Copyright 2007 by Lippincott Williams & Wilkins.)

of interest. Focusing an ultrasound beam with a specific dial on the interface represents the same principle as when you focus on a person's face to take a digital portrait (5). If lateral resolution is poor, the sonographer may not be able to distinguish two structures from one another (e.g., the common peroneal and tibial nerves in the popliteal fossa).

C. **Dropout (acoustic) shadowing.** Acoustic shadowing occurs when a structure blocks ultrasound and causes deeper tissues to appear as absent or less echogenic than normal. This happens when a structure has a larger attenuation coefficient than structures that lie deep to it. This commonly occurs when bone is in the path of the ultrasound beam. Bone has a large attenuation coefficient and therefore creates a dropout shadow below it.

CLINICAL PEARL Acoustic shadowing can be encountered when performing an ultrasound-guided supraclavicular block in a patient with a cervical rib. The rib will create a dropout shadow below it, and this will make it difficult to visualize the pleura deep to the rib (5).

D. **Acoustic enhancement.** This represents the opposite phenomenon to acoustic shadowing. Acoustic enhancement occurs when ultrasound waves pass through tissues that are weak attenuators compared to tissues around them, which results in increased echogenicity (brightness) on the deeper aspect of the weak attenuators. Acoustic enhancement is commonly seen on the deep side of large vessels. Unlike bone, blood is a weak attenuator and therefore more ultrasound waves pass through it and are reflected back when the tissue on the deep side is encountered. This causes the structures deep to the vessel to appear more hyperechoic than similar tissues at the same depth.

CLINICAL PEARL Acoustic enhancement posterior to a reference artery (e.g., axillary) can be mistaken as a neural structure. Depositing local anesthesia near acoustic enhancement artifacts can decrease block efficacy.

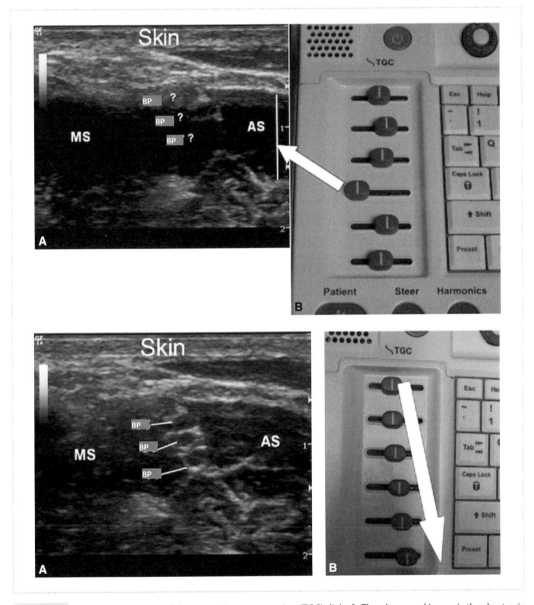

FIGURE 3.8 **(Top)** Incorrect use of the time gain compensation (TGC) dials. **A:** The ultrasound image is the short-axis view of the brachial plexus. The nerve roots/trunks are apparently missing. The arrow points to the band of hypoechoic tissue created by the incorrect use of the fourth time compensation button. **B:** Note the fourth TGC dial is turned down, creating the band of undergain that eliminates the roots/trunks. **(Bottom)** The correct TGC settings. **A:** The roots/trunks of the brachial plexus are now easily seen. **B:** The diagonal arrow indicates the typical pattern for the TGC dials. AS, anterior scalene muscle; MS, middle scalene muscle; BP, brachial plexus roots/trunks. (Adapted from Sites BD, Brull R, Chan VW, et al. Artifacts and pitfall errors associated with ultrasound-guided regional anesthesia. Part II: a pictorial approach to understanding and avoidance. *Reg Anesth Pain Med* 2007;32:420. Copyright 2007 by Lippincott Williams & Wilkins.)

   E. **Blood flow artifact.** Doppler ultrasound technology can be used to detect blood flow and its direction. This is useful in regional anesthesia to detect vascularity that may be in the path of the needle and help to plan the best needle approach. The Doppler principle underlies this technology and can be thought of in analogous fashion to the perceived pitch of sound as an

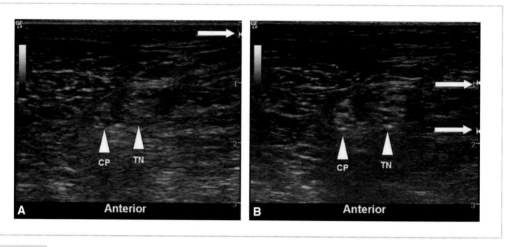

FIGURE 3.9 Impact of lateral resolution on the ability to image the common peroneal nerve (CP) and tibial nerve (TN) in short-axis in the popliteal fossa. **B:** A short-axis image of these nerves. The frequency is set at 12 MHz because the structures are superficial. The beam is electronically focused at the depth of the neural structures. Note that you can clearly delineate two separate nerves. **A:** Inaccurate imaging of the same structures, which were easily seen in (**B**). In this image, the frequency was reduced to 8 MHz and the focus was placed superficial to the nerves. The arrowheads indicate the two nerves. The arrows indicate the focal zone (narrowest point) of the ultrasound beam. (Reprinted from Sites BD, Brull R, Chan VW, et al. Artifacts and pitfall errors associated with ultrasound-guided regional anesthesia. Part II: a pictorial approach to understanding and avoidance. *Reg Anesth Pain Med* 2007;32:421. Copyright 2007 by Lippincott Williams & Wilkins.)

object moves toward or away from a stationary listener. For example, a train whistle moving toward the listener appears to have a higher pitch than the same whistle on a train that is moving away from the listener. This difference in frequency is referred to as the Doppler frequency (2). Doppler technology on an ultrasound machine simply applies a color mapping to this frequency shift. The color is a function of directionality of blood (toward or away from the transducer) and the actual blood velocity.

Doppler equation

$$\text{Doppler shift frequency} = (2 \times F \times v \times \cos \text{angle})/C$$

$$F = \text{ultrasound transmission frequency}$$

$$v = \text{blood cell velocity}$$

$$\cos \text{angle} = \text{angle of incident (angle created between the flow of blood and the ultrasound beam)}$$

$$C = \text{speed of sound in soft tissue (1,540 m/s)}$$

With Doppler analysis, when the ultrasound beam is perpendicular to the flow of blood, the ultrasound image will demonstrate no flow. This is simply a function of solving for blood velocity using the Doppler equation which generates a 0 because the cosine of the angle (at 90 degrees) is 0. This is called a blood flow artifact (Fig. 3.10).

CLINICAL PEARL It is important to tilt the ultrasound beam through different angles when examining the target structures. Such a maneuver will minimize the possibility of failing to detect blood flow when it actually exists (5).

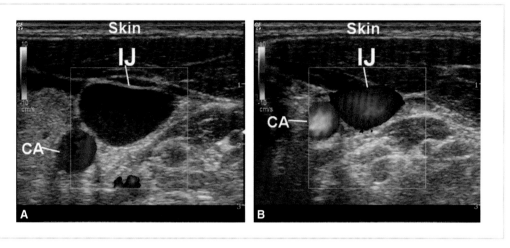

FIGURE 3.10 Ultrasound image of the short-axis view of the internal jugular (IJ) vein being analyzed with color flow Doppler. **A:** There appears to be no flow in the IJ. This artifact was generated because the angle of incidence between the ultrasound beam and the blood flow approached 90 degrees. Blood flow, however, can be visualized by tilting the probe handle toward the patient's head. This will create an angle of incidence greater than 90 degrees, and some blood flow will be revealed **(B)**. CA, carotid artery. (Reprinted from Sites BD, Brull R, Chan VW, et al. Artifacts and pitfall errors associated with ultrasound-guided regional anesthesia. Part II: a pictorial approach to understanding and avoidance. *Reg Anesth Pain Med* 2007;32:425. Copyright 2007 by Lippincott Williams & Wilkins.)

F. Needle reverberation artifact. Reverberation artifact occurs when ultrasound waves bounce back and forth between two strong specular reflectors. This is often seen when waves bounce back and forth between the two walls of a block needle. The waves that have bounced back and forth in the lumen of the needle eventually travel back to the transducer. These waves are perceived to have reflected off a structure at a greater depth because it took longer for them to return. As a result, numerous needle lines appear on the image deeper to the actual location of the needle (Fig. 3.11).

G. Tissue reverberation artifact. Tissues can create reverberation artifacts just like a needle can. This is often seen when the lung is imaged. Ultrasound waves can bounce back and forth between the visceral and parietal pleura and create lines that appear deep to the pleura even though, anatomically, they are not present.

CLINICAL PEARL   A tissue reverberation artifact that occurs when pleura is encountered is referred to as the "comet tail sign" and can be used to help identify (and stay away) from the lung in the supraclavicular region (Fig. 3.12).

H. Bayonet artifact. Bayonet artifact occurs when a needle passes between tissues that have different ultrasound wave velocities (6). It is generally assumed that ultrasound waves travel at 1,540 m/s in the human body, but in fact the speed actually varies from 1,450 to 1,600 m/s depending on tissue medium. If the needle is perpendicular to the ultrasound beam and moves from soft tissue (1,540 m/s) to blood (1,580 m/s), it will appear to bend toward the transducer like a bayonet because the ultrasound waves travel faster in blood and return to the transducer sooner. An example of this can be seen when a needle perpendicular to the ultrasound beam moves from soft tissue to enter the axillary artery. Similarly, when a sciatic nerve block is performed, the needle can appear to bend away from the transducer as it moves from muscle to adipose tissue, because ultrasound waves travel slower in adipose tissue than they do in muscle (Fig. 3.13).

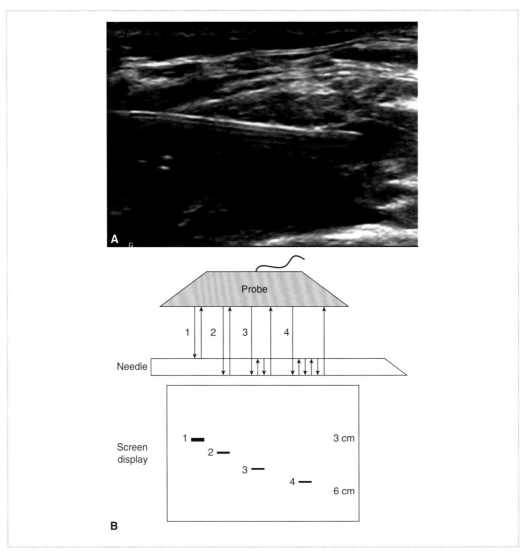

FIGURE 3.11 **A:** Ultrasound image of a needle entering in-plane from the left of the screen. The red arrow is pointing to one of the many linear lines below the needle that represent needle reverberation artifact. **B:** Reverberation artifact, detailed in a stepwise manner. Each number above the needle (**top**) has a corresponding number on the ultrasound screen (**bottom**) to graphically represent the result of different reverberation events. The original ultrasound beam contacts the needle and is reflected back to the probe correctly (1). In addition, part of the ultrasound beam penetrates the hollow needle and is reflected back to the probe from the distal wall of the needle (2). However, a component of the ultrasound beam becomes "stuck" within the needle lumen because the needle walls are highly reflective barriers. This signal component is reflected between the needle walls several times before "escaping" back to the probe (3, 4). Thus, the probe interprets these later occurring signals as objects distal to the needle at intervals which are multiples of the needle diameters. (Part [**B**] Reprinted from Sites BD, Brull R, Chan VW, et al. Artifacts and pitfall errors associated with ultrasound-guided regional anesthesia. Part II: a pictorial approach to understanding and avoidance. *Reg Anesth Pain Med* 2007;32:425. Copyright 2007 by Lippincott Williams & Wilkins.)

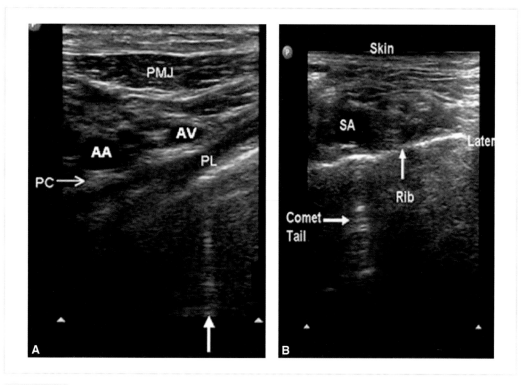

FIGURE 3.12   A: The comet sign visualized during preparation for an infraclavicular block. The streaks ("comets") indicated by the arrows represent multiple reverberations generated by the two layers (visceral and parietal) of pleura of the lung. The unlabeled arrow indicates the comet tail. **B:** Classic comet tail sign involving structures seen during a supraclavicular block. AA, axillary artery; AV, axillary vein; PL, pleura; PMJ, pectoralis major; SA, subclavian artery. (Adapted from Sites BD, Brull R, Chan VWS, et al. Artifacts and pitfall errors associated with ultrasound-guided regional anesthesia. Part II: a pictorial approach to understanding and avoidance. *Reg Anesth Pain Med* 2007;32:426. Copyright 2007 by Lippincott Williams & Wilkins.)

I. **Air artifact.** Air artifact occurs when air is encountered between the ultrasound beam and the target structure. Air does not conduct ultrasound and therefore will create a dropout shadow. This can be seen when air is trapped in an ultrasound transducer cover or after air is injected through the needle and into tissue (Fig. 3.14).

V. **Anatomic errors.** Anatomic errors are often referred to as pitfall errors. They occur when various structures are incorrectly identified as the intended neural target.

A. **Tendons and muscles.** In numerous anatomic locations, tendons and muscles can be mistaken for nerves because they can display similar echogenicity. One common example is the distal forearm. Sonographically, the median nerve and the tendons in this area can have a similar shape and color. In the forearm, the median nerve can be distinguished from a tendon based on the hypoechoic neural fascicles compared to the hyperechoic fibrils of a tendon (7). Another region in the body where this can occur is the popliteal fossa. The common peroneal and tibial nerves can appear similar to the surrounding muscles, especially with the biceps femoris. The distinction between muscle and nerve is easier to make when the patient has significant adipose tissue. Adipose tissue appears hypoechoic and forms a nice interface effect between the hyperechoic nerves and the hyperechoic muscle (5). The most challenging popliteal fossa blocks often occur in athletes with muscular legs and a paucity of adipose tissue.

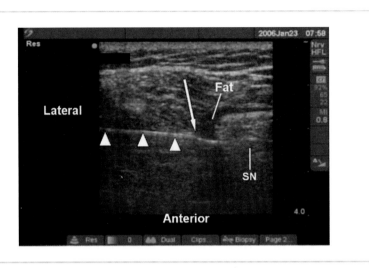

FIGURE 3.13   Ultrasound image of the sciatic nerve (SN) in the popliteal fossa imaged in short-axis. The needle is inserted from the lateral aspect of the patient. As the needle enters the perineural adipose tissue, it appears to bend in an anterior fashion. This is called a bayonet artifact. The artifact is generated by subtle differences of the velocity of ultrasound in adipose and muscle tissue. The arrowheads indicate the needle and the arrow indicates the "bending" point of the needle. (Adapted from Sites BD, Brull R, Chan VW, et al. Artifacts and pitfall errors associated with ultrasound-guided regional anesthesia. Part II: a pictorial approach to understanding and avoidance. *Reg Anesth Pain Med* 2007;32:427. Copyright 2007 by Lippincott Williams & Wilkins.)

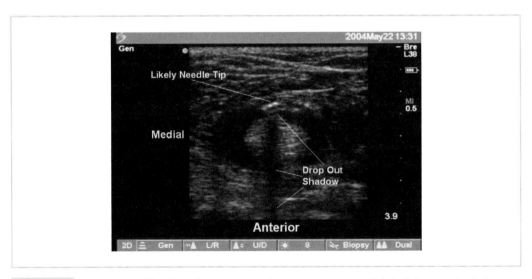

FIGURE 3.14   After 10 mL of local anesthetic injection, the nerve appears to split in half. An acoustic shadow was most likely caused by an air bubble at the needle tip. This acoustic shadow is easy to see passing right through the nerve and into the anterior tissues. (Adapted from Sites BD, Brull R, Chan VW, et al. Artifacts and pitfall errors associated with ultrasound-guided regional anesthesia. Part II: a pictorial approach to understanding and avoidance. *Reg Anesth Pain Med* 2007;32:422. Copyright 2007 by Lippincott Williams & Wilkins.)

CLINICAL PEARL To help confirm that you are actually imaging the target nerve of interest, it is helpful to scan the structure in a proximal and distal direction and confirm that the structure is taking the anticipated anatomic course. For example, if you scan the median nerve of the wrist from distal to proximal, you can trace the nerve back to the antecubital fossa where it is located next to the brachial artery. A flexor tendon of the wrist would not take this course.

B. **Blood vessels.** Throughout most of the body, it is easy to distinguish blood vessels from nerves because the vascular lumen appears anechoic (black), whereas nerves appear either hyperechoic or hypoechoic. This is not the situation when the brachial plexus is targeted above the clavicle. The fascicles of the interscalene brachial plexus in the neck take on an echotexture consisting of 3 to 4 anechoic circles. In this region, it is important to use color flow Doppler to ensure that you are not targeting a blood vessel visualized in cross-section. Blood vessels also have other unique features that could help distinguish them from nerves. Veins are usually compressible and nonpulsatile. Arteries are usually pulsatile but are not compressible. Nerves are neither compressible nor pulsatile (5).

C. **Lymph nodes.** In certain regions of the body, inflamed lymph nodes can resemble nerves or can appear in the pathway of nerves. Inflamed lymph nodes are usually large well-circumscribed structures that are not compressible. Inside, the lymph node may have small hypoechoic areas that represent intranodal necrosis and should not be confused for fascicles. Inflamed lymph nodes are commonly encountered in the cervical, axillary, and inguinal areas. It is important to trace the targeted nerve along its intended path and to use other landmarks to confirm that the targeted structure is the intended nerve (5).

REFERENCES

1. Sites BD, Brull R, Chan VW, et al. Artifacts and pitfall errors associated with ultrasound-guided regional anesthesia. Part I: understanding the basic principles of ultrasound physics and machine operations. *Reg Anesth Pain Med* 2007;32:412–418.
2. Shriki J. Ultrasound physics. *Crit Care Clin* 2014;30:1–24.
3. Marhofer P, Chan VW. Ultrasound-guided regional anesthesia: current concepts and future trends. *Anesth Analg* 2007;104:1265–1269.
4. Kremkau F, Taylor K. Artifacts in ultrasound imaging. *J Ultrasound Med* 1986;5:227–237.
5. Sites BD, Brull R, Chan VW, et al. Artifacts and pitfall errors associated with ultrasound-guided regional anesthesia. Part II: a pictorial approach to understanding and avoidance. *Reg Anesth Pain Med* 2007;32:419–433.
6. Gray AT. Bayonet artifact during ultrasound-guided transarterial axillary block. *Anesthesiology* 2005;102:1291–1292.
7. Gray AT. Ultrasound-guided regional anesthesia: current state of the art. *Anesthesiology* 2006;104:368–373.

Premedication, Monitoring, and Multimodal Analgesia

Rebecca L. Johnson and Michael F. Mulroy

I. **Multimodal therapy**
  A. Goals
  B. Selective components of multimodal therapy

II. **Periprocedural sedation**
  A. Goals
  B. Drugs

III. **Monitoring**

KEY POINTS

1. Preoperative optimization of the patient's perioperative pain management with the use of multimodal analgesia has emerged as a standard tactic to reduce opioid use (1).

2. Multimodal analgesia can be defined as the use of different analgesic agents administered to target various sites along nociceptive pathways.

3. Periprocedural sedation remains a key component for regional anesthesia and analgesia success. Careful titration of sedative agents improves patient cooperation, analgesia, and may promote desirable amnesia.

4. Patients receiving regional anesthesia require the same American Society of Anesthesiologists (ASA) standards of monitoring as those undergoing general anesthesia, including electrocardiogram, blood pressure device, and pulse oximetry.

5. Patients undergoing regional anesthesia must be closely monitored during and after local anesthetic injection for signs and symptoms of local anesthetic systemic toxicity (LAST). The American Society of Regional Anesthesia and Pain Medicine (ASRA) has issued a practice advisory on the prevention, diagnosis, and treatment of LAST (2).

MULTIMODAL ANALGESIA INCORPORATES the use of different analgesic agents that work at targeted sites along the nociceptive pathways (3). **The concept of preemptive oral pain management has emerged as a strategy to significantly decrease postoperative pain and reduce reliance on opioids.** Incorporation of regional anesthesia into a comprehensive, multimodal analgesic clinical pathway promotes early mobilization, shorter hospital stay, and decreased reliance on opioids (4,5). Patients who participate in clinical pathways that include regional anesthesia techniques often report improved pain control and higher overall satisfaction.

Premedication and intraoperative sedation are important components of regional techniques. "Pure" regional anesthesia can be performed without supplementation, especially in ambulatory surgery, but patient acceptance is often enhanced with sedation. Omission of sedation is appropriate in the obstetric suite, where systemic medications must be carefully limited.

The preoperative visit is extremely effective in reducing patient anxiety. Kind attention to the patient's concerns and situation will curtail the need for escalating premedication. Often small gestures, such as comfortable positioning of the bed, a warm blanket, and the practitioner sitting rather than standing while providing tailored patient education, lead to perceptions of more time spent and higher levels of patient satisfaction (6). Music also displays sedative properties. The use of headphones may actually muffle anxiety-provoking sounds and conversations in the induction and operating rooms (7).

In the operating room, successful regional anesthesia for nonobstetric surgery is facilitated by the skillful use of adjuvants to ensure cooperation and acceptance. This may include sedation and analgesia for the performance of the block, as well as sedation during prolonged surgical procedures even in the presence of an adequate block.

I. Multimodal therapy

A. Goals. Multimodal analgesia clinical pathways—the perioperative use of medications and regional anesthesia techniques using local anesthetics to facilitate the recovery process strives to achieve the following **goals**:

1. **To inhibit** the stress response to surgery

2. **To improve** antinociception through the synergistic/additive effects of individual components (Fig. 4.1).

3. **To reduce pharmacologic side effects** by decreasing the overall dose of any individual medication agent, such as opioids.

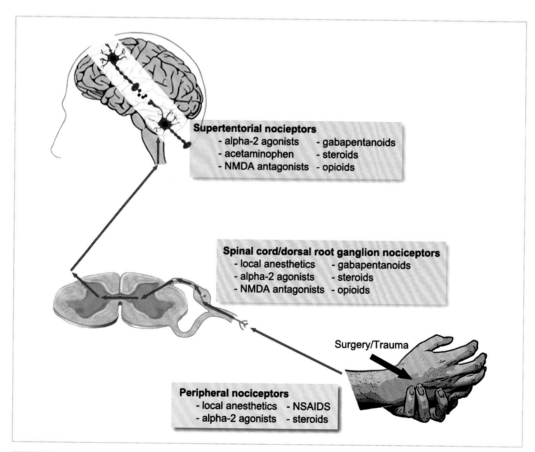

FIGURE 4.1   Targeted sites along nociceptive pathways for multimodal analgesic agents.

B. **Selective components of multimodal therapy (Table 4.1)**

1. **Nonselective and selective cyclooxygenase (COX) nonsteroidal anti-inflammatory drugs (NSAIDs)**

   a. Renowned for their **antipyretic, analgesic, and anti-inflammatory properties**, NSAIDs provide significant pain relief for moderate and severe pain and can reduce the opioid dose required to treat severe pain. They provide an advantage over opioids by decreasing swelling; curtailing the perioperative stress response; and decreasing morbidity, mortality, and resource utilization (3,8).

   b. **Inhibit the COX enzymes** responsible for catalyzing the conversion of arachidonic acid to prostaglandins and thromboxanes.

   c. NSAIDs are categorized by their selectivity in inhibiting the two main isoforms of COX-1 (e.g., aspirin, ketorolac) and COX-2 (e.g., celecoxib).

   d. Consider celecoxib, 400 mg, in single or divided doses for patients >50 kg, who have adequate renal function (creatinine clearance > 50 mL/min) and who are 18 to 64 years of age. Consider reducing the dose to 200 mg or avoiding its use altogether in patients at extremes of age (pediatric or older adults), patients with gastrointestinal bleeding within the past 6 months, or patients afflicted with acute or chronic renal insufficiency (creatinine clearance <30 mL/min).

TABLE 4.1 Common components of multimodal analgesic pathways

Drug (brand name)	Applications	Comments

NSAIDs
    Celecoxib, diclofenac,
    ibuprofen, naproxen
	Antipyretic, analgesic, and anti-inflammatory properties	May result in physiologic disruptions within the gastrointestinal, hematologic, and renal systems

Acetaminophen	Antipyretic and analgesic properties	No anti-inflammatory or peripheral activity
Steroids	Anti-inflammatory, antiemetic, and immunosuppressant effects	Suppression of the hypothalamic–pituitary–adrenal axis after single-dose steroid therapy is unlikely
Alpha-2 receptor agonists Clonidine	Analgesic effects at peripheral, spinal, and brainstem loci and enhanced analgesia with local anesthesia blockade	May cause profound bradycardia and hypotension particularly with neuraxial blocks
Ketamine	Analgesia through noncompetitive NMDA antagonism	Use of subanesthetic or low-dose (<1 mg/kg) ketamine provides analgesia without the dysphoric effects of traditional high-dose methods

Gabapentanoids
    Gabapentin
    Pregabalin
	Prevents release of nociceptive neurotransmitters. Amplifies the analgesia provided by opioids and other multimodal medications	Sedation, dizziness, and nausea side effects may preclude use of gabapentanoids for outpatient surgery or patients older than 70 yr

Opioids (oxycodone, hydrocodone, morphine, hydromorphone, meperidine)	Preoperative use results in prolonged postoperative analgesia	Used with NMDA antagonists and NSAIDs may reduce opioid-induced hyperalgesia and acute tolerance
Local anesthesia	When used during neuraxial and/or peripheral nerve blockade, attenuates or prevents nociceptive signals from reaching central processing centers, thus minimizing the occurrence of hyperalgesia	Local anesthesia agents administered intravenously suppress gastrointestinal reflexes and bowel wall inflammation

NMDA, N-methyl-d-aspartate; NSAIDs, nonsteroidal anti-inflammatory drugs.

e. **All NSAIDs display a ceiling effect for analgesia but not for side effects.** NSAIDs (more COX-1 than COX-2 inhibitors) use may result in gastrointestinal erosions, decreased renal blood flow, and impaired platelet function. Nonselective NSAIDs have been associated with increased blood loss in some surgical procedures. The cause of cardiovascular complications seen with certain selective COX-2 inhibitors became, and remains, a subject of intensive research (9). NSAIDs exposure during orthopedic surgery has further been the subject of intense debate among surgeons and anesthesiologists. High doses of NSAIDs for prolonged periods can increase the risk of bone nonunion. However, there exists no clear contraindication to NSAIDs (e.g., in terms of bone healing) if the latter are dosed appropriately and used during a discrete perioperative episode of care (10).

2. Acetaminophen
   a. **Centrally acting antipyretic and analgesic properties with no anti-inflammatory or peripheral activity.**
   b. Commonly used as an oral premedication in doses ranging from 650 to 1,000 mg every 6 hours to a maximum of 3,500 to 4,000 mg/day based on age. Oral acetaminophen possesses a bioavailability of 80% to 90%; however, in the early postoperative period, individual absorption can be unpredictable because of delayed gastric emptying and may warrant intravenous (IV) administration in special circumstances. Rectal administration results in poor and unpredictable absorption.
   c. Published trials evaluating acetaminophen have demonstrated opioid-sparing effects that are 20% inferior to those of NSAIDs.

3. Gabapentanoids/alpha-2 delta ligands
   a. Gabapentanoids, such as gabapentin and pregabalin, bind to the alpha-2 delta subunit of voltage-gated calcium channels, preventing the release of nociceptive neurotransmitters. Both gabapentin (300 to 600 mg once preoperatively) and pregabalin (50 to 100 mg once preoperatively) have been **shown to decrease postoperative pain and narcotic requirements.**
   b. **Dose-dependent side effects** (e.g., sedation, dizziness, and nausea) are often more pronounced among older adults undergoing general anesthesia (11). Moreover, emerging evidence suggests caution when combining preoperative use of pregabalin with infusions of remifentanil for sedation. Although the combination provides an additive analgesic effect, it seems to result in more pronounced respiratory depression and cognitive decline when compared with that of either agent alone among volunteers (12).

4. Steroids
   a. Inflammation plays a significant role in the development of perioperative pain.
   b. Single perioperative dosing of dexamethasone (dose range 1.25 to 20 mg) in the context of a comprehensive multimodal analgesic regimen in low-risk patients has been shown to lower pain scores, shorten postoperative recovery stay, and has been linked to reduced opioid consumption more than 24 hours after surgery (13). No contemporary evidence exists to show a causal relationship between steroid use and poor wound healing after surgery.

5. Local anesthesia
   a. Local anesthesia can inhibit deleterious inflammatory responses without affecting the normal, necessary inflammatory process, thus making these drugs unique therapeutic agents. Clinical effects may even outlast the presence of the drug.
   b. Additionally, the systemic use of IV lidocaine (1.5 mg/kg IV bolus dose followed by 1 to 2 mg/kg/h infusion) decreases anesthesia requirements (14). As an analgesic, systemic lidocaine reduces pain after major abdominal procedures, outpatient surgery, and may be particularly beneficial for decreasing hyperalgesia in patients with chronic pain (15,16). IV infusions of lidocaine may be as effective as or even better than continuous thoracic

epidural analgesia at promoting the return of bowel function after open colorectal surgery (17). Plasma lidocaine levels from these studies failed to reach toxic thresholds (>5 µg/mL). Levels remained <2 µg/mL even after 24 hours of infusion.

CLINICAL PEARL It is better to prevent rather than treat pain; hence, multimodal strategies should be implemented before surgery.

CLINICAL PEARL Consider the preoperative administration of oral analgesic medications including acetaminophen 1,000 mg, celecoxib 400 mg, and oxycodone 5 to 10 mg for patients >50 kg with adequate renal function. Consider dose reduction or avoiding the use of opioids or NSAIDs altogether in patients at extremes of age (pediatric or older adults), patients with gastrointestinal bleeding within the past 6 months, or patients afflicted with acute or chronic renal insufficiency (creatinine clearance < 30 mL/min).

II. Periprocedural sedation

A. Goals. The supplementation of medication given at the time of procedure to attain **one of these objectives**:

1. To **decrease apprehension and increase the degree of cooperation** in the anxious patient
2. To **provide analgesia** and decrease discomfort associated with the procedure (e.g., needling)
3. To **produce amnesia** or lack of awareness of the intraoperative and perioperative events

CLINICAL PEARL The fourth motive is sometimes incorrectly mentioned: the hope of raising the seizure threshold (in the event of LAST). However, this goal is not attainable with conventional sedative doses of benzodiazepines. Successful reduction in seizure risk would require (1) doses sufficient to produce unconsciousness in most patients, (2) doses associated with elevated risks of respiratory and cardiac depression, and (3) levels of sedation that would mask early warning signs of LAST (18).

CLINICAL PEARL Sedation should be titrated to avoid such deep levels of obtundation that the patient is unable to report paresthesia, which indicate direct nerve contact by the needle.

B. Drugs. A wide spectrum of available sedative agents can be used depending on the patient and clinical situation (Table 4.2).

1. **Opioids**
   a. Medications within this class of drugs **produce analgesia with minimal sedation and, with mindful titration, rarely lead to loss of consciousness**; however, they confer limited **amnesia**. Nonetheless, they are excellent for enhancing patient cooperation and reducing discomfort associated with needle insertion or paresthesia.
   b. Fentanyl is the most popular opioid sedative because of its rapid onset, short duration, and easy titratability. IV increments of 25 to 50 µg provide rapid analgesia lasting 20 to 30 minutes. **Dosage is a function of patient vitality, not body size**; in other words, one dose does not "fit all."
   c. Alternatives to fentanyl include derivatives such as remifentanil; however, the latter's duration of action is too short to facilitate regional techniques. Furthermore, it provides limited analgesic benefits unless administered as an infusion. Morphine provides good

TABLE 4.2 Common sedative medications used to supplement regional anesthetic

Drug (brand name)	Dose range	Applications	Comments
Benzodiazepines			
Midazolam	1–5 mg IV	Rapid-onset sedation in induction and/or operating rooms	Amnesia potential
Narcotics			
Fentanyl	25–200 μg IV	Rapid-onset analgesia in induction and/or operating rooms	Useful adjunct for painful procedures (needle insertion), potential for respiratory depression
Ketamine	Bolus of 10–50 mg IV	Sedation during blocks	Some analgesic properties, supports respiration and blood pressure; risk of confusion and hallucinations with higher doses
Sedative/hypnotics			
Dexmedetomidine	Bolus followed by infusion (0.7 μg/kg/h)	Intraoperative sedation	Potential for bradycardia, hypotension
Propofol	Boluses of 30–60 mg, infusion of 25–100 μg/kg/min	Rapid sedation for procedures in induction room, good sedation intraoperatively	Pain on injection

IV, intravenous.

analgesia and sedation as well, but its long duration of action makes it less ideal for periprocedural sedation in the outpatient setting.

    d. Although rarely encountered in doses used for periprocedural sedation, all of the opioids share the propensity to cause dose-related side effects including nausea and **respiratory depression**. Some respiratory depression is expected regardless of the dose; thus, pulse oximetry and supplemental oxygen are recommended as is monitoring of the patient's level of consciousness.

    e. Side effects may be partially or completely reversed with opioid antagonist therapy (e.g., naloxone), which should be readily available whenever opioids are administered.

  2. Benzodiazepines

    a. Effective, centrally acting **anxiolytics** that confer **amnesia but not analgesia**. Used to treat seizures because of LAST; therefore, additionally beneficial in the event of toxicity.

    b. Midazolam, predictably rapid and short acting, is the most appropriate benzodiazepine in the induction room. Lorazepam (onset time = 30 to 60 minutes) may be appropriate for inpatient premedication but is not as readily titratable.

    c. **Amnestic effects can be variable and unpredictable:** in some patients, benzodiazepines evoke paradoxical confusion and lack of cooperation. Dose-related sedation can be long lasting; therefore, the dosage should be kept to a minimum (0.5 to 1 mg aliquots, rarely higher than 4 mg) especially in outpatients. Intraoperative events and postoperative instructions may not be remembered by an apparently alert outpatient, and there exists a high potential for respiratory depression when benzodiazepines are combined with opioids. Moreover, avoidance (or decreased use) of benzodiazepines has been linked to fewer postoperative dysfunction occurrences in the elderly.

    d. As with opioids, there exists a reversal agent (flumazenil) that should be readily available whenever benzodiazepines are used.

3. **Ketamine**
   a. Ketamine provides **analgesia** while **maintaining cardiovascular stability**. It also produces minimal respiratory depression and obtundation of airway reflexes.
   b. **For sedation and analgesia**, ketamine can be used in low doses (10 to 30 mg) in combination with midazolam for special circumstances (i.e., when hemodynamic stability or spontaneous breathing ventilation is required). In anesthetic doses, ketamine has been associated with hallucinations upon emergence; however, the latter are unlikely to occur in doses used for sedation and in the presence of benzodiazepines (or general anesthesia) (19).

4. **Propofol**
   a. Propofol is primarily administered for general anesthesia because of its profound anxiolytic, sedative, and amnestic potential; however, in lower doses, it can also be used for intraoperative sedation. Benefits include **rapid recovery and antiemetic effects**. However, propofol **lacks the analgesic properties** of opioids and **the subhypnotic amnestic effects** of benzodiazepines.
   b. Common uses: (1) **as a bolus** for brief deep sedation during the performance of selected blocks where consciousness is unnecessary (e.g., retrobulbar block) and (2) **as an infusion** during surgical procedures performed under regional block (usual dose range between 30 and 60 µg/kg/min) (20).

CLINICAL PEARL When combined (in small doses) with midazolam and fentanyl (to enhance the performance of a regional block) and followed by an infusion (for intraoperative sedation), propofol provides an ideal formula for patient satisfaction and rapid recovery. Propofol is easily titratable, and its antiemetic effects make it an ideal sedative option for short outpatient procedures requiring rapid recovery.

5. **Dexmedetomidine**
   a. Dexmedetomidine is **an alpha 2-agonist**, which appears to potentiate analgesia and decrease inhalational anesthesia requirements when used as an IV infusion during surgical procedures or for sedation within intensive care settings (21). It sidesteps respiratory depression but, unlike ketamine, may produce hemodynamic side effects, such as bradycardia and hypotension. Dexmedetomidine displays no amnestic properties.
   b. Commonly used **as intraoperative sedation with peripheral nerve blockade** (an infusion of 0.7 µg/kg/h is equivalent to propofol 35 µg/kg/min). However, the hypotensive effects may make it undesirable for neuraxial blockade.

CLINICAL PEARL Strongly consider titrating small initial doses of sedative agents in opioid-naïve and older adults patients (e.g., midazolam 1 mg IV and fentanyl 25 to 50 µg IV) and subsequently supplementing with additional doses (or agents) if necessary.

CLINICAL PEARL Consider tailoring your sedation plan to fit specific populations:
- **Avoid excessive amounts** of sedation in **outpatients** because oversedation will negate the advantages of rapid recovery and discharge required by ambulatory practices.
- **Heavier sedative doses** that include an amnestic agent may be appropriate in **anxious** patients, **opioid-tolerant** patients, and in **teaching** situations.
- **Children**. Infants usually require a general anesthetic for the performance of a nerve block. Unlike in adult patients (22), the use of general anesthesia to facilitate regional blockade in certain populations (e.g., children, adults with intellectual deficits) is standard practice and apparently not associated with an increased risk of injury (23).

III. Monitoring

4   A. Patients receiving regional anesthesia in the operating room or another location (e.g., induction room) require the same American Society of Anesthesiologists standard of monitoring as those undergoing general anesthesia, including **electrocardiogram**, **blood pressure device**, and **pulse oximetry** (24).

B. **Supplemental oxygen is warranted** when sedatives and analgesics are being delivered.

5   C. Patients undergoing regional anesthesia must be closely **monitored for the signs and symptoms of LAST.** Consider the use of epinephrine-containing solutions (test doses) to objectively identify rising blood levels in the event of intravascular placement. (See Chapter 3.) Specifically, monitoring with continuous verbal contact to detect changes in the patient's mental status is also helpful but less reliable. Sedation levels interfere with this sign and must be titrated to allow for conversation with the patient. Although peak blood levels of local anesthetics manifest rapidly after IV injection, they may not occur until 30 minutes or more after a peripheral nerve block.

D. Monitoring the patient's **block level** should also be a priority, especially for regional anesthesia techniques that result in sympathectomy. Block level and blood pressure should be measured every 3 to 5 minutes for the first 15 minutes and intermittently thereafter to detect unexpected high levels. In particular, neuraxial blocks (i.e., epidural or spinal anesthesia) and deep plexus blocks (e.g., lumbar plexus blockade) may demonstrate significant changes in block level over the first hour.

CLINICAL PEARL   Premonitory signs and symptoms of LAST vary widely. However, alterations in mental concentration or slurring of speech and hemodynamic changes, especially in the first 20 to 30 minutes following the injection of a large quantity of local anesthetic, are important sentinel events, and their detection requires appropriate doses of sedation. In-depth discussion of LAST is provided in Chapter 14.

CLINICAL PEARL   All blocks involving local anesthetic agents should be administered in a location with readily available resuscitation equipment, including access to 20% lipid emulsion therapy.

REFERENCES

1. Practice guidelines for acute pain management in the perioperative setting: an updated report by the American Society of Anesthesiologists Task Force on Acute Pain Management. *Anesthesiology* 2012;116(2):248–273.
2. Neal JM, Mulroy MF, Weinberg GL, American Society of Regional Anesthesia and Pain Medicine. American Society of Regional Anesthesia and Pain Medicine checklist for managing local anesthetic systemic toxicity: 2012 version. *Reg Anesth Pain Med* 2012;37(1):16–18.
3. Kehlet H, Dahl JB. The value of "multimodal" or "balanced analgesia" in postoperative pain treatment. *Anesth Analg* 1993;77(5):1048–1056.
4. Hebl JR, Dilger JA, Byer DE, et al. A pre-emptive multimodal pathway featuring peripheral nerve block improves perioperative outcomes after major orthopedic surgery. *Reg Anesthe Pain Med* 2008;33(6):510–517.
5. Johnson RL, Kopp SL. Optimizing perioperative management of total joint arthroplasty. *Anesthesiol Clin* 2014;32(4):865–880.
6. Johnson RL, Sadosty AT, Weaver AL, et al. To sit or not to sit? *Ann Emerg Med* 2008;51(2):188–193, 193. e1–e2.
7. Mayor S. Listening to music helps reduce pain and anxiety after surgery, review shows. *BMJ* 2015;351:h4398.

8. Ong CK, Lirk P, Tan CH, et al. An evidence-based update on nonsteroidal anti-inflammatory drugs. *Clin Med Res* 2007;5(1):19–34.

9. Cannon CP, Cannon PJ. Physiology. COX-2 inhibitors and cardiovascular risk. *Science* 2012;336(6087):1386–1387.

10. Marquez-Lara A, Hutchinson ID, Nunez F Jr, et al. Nonsteroidal anti-inflammatory drugs and bone-healing: a systematic review of research quality. *JBJS Rev* 2016;4(3).

11. Kinney MA, Mantilla CB, Carns PE, et al. Preoperative gabapentin for acute post-thoracotomy analgesia: a randomized, double-blinded, active placebo-controlled study. *Pain Pract* 2012;12(3):175–183.

12. Myhre M, Diep LM, Stubhaug A. Pregabalin has analgesic, ventilatory, and cognitive effects in combination with remifentanil. *Anesthesiology* 2016;124(1):141–149.

13. Waldron NH, Jones CA, Gan TJ, et al. Impact of perioperative dexamethasone on postoperative analgesia and side-effects: systematic review and meta-analysis. *Br J Anaesth* 2013;110(2):191–200.

14. Benkwitz C, Garrison JC, Linden J, et al. Lidocaine enhances Galphai protein function. *Anesthesiology* 2003;99(5):1093–1101.

15. Kaba A, Laurent SR, Detroz BJ, et al. Intravenous lidocaine infusion facilitates acute rehabilitation after laparoscopic colectomy. *Anesthesiology* 2007;106(1):11–18; discussion 5–6.

16. Kranke P, Jokinen J, Pace NL, et al. Continuous intravenous perioperative lidocaine infusion for postoperative pain and recovery. *Cochrane Database Syst Rev* 2015;16(7):CD009642.

17. Swenson BR, Gottschalk A, Wells LT, et al. Intravenous lidocaine is as effective as epidural bupivacaine in reducing ileus duration, hospital stay, and pain after open colon resection: a randomized clinical trial. *Reg Anesth Pain Med* 2010;35(4):370–376.

18. Mulroy MF, Neal JM, Mackey DC, et al. 2-Chloroprocaine and bupivacaine are unreliable indicators of intravascular injection in the premedicated patient. *Reg Anesth Pain Med* 1998;23(1):9–13.

19. Niesters M, Martini C, Dahan A. Ketamine for chronic pain: risks and benefits. *Br J Clin Pharmacol* 2014;77(2):357–367.

20. Smith I, Monk TG, White PF, et al. Propofol infusion during regional anesthesia: sedative, amnestic, and anxiolytic properties. *Anesth Analg* 1994;79(2):313–319.

21. Kamibayashi T, Maze M. Clinical uses of alpha2-adrenergic agonists. *Anesthesiology* 2000;93(5):1345–1349.

22. Benumof JL. Permanent loss of cervical spinal cord function associated with interscalene block performed under general anesthesia. *Anesthesiology* 2000;93(6):1541–1544.

23. Taenzer AH, Walker BJ, Bosenberg AT, et al. Asleep versus awake: does it matter?: Pediatric regional block complications by patient state: a report from the Pediatric Regional Anesthesia Network. *Reg Anesth Pain Med* 2014;39(4):279–283.

24. American Society of Anesthesiologists Task Force on Sedation and Analgesia by Non-Anesthesiologists. Practice guidelines for sedation and analgesia by non-anesthesiologists. *Anesthesiology* 2002;96(4):1004–1017.

5

Local Anesthetic Pharmacology

Francis V. Salinas

KEY POINTS

1. Local anesthetics must penetrate through several extraneural connective tissue layers to reach the axonal membrane.

2. Local anesthetics provide anesthesia and analgesia by blocking the transmission of painful sensory stimuli along nerve fibers.

3. The action potential is mediated by inward sodium currents and outward potassium currents through their respective voltage-gated ion channels.

4. Local anesthetics bind to the voltage-gated sodium channels, interrupting the rapid inward current of sodium ions and generation of the action potential; thereby inhibiting the transmission of neural impulse.

5. Aminoamide local anesthetics are metabolized in the liver, and aminoester local anesthetics are metabolized by plasma esterase.

6. Local anesthetic potency is related to the physiochemical properties of the specific local anesthetic agent. Increasing lipid solubility increases potency and duration of action.

7. The analgesic efficacy and/or duration of action of local anesthetics may be augmented by the addition of adjuvant agents.

8. Total dose, site of administration, and patient-specific factors (age, cardiovascular and hepatic function, and plasma protein binding) influence subsequent plasma levels and the potential for systemic toxicity.

LOCAL ANESTHETICS ARE A CLASS OF DRUGS that transiently and reversibly inhibit the conduction of sensory, motor, and autonomic neural impulses. They are the primary medications used to provide perioperative regional anesthesia and analgesia. This chapter presents the mechanism of action of local anesthetics, the physiochemical properties that determine their clinical pharmacology, common clinical applications, and potential for toxicity. Karl Koller reported the first clinical use of local anesthetics (cocaine) in 1884 to provide topical anesthesia for ophthalmologic surgery.

I. Clinical anatomy of nerve conduction

A. Anatomy of nerves. The neuron is the basic functional unit responsible for the conduction of neural impulses. It consists of a cell body which is attached to several branching processes (dendrites) and a single axon that transmit neural impulses toward and away from the cell body, respectively (Fig. 5.1). Axons are cylinders of axoplasm encased within a phospholipid bilayer cell membrane that is embedded with various membrane-spanning channel proteins. The most

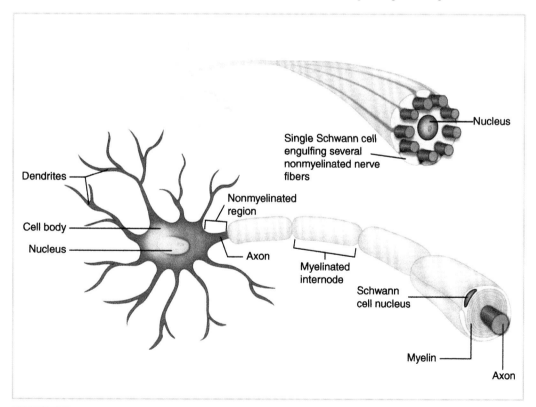

FIGURE 5.1 Representative neuron and myelinated axon and nonmyelinated axon. The neuron consists of a cell body (soma), dendrites, and an axon. Myelinated nerve fibers have a sheath composed of a continuous series of neurolemma (derived from Schwann cells) that surround the axon and form a series of myelin segments. Multiple nonmyelinated nerve fibers are individually encased within a single neurolemma that does not produce myelin. (Adapted from Barash PG, Cullen BF, Stoelting RK, et al. *Clinical Fundamentals of Anesthesia.* 1st ed. Philadelphia, PA: Wolters Kluwer; 2015: 210.)

important of these protein channels include voltage-gated sodium and potassium channels and the sodium–potassium pump. Schwann cells are closely associated with neurons and function to support, insulate, and nourish axons. The cell membrane of Schwann cells (neurolemma) immediately surround axons. A peripheral nerve fiber is composed of an axon, its associated neurolemma, and the surrounding endoneural connective tissue.

B. **Peripheral nerve classification.** Peripheral nerves contain both afferent and efferent nerve fibers that are classified as either myelinated or nonmyelinated (Fig. 5.1). A myelinated nerve fiber is segmentally encased by a continuous series of Schwann cells that produce myelin. Multiple concentric lipid layers of myelin form a specialized neurolemma (myelin sheath) around a single axon. Specific regions (termed nodes of Ranvier), where the voltage-gated sodium channels [VG_{Na}] are concentrated along the axons of myelinated nerve fibers periodically interrupt the myelin sheath. Along myelinated axons, Na^+ conductance is restricted to the nodes of Ranvier. This allows action potential propagation to jump from one node to another via saltatory conduction, which significantly enhances the speed of signal transmission (Table 5.1). In contrast, nonmyelinated nerve fibers consist of multiple axons that are simultaneously encased within the neurolemma of a single nonmyelin producing Schwann cell. VG_{Na} are uniformly distributed along the entire axon of nonmyelinated nerve fibers.

C. **Peripheral nerve fiber microanatomy.** Peripheral nerve fibers are organized within four layers of connective tissue (Fig. 5.2).

1. Individual nerve fibers are encased within *endoneurium*, which contains loose connective tissue that consists of Schwann cells, fibroblasts, and capillaries.

2. A dense layer of collagenous connective tissue, the *perineurium*, encloses bundles of nerve fibers into a fascicle. All but the smallest peripheral nerves are arranged within fascicles. The perineurium functionally provides an effective barrier against penetration of the nerve fibers by foreign substances.

TABLE 5.1 Classification of peripheral nerve fibers

Fiber classification	Diameter (µm)	Myelination	Conduction velocity (m/s)	Anatomic location	Function	Local anesthetic susceptibility
Aα	6–22	Yes	30–120	Efferent to muscles	Motor	++
Aβ	6–22	Yes	30–120	Afferent from skin and joints	Touch and proprioception	++
Aγ	3–6	Yes	15–35	Efferent to muscle spindles	Muscle tone	++++
Aδ	1–4	Yes	5–25	Afferent sensory	Distinct, well-localized (fast) pain, cold temperature, touch	+++
B	<3	Yes	3–15	Preganglionic sympathetic	Autonomic	++
C	0.3–1.3	No	0.7–1.3	Afferent sensory, postganglionic sympathetic	Autonomic, warm temperature, touch, and diffuse (slow) pain	+

+ indicates least susceptible; ++, +++, ++++ indicate most susceptible to conduction blockade.

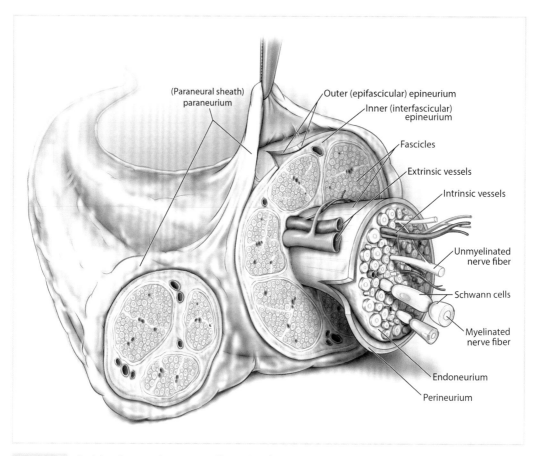

FIGURE 5.2 Peripheral nerve microanatomy illustrating the connective tissues that surround and support peripheral nerve fibers. Individual nerve fibers are encased within *endoneurium*, which contains loose connective tissue that consists of Schwann cells, fibroblasts, and capillaries. A dense layer of collagenous connective tissue, the *perineurium*, encloses bundles of nerve fibers into a fascicle. The *epineurium* is also a dense connective tissue layer that surrounds and encases bundles of fascicles together into a cylindrical sheath structurally resembling a coaxial cable. The *paraneurium* encases peripheral nerves. Together, these tissue layers not only offer protection to peripheral nerves but also present a significant barrier to passive diffusion of local anesthetics toward the axonal cell membrane. (Image Copyright 2017 American Society of Regional Anesthesia and Pain Medicine. Used with permission. All rights reserved).

3. The *epineurium* is also a dense connective tissue layer that surrounds and encases bundles of fascicles together into a cylindrical sheath structurally resembling a coaxial cable.

4. An additional connective tissue layer, *the paraneurium* (*paraneural sheath*), further encases peripheral nerves (1,2). Together, these tissue layers not only offer protection to peripheral nerves but also present a significant barrier to passive diffusion of local anesthetics toward the axonal cell membrane.

II. Electrophysiology of neural conduction and voltage-gated sodium channels

A. **Resting membrane potential** (Fig. 5.3A). Neurons maintain a resting membrane potential of approximately -60 to -70 mV. The Na^+–K^+ (potassium) pump actively cotransports three Na^+ ions out of the cell for every two K^+ ions into the cell. The resulting ionic disequilibrium favors the passive movement of Na^+ ions into the cell and K^+ ions out of the cell. However, despite the concentration gradient for both ions, the resting cell membrane is selectively more permeable to K^+ ions. This facilitates a net passive efflux of K^+ ions out of the cell and leaves a relative net excess of negatively charged ions (polarized) within the axoplasm. This creates the resting electrochemical concentration gradient across the semipermeable cell membrane.

B. The action potential (Fig. 5.3B). Neural impulses are conducted along the axonal cell membrane as action potentials, which are transient membrane depolarizations initiated by various mechanical, chemical, or thermal stimuli. **Depolarization** is mediated primarily via

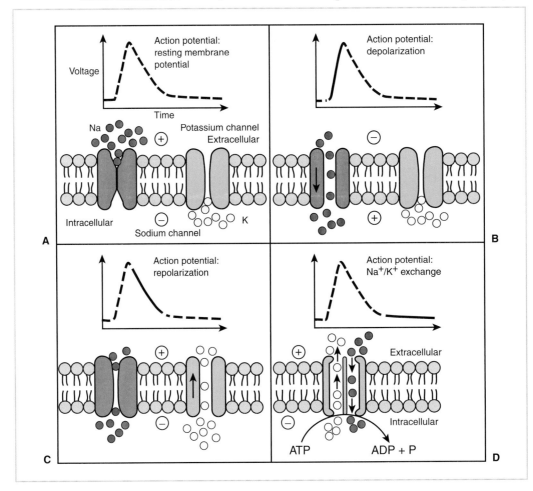

FIGURE 5.3 Sodium and potassium channel functions and ion movements representing the phases of the action potential. **A:** At rest, the sodium channel is in the closed confirmation and there is a relative excess of sodium ions (*red circles*) in the extracellular space and a relative excess of potassium ions in the intracellular space (*yellow circles*). Because there are approximately three positively charged sodium ions in the extracellular space for every two charged potassium ions in the intracellular space, the intracellular space is negative (−50 to −90 mV) relative to the extracellular space. **B:** Following a sufficient stimulus, the voltage-gated sodium channel confirmation changes to the open configuration, and sodium ions flow down their electrochemical gradient into the interior of the neuron, resulting in depolarization. **C:** At the peak of the action potential, the sodium channel conformation changes spontaneously to the inactivated state, which prevents further sodium entry and is refractory to reopening in response to a stimulus. Simultaneously, the voltage-gated potassium channels open, and potassium flows down its concentration gradient to render the neuron interior negative relative to the exterior (repolarization). **D:** The sodium–potassium pump (Na+/K+ adenosine triphosphatase [ATPase]) exchanges three intracellular sodium molecules for every two extracellular potassium molecules, thereby restoring the resting membrane potential and moving the sodium channel to the closed confirmation. ADP, adenosine diphosphate; ATP, adenosine diphosphate; P, phosphate. (Mulroy MF, Bernards CM, McDonald SB, et al. *A Practical Approach to Regional Anesthesia.* 4th ed. Philadelphia, PA: Wolters Kluwer; 2009:6. [Originally Adapted from Barash PK, Clitten S. *Clinical Anesthesia.* 3rd ed. Philadelphia: Lippincott-Raven; 1997:6.])

rapid intracellular influx of Na^+ ions flowing down its electrochemical gradient through VG_{Na}. The VG_{Na} spans the axonal membrane and consists of an α-subunit and one or two varying auxiliary β-subunits. At the resting membrane potential, the VG_{Na} is in a resting (closed) conformation. Upon an initial depolarization, a conformational change results in activation (opening) of the VG_{Na}, inducing a sudden increase in Na^+ ion permeability. The resultant rapid inward Na^+ current activates and opens additional VG_{Na}. This further accelerates depolarization until a threshold membrane potential is reached, triggering an action potential. During the depolarization phase, the inward Na^+ current flows into the axoplasm and spreads to the adjacent (inactive) cell membrane, resulting in a wave of sequential depolarization (and the action potential) propagating along the axon. Although the wave of depolarization spreads from the initial area of excitation in both directions, the just activated membrane behind the impulse is temporarily refractory (owing to inactivation of VG_{Na}) to subsequent depolarization. Thus, the propagation of the impulse is unidirectional.

   C. **Repolarization** (Fig. 5.3C and D). The activated VG_{Na} is inactivated within milliseconds by an additional conformational change. This rapid inactivation process is required for repetitive firing of action potentials in neural circuits and for control of excitability in neurons. Repolarization occurs because of a combination of a progressive decrease in the driving force for the inward Na^+ current and inactivation of VG_{Na}. In addition, membrane depolarization simultaneously activates voltage-gated K^+ channels. This leads to an outward positive current of K^+ ions, which in conjunction with VG_{Na} inactivation, eventually returns the axonal membrane to or just beyond (hyperpolarization) its resting membrane potential.

   D. In **summary**, inward positive currents, mediated by Na^+ ions, depolarize the membrane, and in contrast, outward positive currents, mediated by K^+ ions, repolarize the membrane.

III. **Voltage-gated sodium channels and interactions with local anesthetics.** The prototypical local anesthetic structure consists of a hydrophobic group (typically a lipid-soluble aromatic ring) connected to a tertiary amine group by either an amide or ester linkage (Fig. 5.4). Because the tertiary amine group can accept a proton to become a positively charged quaternary amine, local anesthetics exist in equilibrium as a neutral (base, more hydrophobic form) or the protonated (charged, more hydrophilic form). Local anesthetics must first cross the axonal membrane to reach the local anesthetic binding site. The neutral form more readily crosses the axonal membrane. The charged form is responsible for interacting with the local anesthetic binding site (Fig. 5.4).

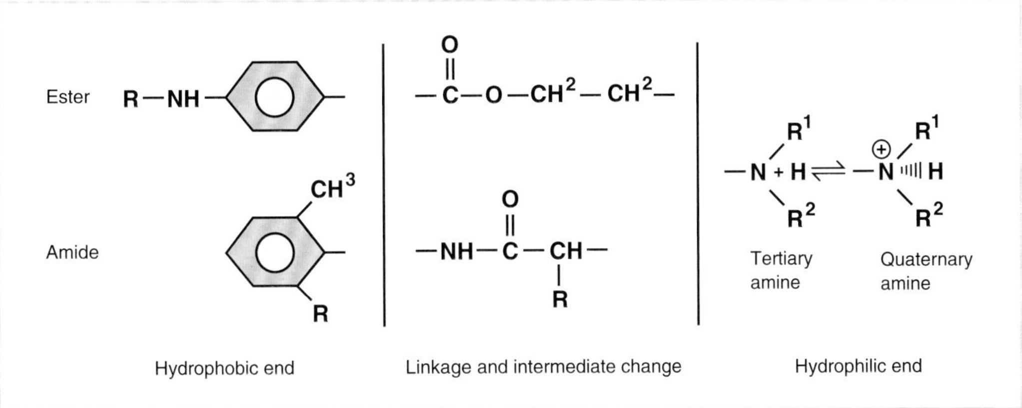

FIGURE 5.4 Typical structures of aminoester and aminoamide local anesthetic molecules. (Mulroy MF, Bernards CM, McDonald SB, et al. *A Practical Approach to Regional Anesthesia*, 4th ed. Philadelphia, PA: Wolters Kluwer; 2009:2.)

4   Local anesthetics act at the axonal membrane by binding to a specific region within the α-subunit of the VG_{Na} (3). This prevents VG_{Na} activation, thus inhibiting the inward Na^+ current that mediates membrane depolarization. The binding site may be approached from two pathways: from the intracellular aspect of the channel pore (hydrophilic pathway) or laterally from within the lipid membrane (hydrophobic pathway) (Fig. 5.4). As the amount of administered local anesthetic increases, an increasing percentage of VG_{Na} can bind to local anesthetics, further inhibiting the inward Na^+ current. Subsequently, the rate of depolarization (in response to stimulation) is attenuated, inhibiting the achievement of the threshold membrane potential. Consequently, achievement of an action potential becomes increasingly difficult. With enough local anesthetic-bound VG_{Na}, an action potential can no longer be generated and impulse propagation is blocked.

    A. Local anesthetics bind more avidly to VG_{Na} in the activated (open) and inactivated (closed) conformations. The difference in binding affinity is attributable to the difference in the availability of the two pathways for local anesthetic to reach the binding site. Local anesthetics produce a concentration-dependent decrease in inward Na^+ current characterized as *tonic blockade*, representing a decrease in the number of open confirmation VG_{Na}.

    B. With repeated depolarization, a greater number of VG_{Na} are in either the activated or inactivated conformations. Therefore, they can be bound at a lower local anesthetic concentration. Additionally, the dissociation rate of local anesthetics from their binding site is slower than the rate of transition from the inactivated to the resting conformation. Thus, repeated stimulation results in accumulation of local anesthetic-bound VG_{Na} characterized as *frequency-dependent blockade*.

  IV. **Mechanisms of nerve block**

    A. **Local anesthetic concentration and volume.** The quality of nerve block is determined not only by the intrinsic potency but also by the concentration and volume of the administered local anesthetic. The potency of a local anesthetic can be expressed as the minimum effective concentration required to establish complete conduction block. The volume of local anesthetic is also important, because a sufficient length of axon or successive nodes of Ranvier must be blocked to inhibit regeneration of the neural impulse. This is caused by the phenomenon of *decremental conduction*. Membrane depolarization passively decays with distance away from the front of the action potential to the point that impulse propagation stops when depolarization falls below the threshold for VG_{Na} activation. If less than a critical length of axon is blocked, the action potential may still be regenerated in the proximal neural membrane segment or node of Ranvier when the decaying depolarization is still above the threshold potential.

    B. **Inherent nerve susceptibility to local anesthetic blockade.** Different types of nerve fibers demonstrate varying minimal blocking concentrations and local anesthetic susceptibilities (Table 5.1). Clinically, there is a predictable progression of sensory and motor function blockade, starting first with loss of temperature sensation, followed by proprioception, motor function, sharp pain, and light touch. Termed *differential block*, this progression was initially attributed to differences in axon diameter, with smaller fibers inherently more susceptible to conduction blockade compared with that of larger fibers. However, small myelinated fibers (Aγ and Aδ) are the most susceptible to conduction blockade. Next in order of block susceptibility are large myelinated fibers (Aα and Aβ), and the least susceptible are small, nonmyelinated C fibers.

CLINICAL PEARL   The afferent fibers that conduct well-localized sharp (surgical) pain and cold temperature sensation share similar conduction velocity and local anesthetic susceptibility. Thus, loss of cold temperature sensation provides a qualitative assessment of the onset and distribution of sensory block.

C. **Anatomic mechanism.** For local anesthetics to bind VG_{Na}, they must initially reach the axonal membrane. Thus, local anesthetics must penetrate through variable amounts of perineural tissue and still maintain a sufficient concentration gradient to diffuse through the phospholipid bilayer.

1. **Peripheral nerve block.** Only a small fraction (1% to 2%) of local anesthetic reaches the neural membrane even when deposited near peripheral nerves. Peripheral nerves that have been desheathed in vitro require about a hundredfold lower local anesthetic concentration than peripheral nerves in vivo. Within peripheral nerves, longitudinal and radial diffusion of local anesthetic will produce varying drug concentrations along and within the nerve during the onset and recovery from clinical block. When local anesthetics are deposited around a peripheral nerve, diffusion progresses from the outer surface (mantle) toward the center (core) along a concentration gradient. Consequently, the nerve fibers arranged in the mantle of mixed peripheral nerves are blocked initially. These outer nerve fibers are typically distributed to more proximal anatomic structures, whereas core fibers innervate more distal structures. This topographic arrangement explains the initial development of proximal, followed by distal anesthesia, because local anesthetic diffuses to the more centrally located core nerve fibers. In summary, the sequence of onset and recovery from peripheral nerve block depends on a combination of the topographic arrangement of the nerve fibers within a mixed peripheral nerve and their inherent susceptibility to local anesthetic blockade.

CLINICAL PEARL   The anatomic distribution of the onset of anesthesia in peripheral nerves is based on the topographic distribution (and subsequent diffusion of local anesthetics) of the nerves from the periphery (mantle) to the innermost (core) of the target peripheral nerve or plexus. This explains why peripheral nerve blocks tend to resolve from distal to proximal.

2. **Neuraxial block.** In contrast, neuraxial nerves are encased in three layers of meninges: the pia mater, arachnoid membrane, and dura mater. The pia mater is adherent to the spinal nerves themselves and is separated from the arachnoid membrane by cerebrospinal fluid that fills the subarachnoid space between these two layers. The *subarachnoid* space, where the spinal nerves are only covered by the pia mater, is the target location for spinal anesthesia. The dura mater further encases the arachnoid membrane, forming the dural sac, a tough covering around the central neuraxis. The epidural space consists of everything located within the vertebral canal but outside the dural sac. The presence of the arachnoid membrane and dura mater result in 10-fold higher local anesthetic dose requirements to produce complete epidural blockade compared with that required in the subarachnoid space.

V. **Local anesthetic pharmacokinetics.** Local anesthetics are most commonly delivered to extravascular tissue near the intended target site. The resulting plasma concentration is influenced by the total dose of administered local anesthetic, the extent of systemic absorption, tissue redistribution, and the rate of elimination. Patient-specific factors such as age, cardiovascular and hepatic function, and plasma protein binding also influence subsequent plasma levels. An understanding of these factors should maximize the clinical application of local anesthetics, while minimizing potential complications associated with potentially toxic systemic drug levels.

A. **Systemic absorption.** The rate and extent of systemic absorption are influenced by several factors, including total local anesthetic dose, site of administration, physiochemical properties of individual local anesthetics, and addition of vasoconstrictors (epinephrine).

1. **Local anesthetic dose**. For any given site of administration, the greater the total dose of local anesthetic, the greater the extent of systemic absorption and peak plasma levels (C_{max}). Furthermore, an increased rate of absorption will also decrease the time to peak plasma levels (T_{max}). Within the clinical range of commonly used doses, the dose–response relationship is nearly linear and is relatively unaffected by anesthetic concentration or speed of injection.

2. **Tissue perfusion.** The extent of perineural tissue perfusion significantly influences systemic absorption, so that local anesthetic administration in highly perfused perineural tissues results in higher C_{max} and shorter T_{max}. Thus, the rate of systemic absorption from highest to lower is intrapleural > intercostal > caudal > epidural > brachial plexus > sciatic/femoral > and subcutaneous tissue.

3. **Physiochemical properties.** The rate of systemic absorption is also influenced by the physiochemical properties of the individual local anesthetic agents. In general, the more potent, lipid-soluble local anesthetics will result in decreased systemic absorption. The greater the lipid solubility, the more likely it will be sequestered in the lipid-rich compartments of both the axonal membrane and perineural tissues.

4. **Vasoconstrictors.** Epinephrine counteracts the inherent vasodilator characteristic of most local anesthetics. The reduction in C_{max} associated with epinephrine is more pronounced for the less lipid-soluble local anesthetics, while increased neural and perineural tissue binding may be a greater determinant of systemic absorption with increased lipid solubility.

5. **General anesthesia with inhaled anesthetics.** Animal data have demonstrated that the plasma concentrations are significantly increased when local anesthetics are administered in the setting of general anesthesia with inhaled anesthetic agents (4).

B. **Distribution.** After systemic absorption, local anesthetics are rapidly distributed throughout all body tissues. The pattern of distribution (and relative tissue concentration) is influenced by the perfusion, partition coefficient, and mass of specific tissue compartments. The highly perfused organs (brain, lung, heart, liver, and kidneys) are responsible for the initial rapid uptake (α-phase), which is followed by a slower redistribution (β-phase) to less perfused tissues (muscle and gut). Because local anesthetics are rapidly extracted by lung tissue, the plasma concentration of local anesthetics decreases significantly as they pass through the pulmonary vasculature.

C. **Biotransformation and elimination.** The chemical linkage determines the biotransformation and elimination of local anesthetics (Fig. 5.4). Aminoamides are metabolized in the liver by cytochrome P-450 enzymes via *N*-dealkylation and hydroxylation. Aminoamide metabolism is highly dependent on hepatic perfusion, hepatic extraction, and enzyme function. Therefore, local anesthetic clearance is decreased by conditions such as cirrhosis and congestive heart failure. Excretion of the aminoamide metabolites occurs by renal excretion, with <5% of unmetabolized local anesthetic excreted by the kidney.

Aminoester local anesthetics are rapidly metabolized by plasma cholinesterase. Procaine and benzocaine are metabolized to *para-aminobenzoic acid* (*PABA*), which has been associated with rare anaphylactic reactions with the use of these local anesthetics. Patients with genetically abnormal plasma cholinesterase or those who are taking cholinesterase inhibitors have decreased aminoester metabolism. They would theoretically be at increased risk for systemic toxic effects, but clinical evidence is lacking.

D. **Clinical pharmacokinetics.** The metabolism of local anesthetics is of significant clinical relevance because systemic toxicity (determined principally by C_{max}) depends on the balance between systemic absorption and elimination.

1. **Plasma protein binding.** Local anesthetics are largely bound to tissue and plasma proteins, yet systemic toxicity is related to the free (unbound) plasma concentration. Thus, plasma protein binding of local anesthetics reduces the free concentration in the systemic circulation and reduces the risk of systemic toxicity. The extent of plasma protein binding is primarily dependent on the plasma levels of α_1-acid glycoprotein and albumin, and it is also influenced by the plasma pH. Clinical conditions that decrease plasma proteins (cirrhosis, pregnancy, and newborn status) decrease binding capacity. Furthermore, the percentage of protein

binding decreases as the pH decreases. Thus, in the presence of acidosis (seizures, cardiac arrest, and renal failure), the amount of unbound drug increases.

2. **Hepatic clearance.** Altered hepatic clearance may also influence the elimination of local anesthetics. For example, neonates have immature hepatic microsomal enzymes, leading to decreased elimination of aminoamide local anesthetics. Some medications such as β-blockers, H_2 receptors antagonists, and fluvoxamine inhibit specific hepatic microsomal enzymes and may also contribute to decreased aminoamide local anesthetic metabolism. Decreased hepatic blood flow can result in a substantial increase of plasma local anesthetic concentration.

   All the previously described factors that influence systemic absorption, distribution, and patient-specific factors should be considered to minimize the risk for systemic toxicity. These factors form the basis for current recommendations of "maximal doses" of local anesthetics (5).
   a. **Clinical conditions that decrease plasma proteins and the extent of plasma protein binding, as well as decrease hepatic blood flow (such as in patients with congestive heart failure) increase the risk for local anesthetic systemic toxicity (LAST).**

VI. **Local anesthetic pharmacodynamics**

A. **Physiochemical properties and relationship to activity and potency.** Local anesthetics in solution are weak bases that typically carry a positive charge at the amine group at physiologic pH. The prototypical local anesthetic structure consists of a hydrophobic group (typically a lipid-soluble aromatic ring) connected to a hydrophilic group (charged amine) by either an amide or ester linkage (Fig. 5.4). The nature of the chemical bond is the basis for classification of local anesthetics as either an aminoamide or aminoester (Table 5.2). The physiochemical properties are largely determined by the nature of the alkyl substitutions on either the aromatic ring or the amine group, the charge of the amine group, or the stereochemistry of the related isomers (Table 5.2). These physiochemical properties largely determine the potency, onset and duration of action, and tendency for differential nerve block.

   1. **Lipid solubility.** Lipid solubility is determined by the degree of alkyl substitutions on either the aromatic ring or the amine group. Lipid solubility is typically expressed by the partition coefficient in a hydrophobic solvent (typically octanol). Compounds with increased octanol solubility are more lipid soluble (Table 5.2). Increased lipid solubility enhances the ability to penetrate the lipid membrane and deliver local anesthetic in closer proximity to the membrane bound VG_{Na}, which in turn correlates with the potency and, to a lesser extent, the duration of action. Although lipid solubility correlates with octanol solubility (and inherent potency in vitro), the minimum in vivo local anesthetic concentration that will block impulse conduction may be affected by numerous factors such as fiber size, type, and myelination, tissue pH (see below), local tissue redistribution and sequestration into lipid-rich perineural compartments, and finally, inherent vasoactive properties of the specific local anesthetic.

   2. **pK_a.** At physiologic pH, local anesthetics are weak bases that exist in equilibrium between either the lipid-soluble (hydrophobic) base form or the water-soluble (hydrophilic) ionized form. The relative percentage of each form is determined by the dissociation constant (pK_a) and surrounding tissue pH. The pK_a is the pH at which the percentage of each form is equal (Table 5.2), which is defined by the Henderson–Hasselbalch equation:

   $$pK_a = pH - \log[BH]/[BH^+]$$

   where $[BH^+]$ is the concentration of the charged (conjugate acid), lipid-insoluble form of local anesthetic, and [B] is the concentration of the uncharged (base) lipid-soluble form of local anesthetic.

TABLE 5.2　Chemical structure and physiochemical properties of clinically useful local anesthetic agents

Local anesthetic	Chemical structure	Partition coefficient (lipid solubility)	pK_a	Percentage ionized at pH 7.4	Percentage protein bound
■ Aminoamides					
Lidocaine		366	7.9	76	65
Prilocaine		129	7.9	76	55
Mepivacaine		130	7.6	61	78
Bupivacaine		3,420	8.1	83	96
Ropivacaine		775	8.1	83	94
■ Aminoesters					
Procaine		100	8.9	97	6
2-Chloroprocaine		810	8.7	95	N/A
Tetracaine		5,822	8.5	93	76

Adapted from Barash PG, Cullen BF, Stoelting RK, et al. *Clinical Anesthesia Fundamentals*, 1st ed. Philadelphia, PA: Wolters Kluwer; 2015:216.

The lower the pK_a for a given local anesthetic, the higher the percentage of the lipid-soluble base form that exists to more readily penetrate the lipid cell membrane, thus speeding the onset of action. After penetration through the cell membrane into the axoplasm, equilibrium between the base form and the charged form is reestablished. It is the charged form within the axoplasm that more avidly binds to local anesthetic binding sites within the channel pore of the VG_{Na}.

3. **Chirality.** Local anesthetics are formulated as either racemic or single-enantiomeric compounds. Racemic compounds (such as bupivacaine) are one-to-one mixtures of a pair of enantiomeric stereoisomers bearing identical chemical composition, but with a different three-dimensional spatial orientation around an asymmetric (chiral) carbon atom. Although enantiomers of local anesthetics have identical physiochemical properties, they exhibit different clinical pharmacodynamics (potency) because of subtle differences in interaction and binding of VG_{Na}. For example, levobupivacaine (the S-enantiomer of bupivacaine) and ropivacaine (the S-enantiomer of bupivacaine, but with a propyl alkyl group rather than the butyl group found in bupivacaine) appear to have equipotent clinical efficacy for neuronal conduction block. However, they have a lower potential for cardiac systemic toxicity than either the R-enantiomer or the racemic mixtures.

B. Additives to augment local anesthetic activity

1. **Sodium bicarbonate.** Local anesthetics are formulated as hydrochloride salts to increase their solubility and stability. The pH of commercially prepared local anesthetic solutions ranges from 3.9 to 6.47 and is especially acidic when prepackaged with epinephrine (see below). Given that the pK_a of the most commonly used local anesthetics ranges from 7.6 to 8.9 (Table 5.2), <3% of the local anesthetic solution is in the lipid-soluble neutral form at physiologic pH. This slows penetration through the cell membrane and delays the onset of conduction block (Fig. 5.5). An even lower lipid-soluble fraction may be encountered clinically when local

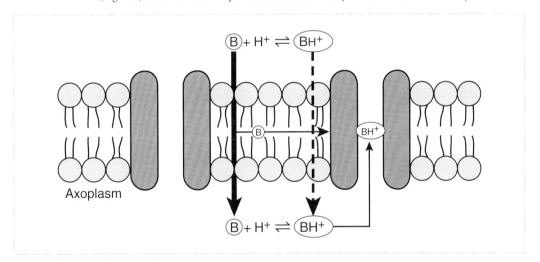

FIGURE 5.5 Model of local anesthetic interaction with the sodium channel. In the extracellular fluid, the local anesthetic molecule is in equilibrium as both a neutral tertiary amine base **(B)** and a positively charged quaternary amine **(BH⁺)**. The uncharged tertiary form of the local anesthetic crosses the cell membrane much more readily than does the charged quaternary form, but the uncharged form does cross to same extent. The same equilibrium between the uncharged tertiary amine and the charged quaternary amine exists within the axoplasm of the nerve as well, although the lower pH within the neuron will tend to favor the quaternary form more than in the extracellular fluid. Only the charged quaternary form is capable of interacting with the local anesthetic binding site within the sodium channel, and it can reach that site only from inside the neuron. Uncharged local anesthetics (e.g., benzocaine) are thought to interact with sodium channels at a separate site that may be reached from within the axonal membrane. Alternatively, uncharged local anesthetics may alter sodium channel function by altering the properties of the axonal membrane and therefore the interaction of the sodium channel with the membrane. (Mulroy M, Bernards, C, McDonald SB, et al. A Practical Approach to Regional Anesthesia. 4th Ed. Philadelphia, PA: Wolters Kluwer; 2009:7).

anesthetics are injected into infected tissues that have a more acidic pH. Thus, alkalinization of local anesthetic solutions by the addition of sodium bicarbonate may potentially increase the onset and the quality of conduction block by increasing the percentage of lipid-soluble base form. Clinical studies demonstrate that the addition of sodium bicarbonate may speed the onset of action, and enhance the depth of sensory and motor block of intermediate-acting local anesthetics (lidocaine and mepivacaine) for lumbar epidural anesthesia and to a much lesser degree, peripheral nerve blocks. Typically, 1 meq of sodium bicarbonate (1 mL of a standard 8.4% solution) is added for every 10 mL of either lidocaine or mepivacaine. In contrast, addition of sodium bicarbonate has minimal effect on the onset of action with the longer acting, more potent amide local anesthetics (bupivacaine or ropivacaine) (6,7).

CLINICAL PEARL   Sodium bicarbonate has been shown to significantly hasten the onset of epidural anesthesia (most commonly for conversion of labor epidural analgesia to surgical anesthesia for cesarean delivery) with lidocaine. However, there appears to be no clinically relevant difference when used with lidocaine or mepivacaine peripheral nerve blocks. The addition of sodium bicarbonate does not hasten the onset of action of the long-acting amide local anesthetics such as bupivacaine or ropivacaine.

2. **Epinephrine.** Epinephrine is commonly added to local anesthetic solutions to induce vasoconstriction at the site of injection. The α_1-adrenoreceptor–mediated vasoconstrictive effect of epinephrine augments local anesthetic activity by antagonizing the inherent vasodilating effect of most local anesthetics. Consequently, decreased vascular absorption facilitates and maintains intraneural local anesthetic uptake. The reported clinical benefits include enhancement of the quality of conduction block and prolongation of the duration of action. It also decreases the peak systemic local anesthetics levels, potentially limiting toxic effects (7,8). The extent to which epinephrine prolongs the duration of conduction block largely depends on the physiochemical properties of the local anesthetic as well as the site of injection. For example, the addition of epinephrine to lidocaine typically extends the conduction block by at least 50%, but the addition of epinephrine to bupivacaine has little to no clinically relevant effect on the duration of blockade. Additional analgesic effects because of epinephrine (and clonidine) may also occur through interaction with α_2-adrenoreceptors in the central nervous system (CNS), directly activating endogenous analgesic mechanisms. The recommended dosing for epidural nerve blocks is 5 µg of epinephrine per mL of local anesthetic. The recommended dosing for peripheral nerve blocks is 2.5 µcg of epinephrine per mL of local anesthetic (8).

3. **Clonidine and dexmedetomidine.** Clonidine is a direct-acting α_2-agonist that inhibits pain transmission by binding to presynaptic and postsynaptic receptors of nociceptive afferent fibers in the dorsal horn of the spinal cord. Clonidine has been shown to block conductance in C and Aδ nerve fibers. Neuraxial administration of clonidine results in selective spinally mediated analgesia, and it is primarily used as an adjunct to local anesthetics. It reduces the concentration of (both intermediate- and long-acting) local anesthetics required for anesthesia and analgesia and increases the duration of both sensory and motor block (7). The analgesic effect of peripherally administered clonidine is not directly attributable to an α_2-agonist effect but instead to blockade of current through hyperpolarization-activated cyclic nucleotide-gated channels, resulting in enhancement of activity-dependent hyperpolarization. This current facilitates return to the resting membrane potential from a hyperpolarized state after an action potential. When this current is blocked, axons are unable to generate subsequent action potentials. Clonidine will improve the duration of sensory block (typically by 2.0 to 2.5 hours), regardless of whether lidocaine or bupivacaine

is used. The most common clinically used dose ranges from 0.5 to 1.0 µg/kg. The potential clonidine-associated side effects (bradycardia, hypotension, and sedation) as well as cost have limited more widespread clinical use. Dexmedetomidine is a highly selective α_2-agonist (α_2:α_1 affinity ratio of 1,620:1, 7 times greater than that of clonidine) has been shown to prolong the duration of peripheral nerve blocks by 2 to 5 hours. Because dexmedetomidine shares similar potential side effects and pharmacoeconomic considerations to clonidine, it has also not gain widespread use for peripheral regional anesthesia–analgesia.

4. **Opioids.** Opioids are the most commonly administered local anesthetic adjuvants for central neuraxial anesthesia and analgesia (9).

   a. **Neuraxial administration.** Opioids synergistically enhance the anesthetic and analgesic effects of local anesthetics by attenuating C-fiber nociception in the dorsal horn of the spinal cord; binding to cerebral opioid receptors from cephalad transport in the cerebrospinal fluid, as well as peripheral and central effects upon vascular absorption. The relative contribution of these antinociceptive actions is influenced by the total dose, site of administration (intrathecal vs. epidural), and physiochemical properties of the specific opioid. Lipophilic agents such as fentanyl demonstrate a rapid onset and shorter duration of action, a narrower band of segmental analgesia owing to rapid uptake by neural tissue, and equally rapid systemic absorption. In contrast, hydrophilic opioids such as morphine penetrate neural tissue less rapidly, resulting in a slower onset and longer duration of action. Uptake and elimination from neural tissue is delayed, allowing more widespread cerebrospinal fluid distribution. The most common potential adverse effects of central neuraxial opioids include respiratory depression, pruritus, and nausea and vomiting.

CLINICAL PEARL Fentanyl is typically used to provide rapid onset of neuraxial analgesia and to augment the depth of local anesthetic-mediated spinal anesthesia. In contrast, morphine is used to provide extended postoperative analgesia well after the resolution local anesthetic-mediated sensory and motor block.

   b. **Peripheral and intra-articular administration.** There is no data to support the administration of the most commonly used opioids for either peripheral nerve block or intra-articular administration (7).

CLINICAL PEARL There is no data to support a locally mediated effect (for peripheral nerve blocks or intra-articular administration) for opioids.

5. **Glucorticoids.** Epidural administration of glucocorticoids has an established history of efficacy and safety for the treatment neck and back pain secondary to spinal nerve root irritation. There has been recent interest in the peripheral perineural administration of dexamethasone because of the consistent increase in the postoperative analgesic duration for both upper and lower extremity peripheral nerve blocks. Although the perineural administration of dexamethasone has consistently been shown to increase the analgesic duration after peripheral nerve blocks, it is not clear that this effect is caused by peripherally mediated and/or systemic analgesic effects. Although perineural dexamethasone has been shown to increase the duration of sensorimotor block and analgesic duration by approximately 20% in some studies, other studies have failed to demonstrate a clinically relevant difference (10–13). Owing to an incomplete understanding of its primary mechanism of action and

the conflicting clinical data, the authors cannot provide any firm clinical recommendations until more is evidence is published.

6. **Liposomal bupivacaine.** Liposomes are microscopic structures consisting of phospholipid bilayer containing an aqueous core. They may be unilamellar (single lipid bilayer enclosing an aqueous core), multilamellar (concentric lipid bilayers), or mutlivesicular (several tightly packed nonconcentric lipid bilayer particles). The nonconcentric nature of multivesicular liposomes confers characteristic drug release patterns from the aqueous core leading to increased stability and an extended duration of drug release. Liposomal bupivacaine consists of particles containing multiple vesicles of bupivacaine loaded in the aqueous chambers. Each particle is composed of a honeycomb-like structure of multiple internal aqueous chambers containing encapsulated bupivacaine. Liposomal bupivacaine is the US Food and Drug Administration (FDA) approved for single-dose wound infiltration in postoperative analgesia, and it is currently not FDA approved for either epidural or peripheral perineural administration. Compared to placebo, liposomal bupivacaine decreased postoperative pain and postoperative opioid requirements in patients undergoing hemorrhoidectomy or bunionectomy. In contrast, liposomal bupivacaine offered no clinically relevant difference in postoperative pain or postoperative opioid requirements compared to plain bupivacaine in patients undergoing breast augmentation or total knee arthroplasty. Liposomal bupivacaine has not been shown to be more neurotoxic or cardiotoxic compared to plain bupivacaine. The limited evidence demonstrates prolonged analgesia compared to placebo, but its increased analgesic efficacy (and pharmacoeconomic advantage) compared to plain bupivacaine warrants further evaluation in rigorously designed prospective trials (14).

VII. Toxicity of local anesthetics. Clinically significant adverse effects of local anesthetics include LAST, local tissue toxicity, allergic reactions, and local anesthetic-specific effects. LAST results from excessive plasma concentrations of local anesthetic, because of either unintentional direct intravascular injection or systemic absorption of larger doses of local anesthetics performed during peripheral nerve blocks, epidural anesthesia, or even large volume infiltration (*tumescent*) anesthesia. As previously discussed, plasma concentration is determined by the balance between systemic absorption and elimination. Clinically significant symptoms of LAST manifest primarily in the CNS and cardiovascular system. LAST, neurotoxicity, and myotoxicity are discussed in more detail in Chapter 14 (Complications Associated with Regional Anesthesia).

A. **Allergic reactions.** Adverse reactions to local anesthetics are relatively common, but true immune-mediated allergic reactions to local anesthetics are rare (15). They are more commonly associated with aminoester local anesthetics, likely because of their metabolism to the recognized allergen, **PABA**. Some preparations of aminoamide local anesthetics also contain methylparaben, which has a similar chemical structure to PABA and is the most likely cause of allergic reactions to aminoamide local anesthetics. Follow-up evaluation with skin prick, intradermal injections, or subcutaneous provocative dose challenges is recommended in any patient suspected of immune-mediated local anesthetic allergy (16).

VIII. Local anesthetic agents and their common clinical applications

A. **Aminoamide local anesthetics**

1. **Lidocaine.** Lidocaine was the first widely used aminoamide local anesthetic and remains the most commonly used local anesthetic. It may be used for infiltration, intravenous regional anesthesia (Bier block), peripheral nerve block, and neuraxial (subarachnoid and epidural) anesthesia. It is characterized by a rapid to intermediate onset of action and intermediate duration of action for peripheral nerve blocks and epidural anesthesia. Although concerns over

transient neurologic symptoms (TNS) have led to decreased use for subarachnoid anesthesia (17), it remains popular for epidural anesthesia. Lidocaine may be applied topically as a jelly, an ointment, a patch, or in aerosol form (to anesthetize the upper airway). Intravenous injections targeting relatively low plasma levels (<5 μg/mL) produce systemic analgesia and have been used as an adjunct to blunt the sympathetic response to laryngoscopy and intubation. One of its most common uses involves intravenous injection to decrease the discomfort associated with intravenous administration of propofol. Lidocaine infusions have been administered to treat chronic neuropathic pain as well as acute postoperative pain.

2. **Mepivacaine.** Mepivacaine has a chemical structure combining the piperidine ring of cocaine with the xylidine ring of lidocaine. It shares a similar clinical profile to lidocaine but with a slightly longer duration of action because it results in less vasodilation. As a spinal anesthetic agent, it appears to have a lower, although not clinically insignificant, incidence of TNS compared with that of lidocaine (17). Metabolism in the fetus and neonate is prolonged and, therefore, it is not used for obstetric analgesia.

3. **Bupivacaine.** Bupivacaine is a more lipid-soluble, structural homologue of mepivacaine owing to a butyl group, rather than a methyl group, on its piperidine ring (Table 5.2). Thus, it is characterized by a relatively slower onset compared with that of lidocaine, but it has an extended duration of action. It provides prolonged sensory anesthesia and analgesia that typically outlasts the duration and intensity of its motor block, especially with the use of lower concentrations in continuous infusions. This characteristic has established bupivacaine as the most widely used local anesthetic for labor epidural analgesia and for acute postoperative pain management. Single injections for peripheral nerve block applications may provide surgical anesthesia for up to 12 hours and sensory analgesia lasting up to 24 hours. It is widely used for subarachnoid anesthesia, typically with duration of action of 2 to 3 hours and, in contrast to lidocaine or mepivacaine, it has rarely been associated with TNS.

4. **Ropivacaine.** Ropivacaine is another structural homologue of mepivacaine and bupivacaine, but with a propyl group on its piperidine ring (Table 5.2), and it is also formulated as an S-enantiomer. Together, these two characteristics result in less potency for sensorimotor blockade and a decreased cardiotoxic profile compared with that for bupivacaine (18–20). Animal studies suggest that the smaller molecular size of ropivacaine, as opposed to steroselectivtiy, maybe the more important factor in reducing the risk for cardiotoxicity (21). It has also an inherent vasoconstriction effect, which may contribute to its reduced cardiotoxic profile and possibly augment its duration of action. Although there is some evidence to suggest that ropivacaine may produce a more favorable sensorimotor differential block compared with bupivacaine, the lack of equivalent potency hinders true comparisons. Overall, the clinical profile for peripheral nerve blocks is similar to bupivacaine, considering its decreased potency compared with that of bupivacaine. In contrast, ropivacaine appears to be 30% to 40% less potent compared to bupivacaine for spinal anesthesia (19,20).

B. **Aminoester local anesthetics**

1. **Procaine.** Procaine was used primarily for infiltration and spinal anesthesia during the first half of the 20th century. Its low potency, relatively slow onset of action (likely owing to its high pK_a), and short duration of action limit the widespread use of procaine. Concerns regarding TNS with lidocaine prompted a renewed interest in the use of procaine for intermediate duration subarachnoid anesthesia. Despite its lower incidence of TNS compared with that of lidocaine, the increased risk of block failure and associated nausea has limited its clinical utility.

2. **2-Chloroprocaine.** Owing to its relative low potency and extremely rapid metabolism by plasma cholinesterases, 2-chloroprocaine may be used in relatively higher concentrations (2% to 3%), yet with the lowest potential for systemic toxicity of all the clinically useful local

anesthetic agents. Despite its relatively high pK_a, the use of relatively higher concentrations results in rapid onset of surgical anesthesia. This characteristic, along with virtually no transmission to the fetus, makes it particularly useful when a rapid onset of surgical epidural anesthesia (i.e., urgent or emergent cesarean delivery) is required. The preservative-free solution of 2-chloroprocaine is gaining increased popularity for ambulatory subarachnoid anesthesia, where a rapid onset of action along with a predictably short duration of action is desired. Furthermore, the use of 2-chlororprocaine has been associated with very low incidence of TNS. Although 2-chloroprocaine has recently been approved for subarachnoid anesthesia in Europe, it has not received FDA approval and its use for this indication in the United States remains off-label.

3. **Cocaine.** Cocaine is the only naturally occurring local anesthetic agent. Current clinical applications for cocaine are largely restricted to topical anesthesia for the ear, nose, and throat procedures, where its intense vasoconstriction is clinically useful to reduce bleeding when instrumenting the nasopharynx. Cocaine inhibits the neuronal reuptake of norepinephrine, mediating its neurogenic vasoconstrictive effects. But it can also result in significant cardiovascular side effects, such as hypertension, tachycardia, and dysrhythmias. Concerns regarding its potential for cardiovascular toxicity, along with its potential for diversion and abuse, have markedly limited its clinical use.

REFERENCES

1. Franco C. Connective tissues associated with peripheral nerves. *Reg Anesth Pain Med* 2012;37:363–365.
2. Prasad NK, Capek S, de Ruiter GC, et al. The subparaneurial compartment: a new concept in the clinico-anatomic classification of peripheral nerve lesions. *Clin Anat* 2015;28:925–930.
3. Scholz A. Mechanisms of (local) anaesthetics on voltage-gated sodium and other ion channels. *Br J Anaesth* 2002;89:52–61.
4. Copeland SE, Ladd LA, Gu XQ, et al. The effects of general anesthesia on the central nervous and cardiovascular toxicity of local anesthetics. *Anesth Analg* 2008;106:1429–1439.
5. Rosenberg PH, Veering BT, Urmey WF. Maximum recommended doses of local anesthetics: a multifactorial concept. *Reg Anesth Pain Med* 2004;29:564–575.
6. Lambert DH. Clinical value of adding sodium bicarbonate to local anesthetics. *Reg Anesth Pain Med* 2002;27:328–329.
7. Bailard NS, Ortiz J, Flores RA. Additives to local anesthetics for peripheral nerve blocks: evidence. Limitations, and recommendations. *Am J Health-Syst Pharm* 2014;71:373–385.
8. Neal JM. Effects of epinephrine in local anesthetics on the central and peripheral nervous system. *Reg Anesth Pain Med* 2003;28:124–134.
9. Rathmell JP, Lair TR, Nauman B. The role of intrathecal drugs in the treatment of acute pain. *Anesth Analg* 2005;101(5 Suppl):S30–S43.
10. Leurcharusmee P, Aliste J, Van Zundert, et al. A multicenter randomized comparison between intravenous and perineural dexamethasone for ultrasound-guided infraclavicular block. *Reg Anesth Pain Med* 2016;41:328–333.
11. Aliste J, Leurcharusmee P, Engsusophon P, et al. A randomized comparison between intravenous and perineural dexamethasone for ultrasound-guided axillary block. *Can J Anaesth* 2017;64:29–36.
12. Abdallah FW, Johnson J, Chan V, et al. Intravenous and perineural dexamethasone similarly prolong the duration of analgesia after supraclavicular brachial plexus block: a randomized, triple-arm, double-blind, placebo-controlled trial. *Reg Anesth Pain Med* 2015;40:125–132.
13. Rahangdale R, Kendall MC, McCarthy RJ, et al. The effects of perineural versus intravenous dexamethasone on sciatic nerve blockade outcome: a randomized, double-blind placebo-controlled study. *Anesth Analg* 2014;118:1113–1119.
14. Tong YC, Kaye AD, Urman RD. Liposomal bupivacaine and clinical outcome. *Best Pract Res Clin Anaesthesiol* 2014;28:15–27.

15. Kvisselgaard AD, Krøgaard M, Mosbech HF, et al. No cases of perioperative allergy to local anesthetics in the Danish Anaesthesia Allergy Centre. *Acta Anaesthesiol Scand* 2017;61:149–155.
16. McClimon B, Rank M, Li J. The predictive value of skin testing in the diagnosis of local anesthetic allergy. *Allergy Asthma Proc* 2011;32:95–98.
17. Zaric D, Pace NL. Transient neurological symptoms (TNS) following spinal anesthesia with lidocaine versus other local anesthetics. *Cochrane Database Syst Rev* 2009;15:CD003006.
18. Graf BM, Abraham I, Eberbach N, et al. Differences in cardiotoxicity of bupivacaine and ropivacaine are the result of physiochemical properties and stereoselective properties. *Anesthesiology* 2002;96:1427–1434.
19. Camorcia M, Capagno G, Berrita C, et al. The relative potencies for motor block after intrathecal ropivacaine, levobupivacaine, and bupivacaine. *Anesth Analg* 2007;104:904–907.
20. Lee YY, Ngan Kee WD, Fong SY, et al. The median effective dose of bupivacaine, levobupivacaine, and ropivacaine after intrathecal injection in lower limb surgery. *Anesth Analg* 2009;109:1331–1334.
21. Groban L, Deal DD, Vernon JC, et al. Does local anesthetic steroselectivtiy or structure predict myocardial depression in anesthetized canines? *Reg Anesth Pain Med* 2002;27:460–468.

6

Spinal Anesthesia

Francis V. Salinas and De Q.H. Tran

KEY POINTS

1. Spinal blocks provide a reliable and rapid onset of dense surgical anesthesia. They should be performed below the L2–L3 intervertebral space to minimize the risk of mechanical trauma to the spinal cord.

2. Knowledge of dermatomal projections is paramount to determine whether the sensory block is adequate for the planned surgical procedure.

3. Subarachnoid **distribution** of local anesthetic agents determines the extent of sensorimotor and sympathetic block. Distribution can be manipulated through the interplay of local anesthetic baricity and patient position (gravity). **Elimination** (vascular absorption) of local anesthetics from the subarachnoid space determines the duration of action.

4. Common adjuncts used to prolong (and intensify) spinal anesthesia include α-adrenergic agonists and opioids.

6. Although preservative-free 2-chloroprocaine offers significant benefits for outpatient surgery, the Food and Drug Administration has not approved its administration for spinal blocks.

7. The midline approach is simple to learn and adequate for most patients. However, in subjects with difficult spinal anatomy, the operator could employ a paramedian approach, lumbosacral method, or ultrasound assistance.

8. Absolute contraindications to spinal anesthesia include patient refusal, infection at the puncture site, untreated hypovolemia, coagulopathy, and increased intracranial pressure.

9. Spinal anesthesia can be associated with major cardiovascular trespass (e.g., bradycardia, hypotension) and serious side effects (e.g., nerve damage, infection, neuraxial hematoma).

1 **ADMINISTRATION OF LOCAL ANESTHETIC** into the subarachnoid space results in a **reliable** and **rapid onset** of **dense surgical anesthesia**. Despite the technical simplicity of spinal blocks, the anesthesiologist should possess a thorough understanding of the anatomy of the lumbosacral spine, the determinants of subarachnoid local anesthetic distribution, and the factors that influence block duration. Furthermore, knowledge of the physiologic effects and potential complications related to spinal anesthesia is paramount to ensure patient safety.

I. Anatomy

A. **Vertebral column.** The vertebral column is composed of 33 vertebrae and 5 ligaments. Together, they form a protective exoskeleton around the spinal cord.

1. There are **7 cervical, 12 thoracic, 5 lumbar, 5 sacral, and 4 coccygeal** vertebral segments (Fig. 6.1). Spinal anesthesia is typically performed in **the lower lumbar region.** The lumbar vertebra is composed of an anterior vertebral body and posterior bony elements. The latter include two pedicles, which project posteriorly from the vertebral body, and two flattened laminae, which connect the pedicles to form the vertebral arch. The anterior and posterior bony elements combine to delineate the **vertebral foramen** (Fig. 6.2). Vertebral foramina of adjoining vertebrae form the longitudinal spinal canal, which houses the spinal cord. The adjoining paired pedicles of each vertebra display superior and inferior notches. The latter form the **intervertebral foramina** through which the paired segmental spinal nerves exit the spinal canal (Fig. 6.2). A single **spinous process** projects posteriorly (and slightly caudally) from the posterior aspect of the vertebral arch at the midline junction of the paired laminae. The bony elements provide sites for muscular and ligamentous attachments

2. **Five ligaments anchor the vertebral column** (Fig. 6.3). The **supraspinous ligament** connects the tips of the spinous processes from the seventh cervical vertebra to the sacrum. The **interspinous ligament** connects adjoining spinous processes. The laminae of adjacent vertebral arches are connected by the tough, wedge-shaped **ligamentum flavum**, which is composed primarily of elastin. The ligamentum flavum binds the paired laminae of adjoining vertebrae together, thereby forming the **posterior wall of the vertebral spinal canal**. It is this posterior ligamentous "opening" (i.e., the intervertebral or interlaminar space) that a spinal needle traverses to reach the subarachnoid space. Anatomic studies demonstrate a 9% to 11% incidence of gaps in the midline of the ligamenta flava.

3. The vertebral column displays **characteristic curvatures in the lumbar and thoracic regions** (Figs. 6.1 and 6.4). Local anesthetic solution injected at the peak height of the lumbar anterior convexity (lumbar lordosis) will distribute both caudad and cephalad to varying degrees depending on the baricity of the solution. The cephalad spread of hyperbaric local anesthetic solutions is typically limited to the mid-to-upper thoracic dermatomes because of pooling within the thoracic concavity (thoracic kyphosis).

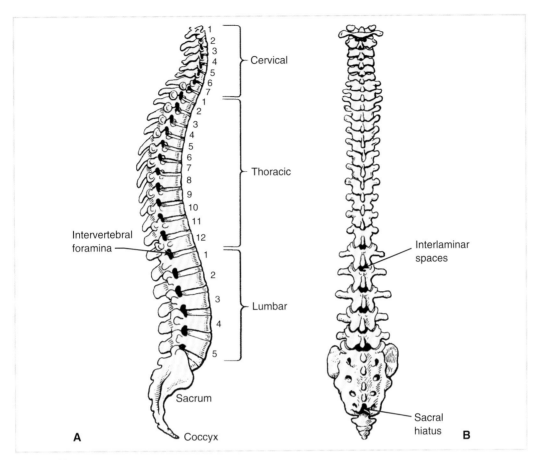

FIGURE 6.1 Vertebral column, lateral **(A)** and posterior **(B)** views, illustrating the cervical, thoracic, lumbar, sacral, and coccygeal segments. Note the curvatures, intervertebral foramina, and interlaminar spaces. (Adapted from Cousins MJ, Bridenbaugh LD, eds. *Neural Blockade in Clinical Anesthesia and Management of Pain*. 3rd ed. Philadelphia: Lippincott Williams & Wilkins; 1998:205.)

B. **Meninges.** The spinal meninges consist of **three membranes** (the *dura mater, arachnoid mater*, and *pia mater*). In conjunction with the cerebrospinal fluid (CSF), the meninges cushion the spinal cord and nerve roots in the subarachnoid space (Fig. 6.5).

1. The **dura mater** ("tough mother"), the outermost and thickest meningeal membrane, is composed primarily of collagen fibrils, interspersed with elastic fibers and ground substance in an anatomic arrangement that allows ready passage of drugs (1). Historically, the dura was (incorrectly) assumed to be the primary barrier for drug diffusion from the epidural to the subarachnoid space. The dura mater forms the **dural sac**, which consists of a long tubular sheath contained within the surrounding spinal canal, which extends from the foramen magnum to the lower border of the second sacral vertebra. At this level, the dural sac fuses with the filum terminale. The dura mater also extends laterally along the spinal nerve roots, becoming continuous with the epineurium of spinal nerves at the level of intervertebral foramina.

2. The **arachnoid mater**, which is closely adherent to the inner surface of the dura mater, is composed of overlapping layers of flattened epithelial-like cells that are connected by frequent tight and occluding junctions (2). The arachnoid is not directly attached to the dura

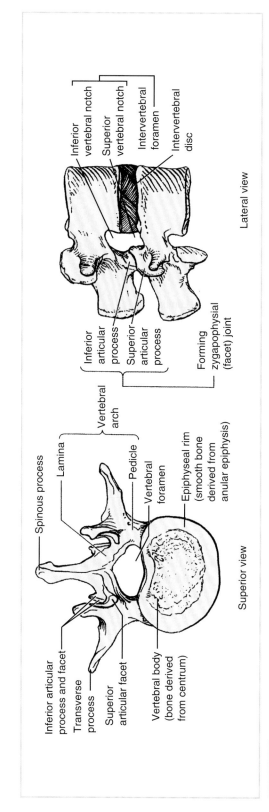

FIGURE 6.2 Typical lumbar vertebra illustrating superior and lateral views of the anterior vertebral body, the elements that form the vertebral arch (the paired pedicles and paired laminae), and single midline spinous process. Note the superior and inferior vertebral notches of the adjoining pedicles, which form the intervertebral foramen. (Adapted from Moore KL, Dalley AF. *Clinically Oriented Anatomy.* 5th ed. Philadelphia: Lippincott Williams & Wilkins; 2006:480.)

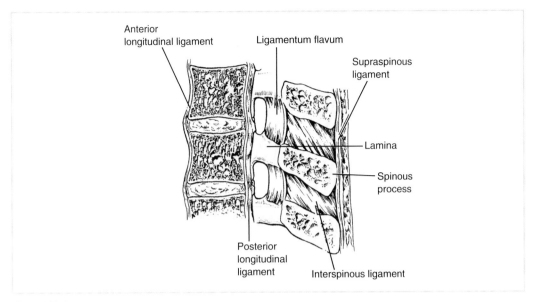

FIGURE 6.3 Sagittal section of vertebral column illustrating the supporting ligaments and their bony attachments. The interspinous ligaments connect adjacent spinous processes, and the ligamentum flavum connects adjacent laminae. (Adapted from Cousins MJ, Bridenbaugh LD, eds. *Neural Blockade in Clinical Anesthesia and Management of Pain*. 3rd ed. Philadelphia: Lippincott Williams & Wilkins; 1998:205.)

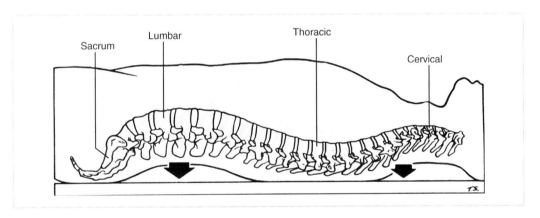

FIGURE 6.4 Normal curvature of the spinal column in the supine horizontal position. Hyperbaric solutions injected at the peak of lumbar lordosis will distribute (through gravity) to the lower sacral and thoracic concavities. (Adapted from Raj PP. *Handbook of Regional Anesthesia*. New York: Churchill Livingstone; 1985:225.)

but is held against its inner surface (dura–arachnoid interface) by the pressure of the **CSF**. During spinal anesthesia, the needle penetrates the dura and arachnoid simultaneously. Functionally, the arachnoid mater accounts for the resistance to drug diffusion through spinal meninges.

3. The **pia mater**, which closely invests the surface of the spinal cord and nerve roots, is composed of three to six layers of cells (3). The **subarachnoid space, which lies between the arachnoid mater and the pia mater and contains the CSF**, constitutes the target compartment for spinal anesthesia. The pia mater extends to the conus medullaris, where it becomes the filum terminale. The latter anchors the spinal cord to the sacrum (Fig. 6.5).

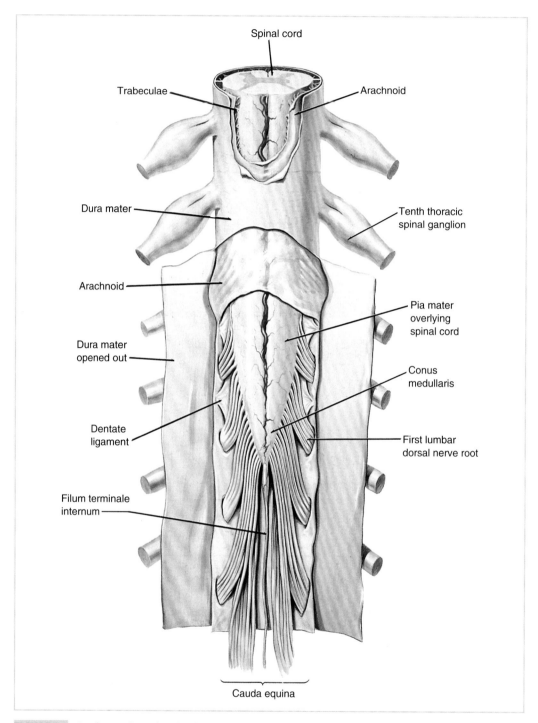

FIGURE 6.5 Lumbosacral spinal cord and the spinal meninges (dura, arachnoid, and pia). Note also the terminal portion of the spinal cord (conus medullaris) and the nerve roots of the lower lumbar and sacral spinal cord segments, giving rise to the cauda equina. (Adapted from Cousins MJ, Bridenbaugh LD, eds. *Neural Blockade in Clinical Anesthesia and Management of Pain*. 3rd ed. Philadelphia: Lippincott Williams & Wilkins; 1998:209.)

C. **Spinal cord**

1. The spinal cord is a **cylindrical structure** that gives rise to 31 pairs of spinal nerves. In turn, each spinal cord segment gives rise to paired **ventral motor and dorsal sensory roots**. Motor and sensory roots cross the subarachnoid space separately before joining together (close to the intervertebral foramina) to form the mixed spinal nerves. Although larger than their ventral counterparts, dorsal nerve roots commonly divide into two or three separate bundles upon exiting the spinal cord. In contrast, most ventral roots exit as a single bundle (4). Moreover, as dorsal nerve root bundles course further laterally, they further subdivide into as many as 10 fascicles before the dorsal root becomes the dorsal root ganglion (5). Therefore, the larger multifilamentous dorsal nerve roots offer a substantially larger surface area for local anesthetic uptake compared to the smaller, unitary ventral roots. This partially explains the faster onset of sensory versus motor blockade.

2. The skin area supplied by a spinal nerve (and its corresponding spinal cord segment) is called a *dermatome* (Fig. 6.6). Dermatomal assessment for the loss of sensory functions (such as temperature, pinprick, and touch) provides a surrogate marker for the segmental distribution of surgical anesthesia.

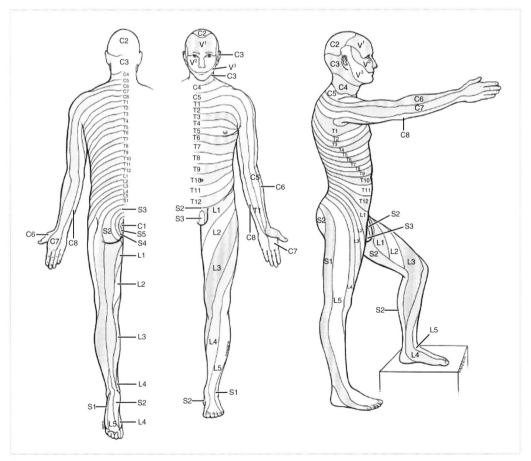

FIGURE 6.6 Sensory dermatomes. (Adapted from Agur AMR, Lee MJ, eds. *Grant's Atlas of Anatomy*. 10th ed. Philadelphia: Lippincott Williams & Wilkins; 1999:296.)

3. In adults, the **spinal cord is shorter than the vertebral column**. The caudal extent of the spinal cord (known as the *conus medullaris* [Fig. 6.5]) usually extends to the **lower third of the first lumbar vertebral body**, but may occasionally reach the upper third of the third lumbar vertebral body (6) and rarely the L4 level. Therefore, attempting spinal anesthesia at or above the L2–L3 intervertebral space (IVS) could result in mechanical trauma to the spinal cord in a small number of patients.

4. The discrepancy in length between spinal cord and vertebral column results in a **progressive obliquity of the lower thoracic, lumbar, and sacral spinal nerve roots**. The collection of spinal nerve roots caudal to the conus medullaris is known as the *cauda equina* (Fig. 6.5). The enlargement of the subarachnoid space containing the cauda equina is termed the *lumbar cistern*. Local anesthetics are deposited within the latter during the performance of spinal anesthesia.

D. **Surface anatomy**

1. Accurate identification of **IVS** levels is paramount for successful spinal anesthesia. The desired level is determined by the palpation of surface landmarks. A **line connecting the iliac crests (i.e., the intercristal or Tuffier's line) most commonly intersects the vertebral column at the L4–L5 IVS** (Fig. 6.7) (6). However, the intercristal line may intersect the vertebral column as cephalad as the L3–L4 IVS and as caudad as the L5–S1 IVS (Fig. 6.8). Even **experienced anesthesiologists incorrectly identify the IVS 70% of the time** (7). Thus, inexperienced operators should preferentially **attempt spinal anesthesia at a lower lumbar (L3–L4 or L4–L5) IVS** to minimize the potential risk for spinal cord injury (8,9). Fortunately, lumbar flexion, which is commonly used to improves access to the intervertebral–interlaminar space, does not alter the position of the intercristal line (10).

II. Indications and contraindications

A. **The injection of local anesthetics into the subarachnoid space results in (afferent) sensory block as well as varying degrees of (efferent) motor block.** The **cephalad extent of spinal anesthesia depends on the baricity of the local anesthetic solution** as well as the patient's position during the spinal block and the surgical procedure. The CSF concentration of local anesthetic decreases as the distance from the injection site starts to increase. This results in a gradient of afferent and efferent conduction block, which stems from the differential sensitivity of spinal nerve fibers to local anesthetic agents (Table 6.1). For instance, **preganglionic efferent fibers are the most sensitive to local anesthetic** conduction block and are commonly anesthetized **two to six dermatome segments more cephalad than afferent sensory block**. In turn, sensory block can be **two to three dermatomes higher than efferent motor block** (11). Although sensory block can be used as a surrogate marker for surgical anesthesia, tolerance to transcutaneous electrical stimulation of 10-mA, 50-Hz continuous square wave for 5 seconds constitutes a more **reliable predictor of tolerance to surgical stimulation** (12).

B. **Knowledge of dermatomal projections is paramount to determine whether the sensory block is adequate for the planned surgical procedure, and to evaluate regression of the spinal block.** For example, the **fourth thoracic dermatome corresponds to the nipples**, the **sixth** thoracic dermatome to the **xyphoid process**, and the **tenth** thoracic dermatome to the **umbilicus** (Table 6.2 and Fig. 6.6). It is also essential to remember that viscera are innervated differently and that anesthesia of an overlying cutaneous region does not inherently confer surgical anesthesia on an underlying visceral organ (Table 6.3).

CLINICAL PEARL

1. Although foot–ankle (S1–L5) and knee surgery (L3–L4) involve lumbosacral dermatomes, the use of thigh tourniquet (and tolerance to tourniquet pain) will often require a peak sensory block height to T10–T8 (13).
2. T6–T4 peak sensory levels are required for lower abdominal surgery such as inguinal herniorrhaphy, appendectomy, abdominal hysterectomy, or cesarean delivery. Nonetheless, patients may still report discomfort associated with (transient) traction on the peritoneum or abdominal viscera.

   C. **There exist absolute and relative contraindications to spinal anesthesia.** Absolute contraindications include **patient refusal, infection at the puncture site, severe untreated hypovolemia, coagulopathy**, and **increased intracranial pressure**. Performance of spinal anesthesia in patients with **preexisting neurologic deficits** such as radicular or peripheral neuropathies (14,15) and demyelinating diseases (e.g., multiple sclerosis) (16) remains **controversial**. This issue is discussed in the chapter pertaining to complications of regional anesthesia (Chapter 14). **Aortic stenosis**, once considered an absolute contraindication to spinal anesthesia, does not necessarily preclude a carefully conducted spinal anesthetic (17). Although spinal blocks should not be performed in patients with untreated systemic infection, subjects with evidence of **systemic infection** may safely undergo spinal anesthesia if appropriate antibiotic therapy has been initiated before dural puncture and response to therapy (e.g., decrease in fever and granulocytosis) demonstrated (18).

III. Determinants of local anesthetic distribution and duration of action

   A. **The clinical pharmacology of local anesthetics and adjuvants is addressed in Chapters 1 and 2.** This section will discuss only the determinants of local anesthetic distribution and duration

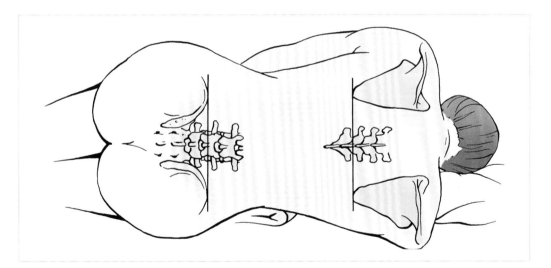

FIGURE 6.7   Patient position for spinal or epidural blockade in the lateral decubitus position. The patient's knees are drawn up toward the chest and the head flexed downward to provide the maximum anterior flexion of the vertebral column. The pillow should be placed under the head but not under the shoulders to avoid rotation of the spine. The hips and shoulders should be perpendicular to the surface of the bed, resisting the usual inclination of the patient to roll the superior shoulder forward. A line drawn between the posterior iliac crests usually crosses the spinal column at the L4–L5 interspace or L4 spinous process. Similarly, for thoracic epidural injection, a line between the inferior tips of the scapulae crosses the T7 spinous process.

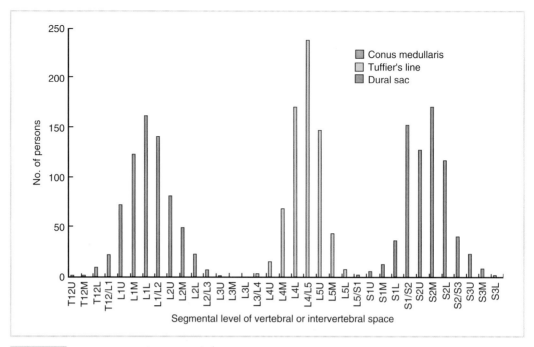

FIGURE 6.8 Distribution of the vertebral level in segments at which the conus medullaris, the intercristal (Tuffier's) line, and the dural sac cross. The segmental levels where the spinal cord ends, Tuffier's line crosses, and the dural sac ends follow a normal distribution. Each vertebra was divided into four segmental thirds of the vertebral body—upper (U), middle (M), and lower (L)—and the intervertebral space. The most caudal distribution of the conus should not cross with the most cephalad level of the actual intercristal line in this patient population. (Adapted from Kim JT, Bahk J, Hung JH. Influence of age and sex on the position of the conus medullaris and Tuffier's line in adults. *Anesthesiology* 2003;99(6):1359–1363.)

TABLE 6.1 Classification of afferent and efferent nerve fibers

Fiber class	Axon diameter (μm)	Myelin	Conduction velocity (m/s)	Innervation	Function
Aα	12–20	+++	75–120	Afferent from muscle spindle proprioceptors Efferent to skeletal muscle	Motor and reflex activity
Aβ	5–12	+++	30–75	Afferent from cutaneous mechanoreceptors	Touch and pressure
Aγ	3–6	++	12–35	Efferent to muscle spindles	Muscle tone
Aδ	1–5	++	5–30	Afferent pain and temperature nociceptors	"Fast" pain, touch, and temperature
B	<3	+	3–15	Preganglionic sympathetic efferent	Autonomic function
C	0.2–1.5	–	0.5–2.0	Afferent pain and temperature	"Slow" pain, temperature

TABLE 6.2   Surface anatomy and dermatomal levels

Surface anatomy	Sensory dermatome
Perineum	S2–S4
Lateral foot	S1
Knee and distal thigh	L3–L4
Inguinal ligament	T12
Umbilicus	T10
Tip of xyphoid process	T6
Nipple	T4
Inner aspect of forearm and arm	T1–T2
Thumb and index finger	C6–C7
Shoulder and clavicle	C5–C4

TABLE 6.3   Common surgical procedures appropriate for spinal anesthesia and recommended peak sensory block height

Surgical procedure	Recommended minimum peak block height

Perirectal and perineal
  Incision and drainage of rectal abscess
  Hemorrhoidectomy
  Transvaginal slings
	L1–L2

Lower extremity surgery with tourniquet use
  Knee replacement
  Knee arthroscopy
  Below-knee amputation
	T10–T8

Transurethral resection of prostate
  Cystoscopy and hysteroscopy
  Vaginal delivery
  Total hip replacement
  Femoral–popliteal bypass
  Varicose vein stripping
	T10

Lower abdominal
  Hysterectomy (low transverse incision)
  Cesarean delivery
  Inguinal herniorrhaphy
  Appendectomy
	T4

for spinal anesthesia. From a pharmacodynamic standpoint, subarachnoid *distribution* of local anesthetic agents determines the extent of sensorimotor and sympathetic block. *Uptake* of local anesthetics dictates the neuronal functions most affected by the spinal block. *Elimination* of local anesthetics from the subarachnoid space determines the duration of action.

3

B. **Determinants of subarachnoid local anesthetic distribution.** Many factors have been proposed to explain the distribution of local anesthetic solutions in the subarachnoid space (19,20). After their injection, local anesthetics will initially spread by simple **bulk flow**. Subsequently, the most important determinant of distribution is the **baricity** of the local anesthetic solution. Other relevant factors include the **total dose**, the IVS selected for injection, and several patient characteristics.

1. **Baricity.** Baricity is defined as the ratio of the density of the local anesthetic solution to the CSF density at 37°C. Local anesthetic solutions that possess the same density as CSF are termed *isobaric*. Local anesthetic solutions that have a greater density than CSF are classified as *hyperbaric*, whereas solutions with a lower density than CSF are termed *hypobaric*. Hyperbaric solutions will sink to the most dependent areas, whereas hypobaric solutions will rise to the nondependent areas of the subarachnoid space. The effects of gravity are determined by the choice of patient position as well as by the natural curvatures of the spine. The mean density of CSF varies significantly among different patient subpopulations (Table 6.4). Thus, local anesthetics (e.g., plain bupivacaine 0.5% and plain lidocaine 2.0%) commonly classified as "isobaric" may in fact behave in a hypobaric manner. Table 6.4 lists the density range and classification of commonly used local anesthetics.

   a. **Hyperbaric spinal anesthesia.** Hyperbaric solutions are commonly prepared by mixing the local anesthetic with **dextrose**. When the patient is placed in the supine position after the injection of a hyperbaric solution, the latter will distribute toward the **lowest points of the thoracic (T6–T7) and sacral (S2) curvatures** (Fig. 6.4) (21). In fact, pooling of hyperbaric local anesthetic solutions within the thoracic kyphosis has been postulated to explain its peak sensory block height in the midthoracic region (22).

      (1) Injection of hyperbaric local anesthetic solutions with the patient in the sitting position (for 5 to 10 minutes) has been (mistakenly) advocated to restrict distribution to the lumbosacral dermatomes, producing a so-called *"saddle block"* (Fig. 6.9). Unfortunately, clinical studies have demonstrated that a hyperbaric spinal anesthetic

TABLE 6.4 Density and baricity of cerebrospinal fluid in different patient subgroups and commonly used local anesthetics

	Mean (SD) density at 37°C	Range within 3 SD of the mean
Patient population		
Men	1.00064 (0.00012)	1.00028–1.00100
Older women	1.00070 (0.00018)	1.00016–1.00124
Younger women	1.00049 (0.00004)	1.00037–1.00061
Pregnant/postpartum	1.00030 (0.00004)	1.00018–1.00042
Hyperbaric solutions[a]		
Lidocaine 5% in dextrose 7.5%	1.02650	1.01300–1.0142
Tetracaine 0.5% in dextrose 5%	1.0136 (0.0002)	1.01300–1.0142
Bupivacaine 0.5%–0.75% in dextrose 8.25%	1.02426 (0.00163)	1.01935–1.029131
Chloroprocaine 3%	1.00257 (0.00003)	1.00248–1.00266
Hypobaric solutions[b]		
Lidocaine 0.5% in water	0.99850	Hypobaric
Bupivacaine 0.35% in water	0.99730	Hypobaric
Tetracaine 0.2% in water	0.99250	Hypobaric
Bupivacaine 0.5%	0.99944 (0.00012)	0.99908–0.99980
Isobaric solutions (plain)		
Lidocaine 2%[c]	1.00004 (0.0006)	0.99986–1.00022
Tetracaine 0.5%[d]	1.0000 (0.0004)	0.99880–1.00120

SD, standard deviation.
[a]Local anesthetic solutions with a baricity of >1.0015 can be expected to predictably behave in a hyperbaric manner.
[b]Local anesthetic solutions with a baricity of <0.9990 can be expected to predictably behave in a hypobaric manner.
[c]May act in an isobaric or hypobaric manner depending on patient population.
[d]Tetracaine 1% diluted 1:1 with 0.9% saline.

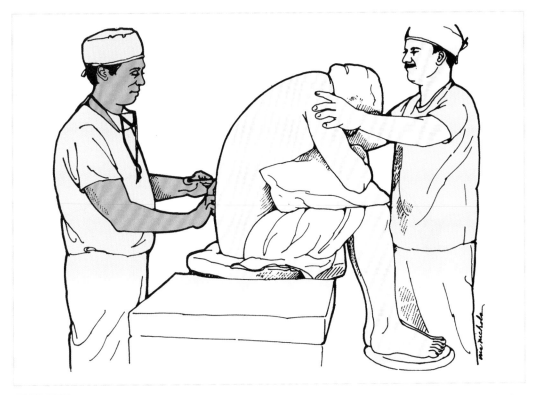

FIGURE 6.9   Sitting position for spinal anesthesia. The patient's legs can hang over the edge of the bed, and the feet are supported on a stool to encourage flexion of the lower spine. The shoulders are hunched forward, and the patient is encouraged to grasp firmly onto a pillow held over the abdomen. If sedation is given, an assistant should maintain the position and monitor the vital signs. This position is optimal for identifying the midline in obese patients or those with unusual spinal anatomy.

block initially restricted to the lumbosacral dermatomes will eventually distribute to a peak thoracic height equivalent to that which would have been achieved had the patient been immediately placed in the supine position (23).

(2) Injection of hyperbaric solutions with a patient in the lateral decubitus position (with the operative side dependent) and maintained in this position for 10 to 15 minutes has been advocated to achieve "unilateral spinal anesthesia" and a decreased incidence of hypotension (24). The major disadvantage of such a strategy stems from the decrease in operating room efficiency, because the patient must be kept in a lateral decubitus position for 15 minutes after the spinal block.

b. **Hypobaric spinal anesthesia.** Hypobaric local anesthetic solutions are prepared by diluting commercially available solutions with **sterile distilled water**. For example, lidocaine 2% diluted with sterile water to lidocaine 0.5% (25) or bupivacaine 0.5% diluted with sterile water to 0.35% (26) will provide "clinically hypobaric" spinal anesthesia. Hypobaric spinal anesthesia is best suited for perineal and perirectal surgical procedures performed with the patient in the prone jackknife position (Fig. 6.10) for two reasons. First, the spinal block is performed with the patient in the operative position. Second, the local anesthetic distribution will be restricted to lumbosacral dermatomes if the patient is maintained in the operative position. However, caution must be exercised, as prematurely returning the patient to a head-up position during the recovery period may cause the block to rise to the thoracic dermatomes (26).

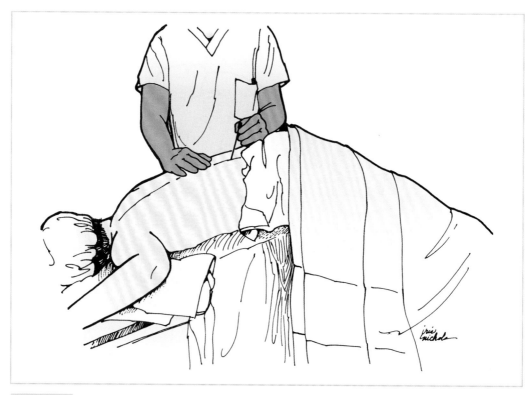

FIGURE 6.10   Jackknife position. Hypobaric spinal anesthesia can be administered with the patient positioned on a flexed operating table, such as for rectal procedures. The flexion point of the table should be directly under the hip joint, and the use of a pillow under the hips will help accentuate the flexion needed to identify the lumbar spinous processes. Aspiration of the spinal needle is often necessary to confirm dural puncture, because the lower cerebrospinal fluid pressure in this position will not necessarily generate a spontaneous flow of fluid.

> **CLINICAL PEARL**   Hypobaric spinal anesthesia may provide significant advantages for hip surgery performed in the lateral decubitus position (with the operative side uppermost) because the same position can be used for the spinal block and the surgical procedure. Moreover, compared with its isobaric bupivacaine counterpart, hypobaric bupivacaine spinal anesthesia demonstrates a significantly delayed onset of sensory regression on the operative side as well as a longer time to first postoperative analgesia (27).

    c. Isobaric spinal anesthesia. The major advantage of truly isobaric solutions is that **patient position during and after injection do not impact subarachnoid distribution.** Since isobaric solutions tend not to distribute far from the site of initial injection, they are particularly useful when the operator aims to limit sensory block to lumbar dermatomes.

  2. Dose, volume, and concentration. Clinical trials attempting to separate the individual impact of dose, volume, and concentration on local anesthetic distribution are notoriously difficult to interpret because manipulating one of these factors invariably affects the other two. In two trials that compared different doses of **plain** local anesthetic solutions (27,28), as well as the same dose administered in lower concentrations and higher volumes, the **predominant factor in increasing the extent of sensory block (peak block height) remains the total dose** (irrespective of volume or concentration). In contrast, total mass becomes secondary for the distribution of **hyperbaric** local anesthetic solutions if patients are positioned supine after the spinal injection (29,30). Conversely, in a dose–response study of hyperbaric bupivacaine 0.75%, 3.75, 7.5, and 11.25 mg yielded peak sensory block heights of T9, T7, and T4, respectively (31).

3. **IVS injection site.** The level of injection site has been purported to impact the cephalad distribution of plain local anesthetic solution. In one study, the mean peak block height decreased from T6 to T10 when plain bupivacaine 0.5% was first injected at L3–L4, followed by a repeat injection in the same patients at the L4–L5 IVS (32). In this study, plain bupivacaine 0.5% was injected at ambient room temperature with the patient in the lateral decubitus position followed immediately by the supine position. In contrast, when plain bupivacaine 0.5% solutions (adjusted to 37°C) were injected with patients placed in the sitting position, no differences were observed in terms of peak sensory block height for injections performed at the L2–L3 versus L3–L4 IVS (33). These conflicting results can be explained by the simple fact that plain bupivacaine 0.5% is hypobaric and not isobaric. Thus, in the first trial, rostral migration of local anesthetic molecules can be explained by the fact that patients were immediately positioned supine following the spinal block. Furthermore, the hypobaric property of bupivacaine 0.5% was accentuated by the room temperature, as density of local anesthetic solutions is inversely proportional to temperature.

4. **Needle aperture direction.** The use of a pencil point needle can selectively divert local anesthetic flow from the longitudinal axis of the needle (34). In one trial, patients were placed in the lateral decubitus position and randomly assigned to spinal anesthesia with plain lidocaine 2% using a needle aperture oriented in a cephalad versus caudad direction (35). Cephalad orientation resulted in a higher peak sensory block (T3 vs. T7), shorter duration of lumbar sensory anesthesia (149 vs. 178 minutes), as well as decreased times to spontaneous urination and discharge.

5. **Patient factors.** Although there exists significant interindividual variation in the extent of local anesthetic distribution (due to interindividual differences in CSF volume), spinal anesthesia is **surprisingly reproducible for the individual subject** (36). Unfortunately, anthropometric factors such as **age, height, body mass index, and gender confer minimal predictive value in terms of local anesthetic distribution from patient to patient.**

C. **Determinants of duration of spinal anesthesia.** Clinically, spinal anesthesia **recedes in a cephalad to caudad direction.** Duration of action can be defined as time to onset of **two-dermatome regression** (from peak sensory block height), or as **time to complete regression** to sacral dermatomes. Clinically, the **duration of surgical anesthesia** depends on the complex interaction between the spatial extent of the block, time-course regression, and anatomic location of the surgical procedure. Block resolution after spinal anesthesia occurs when the CSF neural concentration of local anesthetic falls below the minimum concentration required to blunt neural conduction. Elimination **does not involve metabolism** of local anesthetics but occurs through absorption within meningeal vasculature. Therefore, the **duration of spinal anesthesia is determined by three factors:** the physiochemical properties of the local anesthetic agent (which, in turn, determines its availability for vascular absorption), the total dose administered, and the degree of vascular absorption.

1. **Local anesthetic agent.** Lipid solubility and, to a lesser extent, protein binding determine the time course of vascular absorption (see Table 1.1 in Chapter 1).
   a. **Procaine** is the **shortest acting** local anesthetic for spinal anesthesia. Its short duration of action can be attributed to its very low lipid solubility and protein binding.
   b. **2-Chloroprocaine** is a **short-acting** local anesthetic agent with a comparable anesthetic profile to lidocaine. However, it does not predispose to transient neurologic symptoms (TNS) and possesses a 20% shorter time to complete recovery of sensorimotor function (37).

    c. **Lidocaine** is a **short- to intermediate-acting** local anesthetic agent. Its use has fallen dramatically due to concerns of **TNS** (see discussion on complications). Depending on the type of surgery, the incidence of TNS ranges from 15% to 33%.

    d. **Mepivacaine** is a **short- to intermediate-acting** local anesthetic agent. It provides a similar anesthetic profile and a lower incidence of TNS (3%–6%) compared to lidocaine.

    e. **Bupivacaine** is the prototypical and most commonly used **long-acting aminoamide local anesthetic** agent. The extent and duration of bupivacaine are **dose dependent** (32). Within a clinically relevant range of 3.75 to 11.25 mg of hyperbaric bupivacaine 0.75%, for every additional milligram, the duration of surgical anesthesia increases by 10 minutes, and the time to complete recovery by 21 minutes. Although low doses (5–7.5 mg) have been used for ambulatory anesthesia, they are often hindered by high failure rates and interpatient variability in terms of block resolution.

    f. Although local anesthetic agents may be classified as short, intermediate, and long acting, there exists wide interpatient variability (Table 6.5). In one volunteer study (n = 12), (38) spinal anesthesia was performed on three separate occasions with three different hyperbaric local anesthetic agents (lidocaine 100 mg, bupivacaine 15 mg, and tetracaine 15 mg) in the same subject. Not only was the average time to complete sensory resolution different between the three agents, but it also varied significantly within each local anesthetic agent group: lidocaine (234 minutes, range 137 to 360 minutes), bupivacaine (438 minutes, range 180 to 570 minutes), and tetracaine (546 minutes, range 120 to 720 minutes).

TABLE 6.5   Doses and duration of commonly used local anesthetic solutions for spinal anesthesia

Local anesthetic solution	Dose (mg)	Mean peak block height	Onset of two-dermatome regression (min) (SD)	Time to regression to L1–L2 (min) (SD)	Complete regression (min) (SD)
Hyperbaric chloroprocaine	30	T8[a]	40 (20)	42 (10)	103 (12)
Hyperbaric chloroprocaine	40	T7[a]	45 (20)	64 (10)	114 (14)
Plain lidocaine	50	T6	56 (5)	104 (5)	130 (18)
Hyperbaric lidocaine	50	T4	50 (16)	104 (5)	130 (18)
Plain mepivacaine	60	T4	95 (21)	150 (32)	210 (18)
	80	T4	100 (20)	160 (20)	225 (23)
Plain bupivacaine	10	T7	33 (16)	127 (41)	178 (20)
Hyperbaric bupivacaine	8	T5	59 (13)	135 (51)	198 (33)
	12	T5	65 (32)	123 (44)	164 (30)
	15	T10[b]	159 (49)	253 (64)	>360
	15	T4[b]	110 (30)	216 (46)	360

SD, standard deviation.
[a]Kopacz DJ. Spinal 2-chloroprocaine: minimum effective dose. *Reg Anesth Pain Med* 2005;30:36–42.
[b]Hyperbaric bupivacaine 15 mg with two patient groups (supine position with peak block height of T4 compared with 30-degree head elevation position with peak block height restricted to T10). Note the significant difference in onset of two-dermatome regression, duration of lumbar anesthesia, and complete regression with the same dose of hyperbaric bupivacaine but with different initial peak blocks.
From Kooger-Infante NE, Van Gessel E, Forster A, et al. Extent of hyperbaric spinal anesthesia influences duration of block. *Anesthesiology* 2000;92:1319–1323.

5 **CLINICAL PEARL**   For short outpatient, surgical procedures (e.g., knee arthroscopy and perianal surgery), preservative-free 2-chloroprocaine offers significant benefits. It provides a predictable, short-acting duration with minimal risks of TNS. Currently, the Food and Drug Administration has approved 2-chloroprocaine only for peripheral nerve blocks and epidural anesthesia. Thus, its use in the context of spinal anesthesia remains off label in the United States. In contrast, 2-chloroprocaine has been recently approved by the European Medicine Agency for spinal anesthesia (39).

2. **Local anesthetic dose.** For any given local anesthetic agent, **increasing the dose increases the duration** of action. See Table 6.5 for details.

3. **Block distribution.** For a given dose of local anesthetic, spinal anesthesia **will regress more quickly with a higher compared to a lower peak sensory block** (40). The most likely explanation stems from the wider distribution within the CSF, which results in a lower local anesthetic CSF concentration throughout the subarachnoid space, as well as a larger surface area, leading to more rapid vascular absorption (41).

4 4. **Anesthetic adjuncts. Common adjuncts used to prolong (and intensify) spinal anesthesia include** α-**adrenergic agonists and opioids**.

a. α-**Adrenergic agonists. Epinephrine** prolongs the duration of spinal anesthesia through α-adrenergic–mediated **vasoconstriction**, which leads to decreased vascular absorption. The clinical impact of intrathecal epinephrine may depend on the local anesthetic agent. For instance, although epinephrine 0.2 mg does not prolong the duration of thoracic anesthesia when added to lidocaine, it does increase the duration of lumbosacral anesthesia by 25% to 30% (42). Similarly, epinephrine 0.2 mg, when added to plain bupivacaine 15 mg, does not prolong thoracic anesthesia, but increases the duration of lumbar anesthesia by 20% (43). In contrast, epinephrine 0.2 to 0.3 mg significantly prolongs the duration of tetracaine spinal anesthesia by 30% to 50% at all dermatomal levels (44,45).

CLINICAL PEARL   Because it significantly delays the return of sacral autonomic function (the ability to spontaneously void), epinephrine increases the risk of urinary retention and bladder overdistention (46). Thus, it should not be used for outpatient spinal anesthesia.

b. **Opioids.** Opioids bind to receptors located within the gray matter of the substantia gelatinosa in the dorsal horn of the spinal cord. Spinally mediated analgesia occurs through several mechanisms: (i) increased K^+ conductance, which hyperpolarizes ascending postsynaptic second-order projecting neurons, (ii) release of spinal adenosine, and (iii) inhibition of the release of excitatory neurotransmitters (e.g., glutamate and substance P) from primary afferent neurons (47,48).

(1) **Fentanyl** is the most commonly used intrathecal opioid. The lipophilic profile of fentanyl explains its **rapid onset** (5 to 10 minutes) and **intermediate duration** of action (60 to 120 minutes). Clinical studies have demonstrated that 20 to 25 µg of fentanyl added to lidocaine (49) or bupivacaine (50) increases the duration of spinal anesthesia without prolonging the time to complete recovery of sensorimotor and bladder function.

(2) **Morphine** is the most commonly used hydrophilic opioid. Its physiochemical characteristics result in a **slow onset** (30 to 60 minutes), coupled with a **prolonged**

duration of action, which makes it well suited for postoperative analgesia. Doses of morphine in the range of 100 to 200 µg provide extended analgesia (up to 24 hours) for surgical procedures such as cesarean delivery, abdominal hysterectomy, radical prostatectomy, and total hip arthroplasty (51). With such low doses, the risk of respiratory depression is minimal. In contrast, the minimum effective analgesic dose required for total knee arthroplasty is 300 to 500 µg (52). With such doses, the occurrence of **side effects (e.g., nausea, vomiting, urinary retention, pruritus, respiratory depression)** increases significantly.

IV. Technique. Spinal anesthesia should be performed only in locations equipped with an oxygen source, modalities to administer positive pressure ventilation, airway management equipment, as well as immediate access to emergency drugs for resuscitation and endotracheal intubation. Patient preparation includes proper monitoring of heart rate and rhythm, blood pressure, and oxygen saturation. Furthermore, intravenous sedation may be judiciously administered to ensure that the patient is comfortable, cooperative, and communicative.

A. Patient position. The choice of patient position is dictated by the combined influence of the operator's preference, the patient's characteristics (e.g., obesity, hemodynamic status, presence of trauma such as hip fracture), and the baricity of the local anesthetic solution.

1. **Lateral decubitus position** (Fig. 6.7). The lateral decubitus position is especially useful for **lower extremity surgery**. For instance, hyperbaric solutions will allow preferential migration of local anesthetic to the surgical limb if patients are placed (and kept) in the lateral decubitus position with the operative side dependent. Hypobaric solutions are ideally suited for hip surgery, such as total or hemiarthroplasty, because the lateral decubitus position (with the surgical limb nondependent) can be used for the duration of the spinal anesthetic and the operation. Ideally, the patient's back is positioned parallel to the edge of the operating table to allow easy access to the lumbar spine. The hips and knees are flexed. The hips and shoulders should be aligned so that they are perpendicular to the edge of the bed, thereby preventing rotation of the spine. The head and lower legs may need to be supported with pillows. The patient should also be encouraged to actively curve the lower back toward the anesthesiologist. These maneuvers will contribute to widening of the lumbar intervertebral and interlaminar spaces.

2. **Sitting position** (Fig. 6.9). The sitting position **facilitates identification of the midline**. The patient should be seated with the legs hanging off the operating table and the feet supported by a footrest. A pillow placed on the patient's thighs will encourage the patient to maintain forward flexion of the lumbar spine. An assistant can prove invaluable to ensure that the patient keeps the desired position.

3. **Prone jackknife position** (Fig. 6.10). For procedures that require a prone jackknife position (e.g., **rectal or perineal surgery),** spinal anesthesia may be accomplished by the injection of a **hypobaric** local anesthetic solution with the patient placed in the jackknife position. The patient's hips should be placed directly over the break in the operating table (Fig. 6.10). Moreover, a pillow, placed under the lower abdomen, enhances flexion of the lumbar spine.

B. Conventional approach to the subarachnoid space. Spinal anesthesia should not be attempted at or above the L1–L2 IVS to minimize the risk of needle trauma to the conus medullaris (Fig. 6.8). All antiseptic solutions are neurotoxic: thus, care must be taken to avoid contamination of spinal needles and local anesthetic solutions with the disinfectant. Current recommendations from both the American Society of Anesthesiologists and American Society of Regional Anesthesia support the use of chlorhexidine-alcohol solutions for decreasing the risk of infectious complications associated with neuraxial anesthesia (53).

1. **Midline approach.** For the midline approach, the needle **insertion is located between contiguous spinous processes** (Figs. 6.3 and 6.11).

   a. Using a 25-gauge 5/8-inch hypodermic needle, the operator infiltrates the skin and subcutaneous tissues with local anesthetic. The needle is then advanced with a 10- to 15-degree cephalad angulation (while injecting local anesthetic) through the supraspinous and interspinous ligament (Fig. 6.11). Care must be taken not to insert the hypodermic needle too far in thin patients, because it may inadvertently penetrate the dura–arachnoid membrane.

   b. The 19- or 20-gauge **introducer needle** is then inserted (Figs. 6.11 and 6.12). The use of an introducer is required with smaller-gauge spinal needles (i.e., 24- to 27-gauge) to reduce the deflection of the needle tip away from the midline (54). The introducer also **reduces cross-contamination** of the spinal needle with the disinfectant solution, epidermis, and skin bacteria. If properly positioned, the introducer should be firmly anchored in the interspinous ligament.

   c. The operator stabilizes the introducer needle by holding its hub between the thumb and the index finger of the nondominant hand. The operator then grasps the spinal needle with the thumb and index finger of the dominant hand and inserts it through the introducer (Fig. 6.13).

   d. If the needle stays on the correct course, the operator will sense a subtle change in resistance (often perceived as a loss of resistance or "pop"). This usually indicates that the spinal needle tip has penetrated the dura–arachnoid complex and entered the subarachnoid space. The stylet of the spinal needle is withdrawn to verify **backflow of CSF**. If free flow of CSF does not occur, the hub of the spinal needle is rotated 90 degrees, in the event that a small dural or arachnoid flap obstructs the aperture. If no fluid is obtained, the stylet is replaced and the needle gently advanced until another "pop" can be appreciated. The stylet is removed and the preceding steps repeated until CSF return.

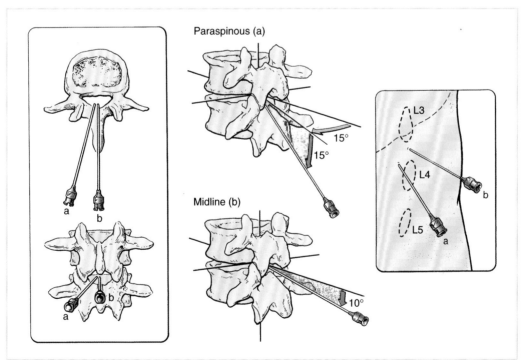

FIGURE 6.11   The needle insertion point and angulation of needle advancement are illustrated for paraspinous (*a*) and midline (*b*) approaches. (Adapted from Cousins MJ, Bridenbaugh LD, eds. *Neural Blockade in Clinical Anesthesia and Management of Pain*, 3rd ed. Philadelphia: Lippincott Williams & Wilkins; 1998:231.)

CLINICAL PEARL If, at any time, the patient reports a paresthesia or pain, needle advancement should be immediately halted. Paresthesias are usually transient and indicate needle tip contact with the cauda equina in the subarachnoid space. Thus, the stylet is removed to confirm CSF backflow through the spinal needle. If a paresthesia occurs without CSF return, the needle may have contacted nerve roots traversing the epidural space, thereby suggesting that it has deviated away from midline. In such an event, the needle should be withdrawn and gently redirected toward the contralateral side. If pain or paresthesia recurs with either aspiration or injection, *under no circumstances should the injection be carried out!* The spinal needle should be withdrawn (9).

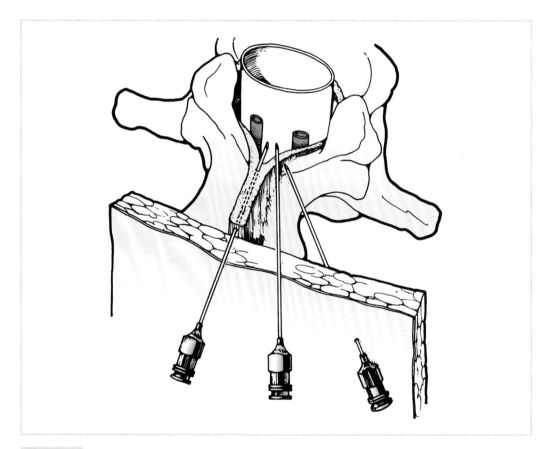

FIGURE 6.12 Spinal needle insertion, lateral and paramedian approach. In the classic midline approach, the needle traverses the entire interspinous ligament in a slight cephalad direction and exits through the triangular ligamentum flavum into the epidural space before puncturing the dura. In elderly patients with calcified interspinous ligaments, the entry point can be moved one fingerbreadth lateral to the ligament, still passing in the midline of the interspace, but approaching the ligamentum flavum from a slightly oblique angle. A third alternative is to enter the skin much further laterally and inferior to the interspace (a fingerbreadth opposite the inferior spinous process) and pass the needle directly perpendicular onto the lamina, and then "walk" superior and medially until the ligament is contacted. All three of these approaches are suitable for spinal or epidural blockade.

    e. Once free flow of CSF is obtained, the syringe containing the local anesthetic solution is attached to the hub of the spinal needle. During the injection process, the latter is stabilized by placing the dorsum of the nondominant hand against the patient's back and by grasping the hub between the thumb and the index finger (Fig. 6.13). **Gentle aspiration of 0.1 to 0.2 mL of CSF** confirms subarachnoid position of the needle tip.

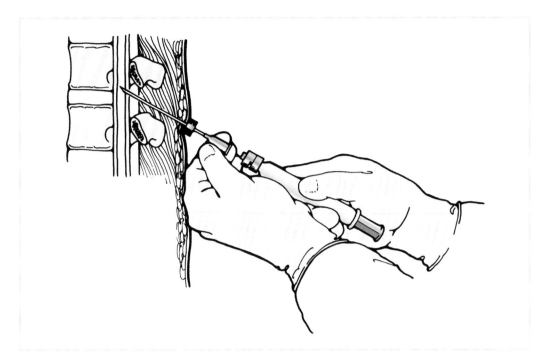

FIGURE 6.13   Spinal needle and introducer. The spinal needle is inserted through a larger-gauge introducer. The use of the introducer avoids the problem of contamination of the tip of the spinal needle with prep solution, epidermis, or skin bacteria and allows a rigid channel for the smaller-gauge needles frequently used to reduce the incidence of headaches. Whenever the syringe is attached or removed from the needle hub, the opposite hand rests firmly against the back and grasps the hub firmly, preventing unintentional advancement or withdrawal.

The **local anesthetic solution is injected slowly (0.5 mL/s).** Some anesthesiologists repeat aspiration midway through the injection or at the end of the latter to confirm that the needle tip remains in the subarachnoid space. Once the injection is complete, the spinal needle and introducer are removed together as a unit.

CLINICAL PEARL   If bone is encountered, a mental note is made of its depth. The spinal needle is partially withdrawn and reinserted in a slightly more cephalad direction. If bone is contacted again, the depth is compared to the first one encountered (Fig. 6.14). **Deeper bone contact** indicates that the needle is most likely progressing along the superior crest of the spinous process below the IVS. Thus, it should be angled more cephalad and advanced further. **If bony contact is more superficial** than previously encountered, the needle tip has encountered the inferior surface of the spinous process above the IVS, and less cephalad angulation is required. If bony contact repeatedly occurs at the **same depth,** the operator has most likely encountered lamina. This suggests that the needle is not in the true midline. The most frequent misdirection occurs when the patient, placed in the lateral decubitus position, rolls slightly forward away from the operator during attempts to flex the spine. In such a scenario, although the needle may be advanced parallel to the floor, it will not be perpendicular to the spinal column, and the needle tip will deviate from the midline (Fig. 6.15).

CLINICAL PEARL   The technique for the midline approach is similar for patients placed in the prone jackknife position. However, CSF return may not be as brisk because of the lower CSF pressure. Thus, the operating table can be adjusted to transiently raise the head in order to augment CSF pressure.

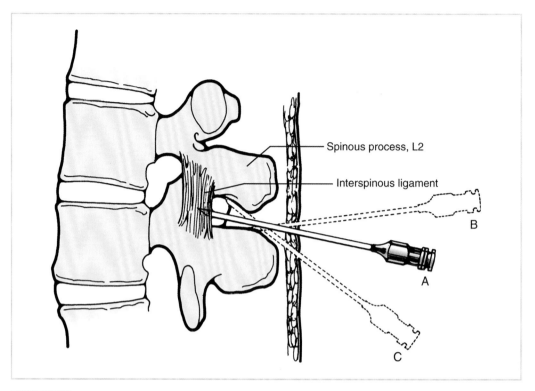

FIGURE 6.14   Spinal needle insertion, lateral view. For the classic midline approach, the needle is introduced in the middle of the interspace and advanced with a slight cephalad angulation. If correctly angled (*A*), it will enter the interspinous ligament, ligamentum flavum, and epidural space. If bone is contacted, it may be the inferior spinous process (*B*), and cephalad redirection will identify the correct path. If angling cephalad causes bony contact at a shallower depth (*C*), it is probably the superior spinous process. If bone is encountered at the same depth after several attempts at redirection (not shown), the needle is most likely on the lamina lateral to the interspace, and the position of the true midline should be reassessed.

2. **Paramedian.** The midline approach is simple to learn and adequate for most patients. However, if the patient cannot flex the lumbar spine, the spinous process can be efficiently bypassed with the paramedian approach. The latter can be performed **just slightly lateral from the midline or farther away from the midline**.
   a. In the paramedian-lateral approach, the initial puncture site is situated **one to one-half fingerbreadths from the midline** while staying in the **same IVS**. The needle is introduced with a slight medial angle coupled with the usual cephalad angulation (Figs. 6.11 and 6.12). The anesthesiologist must develop a **three-dimensional image** during needle advancement to ensure that the needle tip ends up in the midline IVS on reaching the subarachnoid space.
   b. The **paramedian-lateral oblique approach** begins lateral to the midline, but from a **level opposite the spinous process below the interspace** (Figs. 6.11 and 6.12). The needle is advanced approximatively 45 degrees to the midline and 45 degrees cephalad to enter the subarachnoid space in the midline.
3. **Lumbosacral (Taylor) approach.** Occasionally, neither the midline nor the paramedian approach allows entry into the spinal canal because of extensive calcification or fusion of the IVS. In such an event, the lumbosacral (L5–S1) vertebral foramen offers the **largest interlaminar target**. The lateral oblique approach to the L5–S1 IVS is called the *Taylor approach* in recognition of the urologist who helped popularize this technique.
   a. The **posterior–superior iliac spine** (**PSIS**) is identified, and a skin mark is made **1 cm medial and 1 cm caudad to the PSIS**. The midline L5–S1 IVS is also identified and

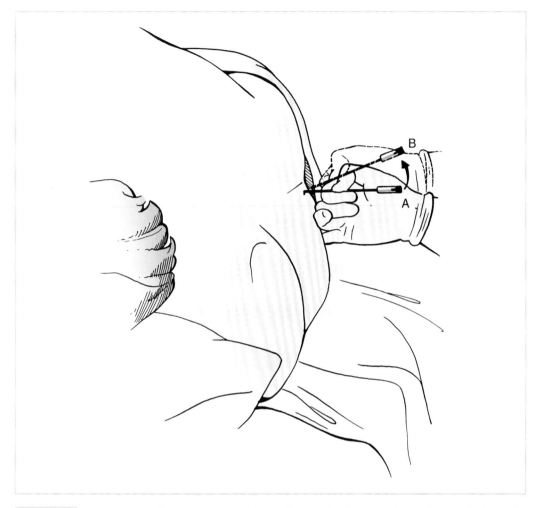

FIGURE 6.15 Patient position lateral view. Most patients will rotate their body anteriorly to flex their back, and the initial spinal (or epidural needle) orientation (*A*) will therefore need to be redirected slightly downward toward the plane of the floor (*B*) to be truly perpendicular to the midline of the patient.

marked. A longer spinal needle (120 to 125 mm) is usually required because the pronounced oblique angulation creates a greater distance to reach the subarachnoid space.

b. After local infiltration, the operator inserts the introducer and directs the latter approximately 45 degrees cephalad and 45 degrees medially, while aiming for the midline L5–S1 IVS (Fig. 6.16).

C. Ultrasound approach to the subarachnoid space. Ultrasonography has revolutionized the practice of regional anesthesia by enabling the operator to visualize the needle, nerve, and spread of local anesthetic agents. Increasingly, ultrasonography is also being used for neuraxial blocks. Currently, most operators favor ultrasound *assistance* over true *guidance*: in other words, preprocedural ultrasound scanning is used solely to refine cutaneous landmarks, and the spinal needle is subsequently advanced in standard blind fashion. Compared to conventional palpation of landmarks, ultrasound assistance results in fewer needle passes/insertions and skin punctures for neuraxial blocks in obstetric and surgical patients. These benefits seem most pronounced when expert operators carry out the sonographic exam and for patients displaying difficult spinal anatomy (55,56).

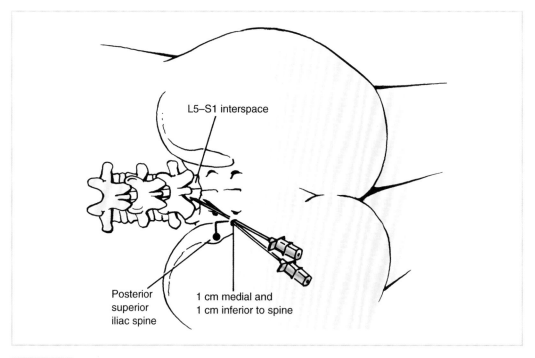

FIGURE 6.16   Taylor approach for spinal anesthesia. The needle is introduced 1 cm medial to and 1 cm caudad to the posterior–superior iliac spine and advanced at an angle of 45 degrees to the midline and 45 degrees cephalad. On contacting the lamina, the needle is then walked upward and medially to enter the L5–S1 interspace.

CLINICAL PEARL   Conventional neuraxial blocks can be performed using a midline or paramedian approach. Similarly, the neuraxial space can be insonated through a transverse (midline) or parasagittal (paramedian) window. To date, no trial has compared both ultrasound-assisted techniques. Because of simplicity, most operators employ the midline method for ultrasound-assisted spinal blocks (55,56).

1. The operator insonates the lumbar spine using a curved array transducer and a parasagittal (oblique) window (Fig. 6.17). The sacrum appears as a continuous hyperechoic line. Cephalad to the latter, the laminae appear as hyperechoic structures resembling a "sawtooth pattern." Between consecutive laminae, the operator identifies the sonographic "gaps," which correspond to the IVSs. The anterior complex (i.e., the composite image of the anterior dura, the posterior longitudinal ligament, and the posterior surface of the vertebral body) can be visualized inside each IVS (Fig. 6.17).

2. Using a skin marker, the operator identifies the spinal levels from L1 to L5 (Fig. 6.18).

3. The operator then proceeds to insonate the L3–L4 or L4–L5 IVS in a transverse axis. In this view, the posterior complex (i.e., the composite image of the ligamentum flavum, the epidural space, and the dura) can be easily identified (Fig. 6.19).

4. The operator delineates the midpoint of the long and short sides of the ultrasound transducer. The probe is then set aside and the lines are connected (Fig. 6.20). The intersection of the horizontal and vertical lines represents the puncture site.

5. The operator proceeds with disinfection/draping, local infiltration, and introducer/spinal needle insertion in the usual fashion.

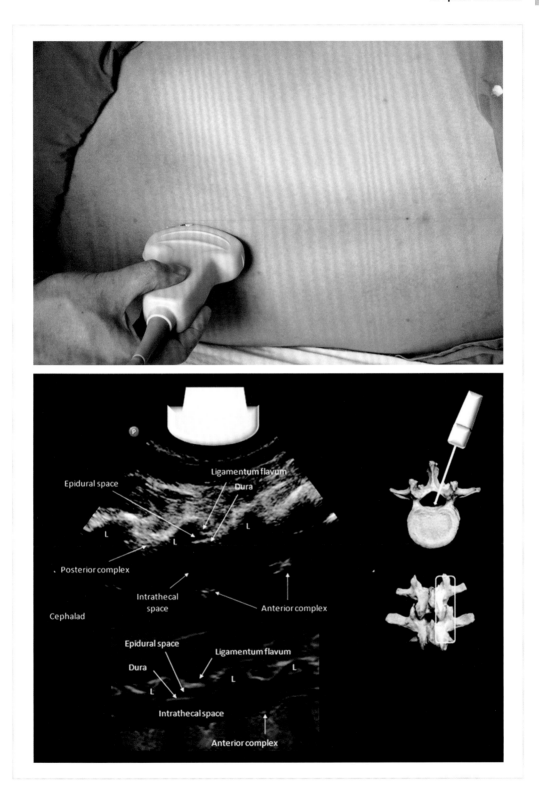

FIGURE 6.17   Position of the ultrasound transducer to obtain a parasagittal oblique sonographic window. (Adapted from Chin KJ, Karmakar MK, Peng PW. Ultrasonography of the adult thoracic and lumbar spine for central neuraxial blockade. *Anesthesiology* 2011;114(6);1459–1485.)

CLINICAL PEARL In the transverse window, the operator can measure the distance from the skin to the posterior complex. This will estimate the depth of the subarachnoid space. However, as a result of compression of the underlying skin and soft tissues by the transducer, the measured distance on the US image will slightly underestimate the true depth.

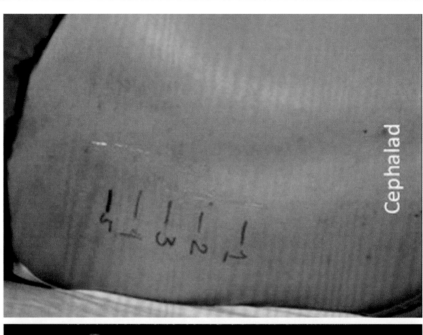

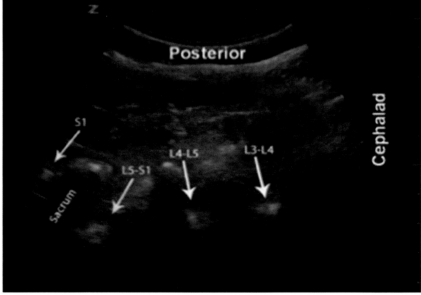

FIGURE 6.18 L1–L5 spinal levels are marked on the patient's back.

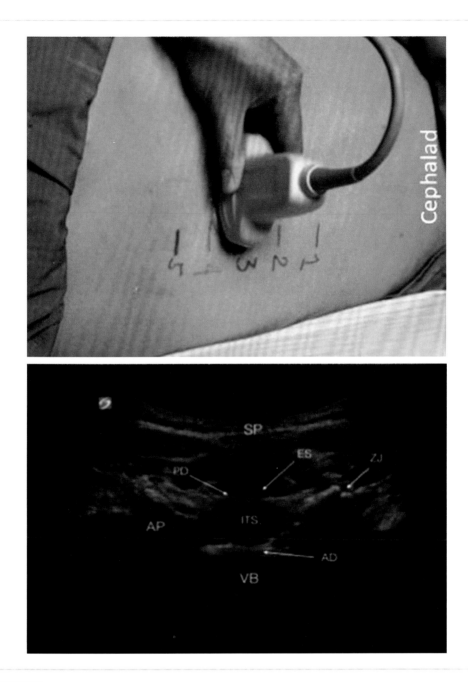

FIGURE 6.19   The L3–L4 interspace is insonated in a transverse axis. AD, anterior dural complex; AP, articular process; ES, epidural space; ITS, intrathecal space; PD, posterior dural complex; SP, spinous process; VB, vertebral body; ZJ, zygapophyseal joint.

D. **Patient management after spinal injection.** When positioning the patient after spinal anesthesia, care must be taken to **avoid compression on peripheral nerves or bony prominences**, because the patient will no longer be able to report uncomfortable pressure points.

1. The **heart rate and blood pressure are checked** as soon as possible because the sympathetic fibers are anesthetized very quickly, and venous pooling in the lower extremities begins

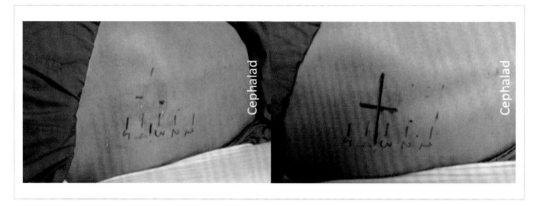

FIGURE 6.20 Delineation of the midpoints of the ultrasound probe. The intersection of the vertical and horizontal lines indicates the cutaneous puncture site.

almost immediately. The loss of venous return can lower heart rate and blood pressure, particularly in patients who are volume depleted or taking ACE inhibitors, angiotensin receptor blockers, or beta-blockers. The **peak sensory block height may continue to increase even 30 to 60 minutes** after local anesthetic injection. Blockade of the upper thoracic sympathetic efferent fibers may manifest as profound **bradycardia** due to blockade of the T1–T4 cardio-accelerator fibers. Therefore, frequent blood pressure readings and continuous heart rate monitoring are mandatory for the safe conduct of spinal anesthesia.

2. **Temperature sensation is tested** with an alcohol swab approximately 2 to 3 minutes after the spinal block. This early assessment confirms the presence of successful spinal anesthesia and provides an estimate of the ultimate peak sensory block height. If temperature sensation is difficult to evaluate, **pinch or pinprick may be employed** to assess sensory block distribution.

3. With hyperbaric local anesthetic agents, the block level may be manipulated by utilizing the Trendelenburg (to increase the peak sensory height) or reverse Trendelenburg (to limit the peak sensory height) position. However, if the level of injection is caudad to the peak lumbar lordosis, the Trendelenburg maneuver may be inadequate to promote rostral spread of hyperbaric local anesthetic, because the latter will preferentially pool in the sacral kyphosis. Because hip flexion attenuates the normal lumbar lordosis, it could be used to curtail pooling of local anesthetic in the sacral kyphosis. Thus, the combination of hip flexion and Trendelenburg position has been shown to effectively increase the peak sensory height of spinal anesthesia compared to the Trendelenburg position alone (57). The early use of reverse Trendelenburg position may limit the cephalad spread of hyperbaric solutions but will not promote their regression once they have reached the higher thoracic segments. In fact, it may compound the hypotension associated with high spinal blockade.

4. Intraoperatively, **supplemental oxygen** is recommended, especially for older patients or those with high blocks or deeper levels of intravenous sedation. **End tidal carbon dioxide monitoring** (through nasal cannulae or face mask) can be used to assess the rate of spontaneous ventilation. Supplemental intravenous **opioids, benzodiazepines, or hypnotics** may be titrated for anxiolysis and positional comfort. A warming blanket is indicated for longer procedures.

5. Postoperatively, the patient should be monitored until the spinal anesthetic recedes. Sympathetic efferent block usually dissipates with the return of sensorimotor function (such as proprioception of the great toe). In contrast, **the functional balance required for unassisted ambulation may still be impaired 90 to 120 minutes after the recovery of**

gross motor function (58). Therefore, unassisted ambulation constitutes a major determinant of home readiness after outpatient spinal anesthesia.

V. Complications. A detailed discussion of complications related to spinal anesthesia can be found in Chapter 14.

A. **Cardiovascular.** Hypotension, bradycardia, and cardiovascular collapse are potential side effects associated with spinal anesthesia.

B. **Total spinal.** *Total spinal anesthesia* refers to a sensory **block that rises above the cervical region**. This level of blockade is usually unintentional, resulting from unanticipated patient movement, inappropriate positioning, or inappropriate doses of local anesthetic. Total spinal anesthesia manifests as rapidly **ascending sensorimotor block, bradycardia, hypotension, and dyspnea** with difficulty swallowing and phonating. **Respiratory arrest and loss of consciousness may be imminent**.

C. **Subdural anesthesia.** The subdural space corresponds to the **potential space between the inner surface of the dura and the arachnoid membrane**. On rare occasions, local anesthetic can be inadvertently injected in this virtual space. If the dose was intended for spinal injection (i.e., relatively small dose), the resulting distribution of local anesthetic results in **widespread but patchy anesthesia** and may explain many cases of "failed spinal anesthesia" despite initial backflow of CSF.

D. **Central neuraxial (epidural or spinal) hematoma.** Epidural or spinal hematoma is a **rare but catastrophic** complication following spinal anesthesia. Although they can occur in healthy subjects, spinal epidural hematomas are usually seen in **patients with altered primary or secondary hemostasis** (59). A hematoma should be suspected when a spinal anesthetic (sensorimotor impairment) is unusually long in duration. Other possible signs and symptoms include a new onset of back pain and bowel or bladder dysfunction. Prompt imaging and neurosurgical consultation are required, as neurologic outcome is poor if more than 6 to 8 hours have elapsed between the onset of paralysis and surgical decompression (60).

E. **Infectious complications.** Bacterial infection after spinal anesthesia may present as localized skin infection, **spinal epidural abscess, or meningitis**. The most common source of infection stems from the patient's (or anesthesiologist's) normal skin flora. The **diagnosis of abscess is confirmed with magnetic resonance imaging**. Therapeutic options include **intravenous antibiotics and surgical drainage/decompression**.

F. **Nerve injury secondary to spinal anesthesia can be caused by drug toxicity (i.**e., local anesthetic or adjunct) or direct needle trauma.

G. **Hearing loss has been increasingly described after spinal anesthesia (61)**. Its **duration is typically less than 1 week**. The postulated mechanism involves **loss of CSF after dural puncture**: the decrease in CSF pressure is transmitted to the perilymph within the cochlea, thus leading to a disruption of hair cell function.

H. **Nausea.** The most common etiologies are hypotension and the use of **intrathecal opioids**. **Hypotension** causes nausea through hypoxemia or hypoperfusion of the chemoreceptor trigger zone in the medulla (62). Furthermore, spinal anesthesia may promote **sympathetic–vagal imbalance**: the unopposed vagal tone thus results in gastrointestinal hyperactivity. The therapeutic efficacy of **vagolytic agents (e.g., glycopyrrolate or atropine)** seems to support this mechanism.

I. **PDPH (63).** The incidence of PDPH after spinal anesthesia is approximately 0.4% to 1.0%. However, the risk increases significantly with the use of larger cutting needles (e.g., 17- to 18-gauge epidural needle) and can be as high as 75%.

REFERENCES

1. Fink BR, Walker S. Orientation of fibers in the human dorsal lumbar dura mater in relation to lumbar puncture. *Anesth Analg* 1989;69:768–772.
2. Vandenabeele F, Creemers J, Lambrichts I. Ultrastructure of the human spinal and dura mater. *J Anat* 1996;189:417–430.
3. Reina MA, De Leon Casasola O, Villanueva MC, et al. Ultrastructural findings in human spinal pia mater in relation to subarachnoid anesthesia. *Anaesth Analg* 2004;98:1479–1485.
4. Hogan Q. Size of human lower thoracic and lumbosacral nerve roots. *Anesthesiology* 1996;85:37–42.
5. Hogan Q, Toth J. Anatomy of the soft tissues of the spinal canal. *Reg Anesth Pain Med* 1999;24:303–310.
6. Kim JT, Bahk JH, Sung J. Influence of age and sex on the position of the conus medullaris and Tuffier's line in adults. *Anesthesiology* 2003;99:1359–1363.
7. Broadbent CR, Maxwell WB, Ferrie R, et al. Ability of anaesthetists to identify a marked lumbar interspace. *Anaesthesia* 2000;55:1122–1126.
8. Reynolds F. Damage to the conus medullaris following spinal anaesthesia. *Anaesthesia* 2001;56:238–247.
9. Hamandi K, Mottershead J, Lewis T, et al. Irreversible damage to the spinal cord following spinal anesthesia. *Neurology* 2002;59:624–626.
10. Kim JT, Jung CW, Lee JR, et al. Influence of lumbar flexion on the position of the intercristal line. *Reg Anesth Pain Med* 2003;28:509–511.
11. Rocco AG, Raymond SA, Murray E, et al. Differential spread of blockade of touch, cold, and pinprick during spinal anesthesia. *Anesth Analg* 1985;64:917–923.
12. Sakura S, Sakaguchi Y, Shinzawa M, et al. The assessment of dermatomal level of surgical anesthesia after spinal tetracaine. *Anesth Analg* 2000;90:1406–1410.
13. Kouri ME, Kopacz DJ. Spinal 2-chloroprocaine: a comparison with lidocaine in volunteers. *Anesth Analg* 2004;98:75–80.
14. Hebl JR, Horlocker TT, Schroeder DR. Neuraxial anesthesia and analgesia in patients with preexisting central nervous system disorders. *Anesth Analg* 2006;103:223–228.
15. Hebl JR, Kopp SL, Schroeder DR, et al. Neurological complications after neuraxial anesthesia or analgesia in patients with preexisting peripheral sensorimotor neuropathy or diabetic polyneuropathy. *Anesth Analg* 2006;103:1294–1299.
16. Perlas A, Chan VW. Neuraxial anesthesia and multiple sclerosis. *Can J Anaesth* 2005;52:454–458.
17. McDonald SB. Is neuraxial blockade contraindicated in patients with aortic stenosis? *Reg Anesth Pain Med* 2004;29:496–502.
18. Wedel DJ, Horlocker TT. Regional anesthesia in the febrile or infected patient. *Reg Anesth Pain Med* 2006;31:324–333.
19. Green NM. Distribution of local anesthetics within the subarachnoid space. *Anesth Analg* 1985;64:715–730.
20. Hocking G, Wildsmith JAW. Intrathecal drug spread. *Br J Anaesth* 2004;93:568–578.
21. Hirabayshi Y, Shimizu R, Saitoh K, et al. Anatomical configuration of the spinal column in the supine position. I. A study using magnetic resonance imaging. *Br J Anaesth* 1995;75:3–5.
22. Hirabayshi Y, Shimizu R, Fukuda H, et al. Anatomical configuration of the spinal column in the supine position. II. Comparison of pregnant and non-pregnant women. *Br J Anaesth* 1995;75:6–8.
23. Veering BT, Immink-Speet TT, Burm AG, et al. Spinal anaesthesia with 0.5% hyperbaric bupivacaine in elderly patients: effects of duration of spent in the sitting position. *Br J Anaesth* 2001;77:738–742.
24. Casati A, Fanelli G, Aldegheri G, et al. Frequency of hypotension during conventional or asymmetric hyperbaric spinal block. *Reg Anesth Pain Med* 1999;24:214–219.
25. Bodily MN, Carpenter RL, Owens BD. Lidocaine 0.5% spinal anesthesia: a hypobaric solution for short-stay perirectal procedures. *Can J Anaesth* 1992;39:770–773.
26. Faust A, Fournier R, Van Gessel E, et al. Isobaric versus hypobaric spinal bupivacaine for total hip arthroplasty in the lateral position. *Anesth Analg* 2003;97:589–594.
27. Sheskey MC, Rocco AG, Bizzarri-Scgmid M, et al. A dose-response study of bupivacaine for spinal anesthesia. *Anesth Analg* 1983;62:931–935.
28. Van Zundert AA, Grouls RJ, Korsten HH, et al. Spinal anesthesia. Volume or concentration: what matters? *Reg Anesth* 1996;21:112.

29. Brown DT, Wildsmith JAW, Covino BG, et al. Effect of baricity on spinal anesthesia with amethocaine. *Br J Anaesth* 1980;52:589–596.

30. Wildsmith JAW, McClure J, Brown DT, et al. Effects of posture on spread of isobaric and hyperbaric amethocaine. *Br J Anaesth* 1981;53:273–278.

31. Liu SS, Ware PD, Allen HW, et al. Dose-response characteristics of spinal bupivacaine in volunteers. Clinical implications for ambulatory anesthesia. *Anesthesiology* 1996;85:729–736.

32. Touminen M, Pitkanen M, Taivainen T, et al. Predictors of spread of repeated spinal anesthesia with bupivacaine. *Br J Anaesth* 1992;68:136–138.

33. Olson KH, Nielsen TH, Kristofferson E, et al. Spinal anesthesia with plain bupivacaine 0.5%administered at interspace L2/L3 or L4/L5. *Br J Anaesth* 1990;64:170–172.

34. Serpell MG, Gray WM. Flow dynamics through spinal needles. *Anaesthesia* 1997;52:229–236.

35. Urmey WF, Stanton J, Bassin P, et al. The direction of the Whitacre needle aperture affects the extent and duration of isobaric spinal anesthesia. *Anesth Analg* 1997;84:337–341.

36. Taivainen T, Touminen M, Kuulasmaa KA, et al. A prospective study on reproducibility of the spread of spinal anesthesia using plain bupivacaine 0.5%. *Reg Anesth* 1990;15:12–14.

37. Casati A, Fanelli G, Danelli G, et al. Spinal anesthesia with lidocaine or preservative-free 2-chloroprocaine for outpatient knee arthroscopy: a prospective, randomized, double-blind comparison. *Anesth Analg* 2007;104:959–964.

38. Frey K, Holman S, Mikat-Stevens M, et al. The recovery profile of hyperbaric spinal anesthesia with lidocaine, bupivacaine, and tetracaine. *Reg Anesth Pain Med* 1998;23:159–163.

39. Ghisi D, Bonarelli S. Ambulatory surgery with chloroprocaine spinal anesthesia: a review. *Ambulatory Anesth* 2015;2: 111–120.

40. Kooger-Infante NE, Van Gessel E, Forster A, et al. Extent of hyperbaric spinal anesthesia influences duration of block. *Anesthesiology* 2000;92:1319–1323.

41. Burm AG, Van Kleef JW, Gladines MP, et al. Plasma concentrations of lidocaine and bupivacaine after subarachnoid administration. *Anesthesiology* 1983;59:191–195.

42. Chiu AA, Liu SS, Carpenter RL, et al. The effects of epinephrine on lidocaine spinal anesthesia: a crossover study. *Anesth Analg* 1995;80:735–739.

43. Racle JP, Benkhadra A, Poy JY, et al. Prolongation of isobaric spinal anesthesia with epinephrine and clonidine for hip surgery in the elderly. *Anesth Analg* 1987;66:442–446.

44. Armstrong IR, Littlewood DG, Chambers WA. Spinal anesthesia with tetracaine-effect of added vasoconstrictors. *Anesth Analg* 1983;62:793–795.

45. Concepcion M, Maddi R, Francis D, et al. Vasoconstrictors in spinal anesthesia with tetracaine-comparison of phenylephrine and epinephrine. *Anesth Analg* 1984;63:134–138.

46. Moore JM, Liu SS, Pollock JE, et al. The effect on epinephrine on small-dose hyperbaric bupivacaine spinal anesthesia: clinical implications for ambulatory surgery. *Anesth Analg* 1998;86:973–977.

47. Chiari A, Eisenach JC. Spinal anesthesia: mechanisms, agents, methods, and safety. *Reg Anesth Pain Med* 1998;23:357–362.

48. Hamber EA, Viscomi CM. Intrathecal lipophilic opioids as adjuncts to surgical spinal anesthesia. *Reg Anesth Pain Med* 1999;24:255–263.

49. Liu SS, Chiu AA, Carpenter RL, et al. Fentanyl prolongs lidocaine spinal anesthesia without prolonging recovery. *Anesth Analg* 1995;80:730–734.

50. Singh H, Yang J, Thornton K, et al. Intrathecal fentanyl prolongs sensory bupivacaine spinal block. *Can J Anaesth* 1995;42:987–991.

51. Rathmell JP, Lair TR, Nauman B. The role of intrathecal drugs in the treatment of acute pain. *Anesth Analg* 2005;101:S30–S43.

52. Rathmell JP, Pino CA, Taylor R, et al. Intrathecal morphine for postoperative analgesia: a randomized, controlled, dose-ranging study after hip and knee arthroplasty. *Anesth Analg* 2003;97:1452–1457.

53. American Society of Anesthesiologists Task Force on infectious complications associated with neuraxial techniques. Practice advisory for the prevention, diagnosis, and management of infectious complications associated with neuraxial techniques: a report by the American Society of Anesthesiologists Task Force on infectious complications associated with neuraxial techniques. *Anesthesiology* 2010;112:530–545.

54. Ahn WS, Bahk JH, Lim YJ, et al. The effect of introducer gauge, design, and bevel direction on the deflection of spinal needles. *Anaesthesia* 2002;57:1007–1011.

55. Chin KJ, Karmakar MK, Peng P. Ultrasonography of the adult thoracic and lumbar spine for central neuraxial blockade. *Anesthesiology* 2011;114:1459–1485.
56. Elgueta MF, Duong S, Finlayson RJ, et al. Ultrasonography for neuraxial blocks. *Minerva Anestesiol* 2017;83:512–523.
57. Kim JT, Shim JK, Kim SH, et al. Trendelenburg position with hip flexion as a rescue strategy to increase spinal anaesthetic level after spinal block. *Br J Anaesth* 2007;98:396–400.
58. Imarengiaye CO, Song D, Prabhu AJ, et al. Spinal anesthesia: functional balance is impaired after clinical recovery. *Anesthesiology* 2003;98:511–515.
59. Cullen DJ, Bogdanoiv E, Htut N. Spinal epidural hematoma occurrence in the absence of known risk factors: a case series. *J Clin Anesth* 2004;16:3786–3781.
60. Lee LA, Posner KL, Domino KB, et al. Injuries associated with regional anesthesia in the 1980s and 1990s: a closed claims analysis. *Anesthesiology* 2004;101:143–152.
61. Cosar A, Yetiser S, Sizlan A, et al. Hearing impairment associated with spinal anesthesia. *Acta Otolaryngol* 2004;124:1159–1164.
62. Borgeat A, Ekatodramis G, Schenker CA. Postoperative nausea and vomiting in regional anesthesia. *Anesthesiology* 2003;98:530–547.
63. Harrington BE. Postdural puncture headache and the development of the epidural blood patch. *Reg Anesth Pain Med* 2004;29:136–163.

7 Epidural Anesthesia and Analgesia

De Q.H. Tran and Julian Aliste

KEY POINTS

1. In clinical practice, continuous thoracic and lumbar epidural blocks are routinely used to provide postoperative analgesia for major thoracic/abdominal surgeries and labor, respectively (1). Since the implementation of peripheral nerve blocks in orthopedic pathways, epidural analgesia is less frequently employed for lower limb surgery.

2. The epidural space is most commonly identified with loss-of-resistance (LOR). Though sensitive, the latter lacks specificity, because ligamentous cysts, gaps in ligamenta flava, thoracic paravertebral spaces, and intermuscular planes can yield a nonepidural (i.e., false) LOR (2).

3. Various adjuncts (e.g., epidural waveform analysis [EWA], neurostimulation) can be used to differentiate between epidural and nonepidural LOR (3).

4. Although epidural blocks provide substantial clinical benefits (e.g., optimal pain control, decreased pulmonary complications after thoracic/upper abdominal surgery and trauma, and decreased ileus after abdominal surgery), they can also lead to complications, which range from the common (e.g., hypotension) to the rare (e.g., dural puncture) to the potentially catastrophic (e.g., epidural hematoma). Thus, the prudent anesthesiologist should possess a firm grasp of the anatomy, pharmacology, and techniques underlying the safe conduct of epidural anesthesia and analgesia.

I. Anatomy. The reader is referred to Chapter 6 (Spinal Anesthesia) for an in-depth discussion of neuraxial anatomy. For epidural blocks, one needs to remember certain key facts:

   A. Surface landmarks can be used to estimate spinal levels and to select the optimal insertion site for continuous epidural blocks. For instance, the scapular spine, the inferior angle of the scapula, and the intercristal line correspond to the T3 level, T8 level, and L4–L5 intervertebral space, respectively (Fig. 7.1). However, significant interindividual variation exists. Thus, correlation between surface landmark and spinal level is approximate at best.

   B. Spinous processes are almost horizontal in the cervical and lumbar levels. In contrast, they possess a moderate caudal angulation in the upper and lower thoracic levels. In the midthoracic spine, spinous processes display a notoriously sharp caudal angulation (Fig. 7.2). To further compound the technical challenge, the interlaminar spaces can be narrow, and laminae can sometimes overlap between T4 and T7.

   C. The interspinous ligament, which connects adjacent spinous processes, displays a high incidence of age-related cysts.

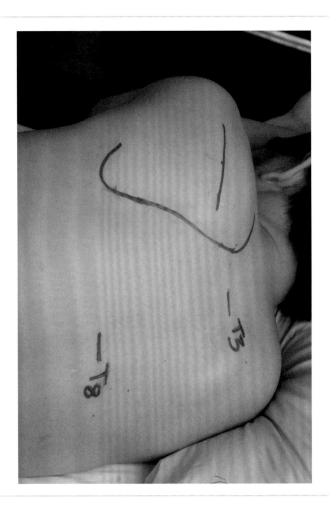

FIGURE 7.1   Surface landmarks.

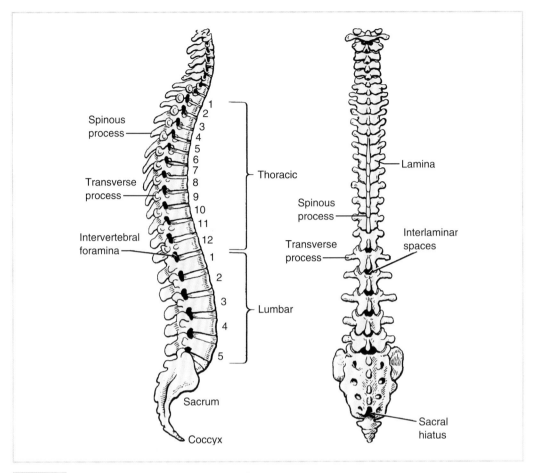

FIGURE 7.2   Comparative lumbar and thoracic spinal anatomy.

D. **Midline gaps can often be found in ligamenta flava in the cervical, thoracic, and lumbar levels.**

E. **The epidural space contains loose connective tissues, fat, arterial vessels, a plexus of veins, as well as nerve roots.** Pockets of epidural adipose tissue are commonly found in the posterior and anterolateral epidural spaces (Fig. 7.3). Their pharmacokinetic importance stems from the fact that they act as a reservoir for lipophilic (opioid) drugs, thereby slowing the latter's onset and/or increasing their duration of action. Epidural veins are usually confined to the anterior epidural space and rarely does one find a prominent vein posterior to the intervertebral foramen. The distance between ligamentum flavum and dura (i.e., the width of the epidural space) varies between 2 and 25 mm, with an average of 7 mm. The epidural space is largest at the lumbar level and progressively narrows as it ascends rostrally.

F. **The dura mater is composed of multiple layers of collagen and elastic fibers.** The latter do not display any specific orientation. The dura is closely adherent to the arachnoid mater, a 5- to 6-cell-thick layer whose fibers run parallel to the spinal axis. Contrary to popular belief, the arachnoid mater (and not the dura) is responsible for containing the cerebrospinal fluid inside the intrathecal space.

> **CLINICAL PEARL** For midthoracic epidural blocks, a paramedian approach should be used (*vide infra*) because it allows the operator to circumvent the caudal angulation of the spinous processes.

> **CLINICAL PEARL** Cysts in interspinous ligaments and midline gaps in ligamentum flavum can explain the occurrence of false loss-of-resistance (i.e., nonepidural loss-of-resistance) with the midline technique (*vide infra*).

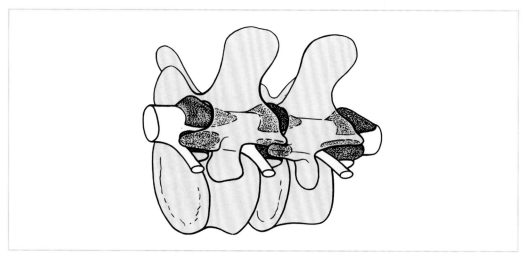

FIGURE 7.3 Epidural fat (stippled area) is discontinuously distributed within the epidural space. In areas where fat is absent, the dura mater abuts the ligamentum flavum and represents a "potential space." (Adapted from Hogan Q. Lumbar epidural anatomy: a new look by cryomicrotome section. *Anesthesiology* 1991;75(5):767.)

II. Pharmacology

A. Site of action. Although local anesthetics can penetrate the spinal meninges to reach the cerebrospinal fluid, spinal cord transmission remains intact, thus indicating that the spinal cord itself is not the primary site of action. Instead, animal studies suggest that epidural blocks target the extradural spinal nerves (which traverse the epidural space) as well as the spinal nerve rootlets (within the subarachnoid space).

B. Local anesthetic agents. Only preservative-free local anesthetic solutions should be used in the epidural space. Local anesthetics are commonly classified according to their duration of action. The latter can be defined in terms of "two-dermatome regression" (i.e., the time it takes a block to recede by two dermatomes from its maximum extent), which estimates the duration of effective surgical block, or "complete resolution," which approximates the time required for outpatient discharge (Table 7.1).

1. **Short duration. Chloroprocaine** (2% or 3%) provides the fastest onset and the shortest duration for epidural blockade (Fig. 7.4). Large doses of preservative-free chloroprocaine have been associated with back pain, whereas lower doses (900 mg) may result in mild back pain. The latter usually appears immediately unlike the back pain associated with Transient Neurologic Symptoms. For reasons unknown, epidural chloroprocaine decreases the efficacy of subsequently administered epidural morphine and clonidine.

2. **Intermediate duration.** These agents provide an onset that is comparable to that of chloroprocaine. However, their slower rate of resolution may delay outpatient discharge. **Lidocaine**

TABLE 7.1 Local anesthetics used for surgical epidural block

| | Duration of sensory block | | |
Drug[a]	Two-dermatome regression (min)	Complete resolution (min)	Prolongation by epinephrine (%)
Chloroprocaine 3%	45–60	100–160	40–60
Lidocaine 2%	60–100	160–200	40–80
Mepivacaine 2%	60–100	160–200	40–80
Ropivacaine 0.5%–1.0%	90–180	240–420	No
Etidocaine 1%–1.5%	120–240	300–460	No
Bupivacaine 0.5%–0.75%	120–240	300–460	No

[a]These concentrations are recommended for surgical anesthesia; more dilute concentrations are appropriate for epidural analgesia.

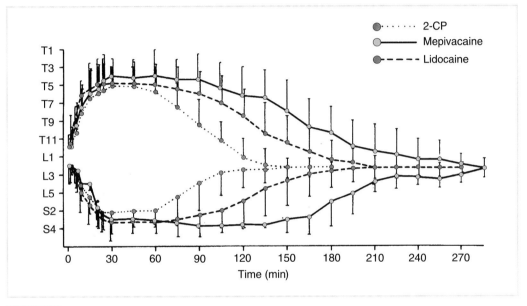

FIGURE 7.4 Onset and duration of epidural anesthesia. Sensory dermatomal blockade level (with standard deviations) versus time following the injection of 20 mL of 3% 2-chloroprocaine (CP), 1.5% lidocaine, or 1.5% mepivacaine with 1:200,000 epinephrine at the L2 interspace. Average total durations were 133, 182, and 247 minutes, respectively. (Adapted from Kopacz DJ, Mulroy MF. Chloroprocaine and lidocaine decrease hospital stay and admission rate after outpatient epidural anesthesia. Reg Anesth 1990;15:19.)

(1.5% or 2.0%) provides excellent anesthesia for 60 to 90 minutes (as a single injection) but can result in tachyphylaxis (i.e., decreasing duration with repeated injection) when (repeatedly) administered through an epidural catheter. The mechanism behind tachyphylaxis remains poorly understood, but may stem from changes in drug distribution/elimination from the epidural space. **Mepivacaine** (1% or 1.5%) can produce a slightly longer block than lidocaine.

3. **Long duration. Bupivacaine** (0.5% or 0.75%), which is supplied as a racemic mixture of the levo- and dextrorotatory optical isomers, produces a denser sensory than motor block. This property explains its popularity (in dilute concentrations) for continuous epidural blocks. Bupivacaine displays a slower uptake from the epidural space than intermediate-duration local anesthetics, and thus has less potential for systemic toxicity caused by local anesthetic absorption. However, because of its inherent cardiotoxicity, bupivacaine should not be used

in high doses, and inadvertent intravascular injection should be avoided by using a test dose and incremental injection. **Ropivacaine**, a single optical isomer, is less cardiotoxic but also 40% less potent than bupivacaine in the epidural space. If one accounts for this difference in potency, contrary to popular belief, it does not have greater "motor sparing" effects than bupivacaine despite its increased cost.

C. **Adjuvants.** The duration of sensory and/or motor block produced by local anesthetic agents can be "fine-tuned" with various adjuvants.

  1. **Epinephrine.** A 5 µg/mL concentration of epinephrine prolongs the duration of sensorimotor block produced by short- and intermediate-duration local anesthetics, but not by long-duration drugs. In addition to this pharmacokinetic effect, epinephrine also displays α_2-adrenergic agonistic properties and may decrease pain transmission in the spinal cord. Compared to plain local anesthetic agents, the addition of epinephrine results in a greater decrease in the mean arterial pressure (MAP) (Fig. 7.5). The lower MAP is caused by a reduction in systemic vascular resistance (SVR), which seems to be mediated by the vasodilatory β_2-adrenergic properties of low-dose epinephrine. The decrease in SVR also leads to a significantly higher cardiac output and a modestly elevated heart rate. Animal studies reveal that the presence

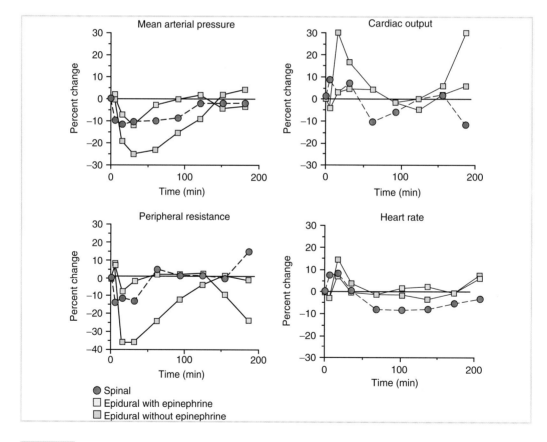

FIGURE 7.5   The cardiovascular effects of spinal and epidural anesthesia in volunteers with T5 blocks. The effects of spinal anesthesia and epidural anesthesia without epinephrine were generally comparable and are both qualitatively and quantitatively different from the effects of epidural anesthesia with epinephrine. (Republished with permission of John Wiley and Sons Inc, from Bonica JJ, Kennedy WF Jr, Ward RJ, et al. A comparison of the effects of high subarachnoid and epidural anesthesia. Acta Anaesthesiol Scand Suppl 1996;23:429-37; permission conveyed through Copyright Clearance Center, Inc.)

of epinephrine in the local anesthetic solution does not decrease cardiovascular toxicity in the event of accidental intravascular injection. However, epinephrine will decrease the plasmatic levels of local anesthetics (through its α_1-vasoconstrictive properties) and provide a marker for intravascular injection (through its β_1-chronotropic properties).

2. **Opioids.** The addition of opioids to epidural local anesthetics increases the duration of sensory, but not motor block. The magnitude (and duration) of sensory prolongation depends on the dose administered and the opioid chosen. For instance, hydrophilic opioids (e.g., morphine) provide a greater effect than their hydrophobic counterparts (e.g., fentanyl). Moreover, they display greater rostral spread in the epidural space.

3. **Clonidine.** Epidural clonidine (150 to 300 µg) prolongs sensory, but not motor block. Unlike epinephrine, its effect occurs with long-acting local anesthetic agents. Epidural clonidine can result in sedation as well as a decrease in blood pressure. Unlike epinephrine, epidural clonidine is associated with a modest decrease in heart rate.

4. **Bicarbonate.** Addition of sodium bicarbonate (0.1 mEq/mL) to local anesthetic agents has been historically advocated to hasten the onset of epidural block. This effect is unreliable at best.

D. **Dose.** Within the epidural space, local anesthetic solutions spread cephalad and caudad from the initial injection site (Fig. 7.6). Unfortunately, it is impossible to predict with certainty the dose required to produce a given extent of epidural blockade. Consequently, clinicians must be cognizant of the major and minor factors that determine the spread of epidural blocks (Table 7.2).

1. **Dose, volume, and concentration.** Dose and volume constitute independent predictors of the spread of epidural blockade. In other words, increasing the dose while keeping the volume constant (i.e., increasing the drug concentration) and increasing the drug volume while keeping the dose constant (i.e., decreasing concentration) will both increase the extent of epidural blockade. Unfortunately, the relationship is not linear: as the dose is increased, the *spread per milliliter injected* decreases so the net increase in spread is only a few dermatomes.

2. **Technique.** Because local anesthetic can spread cephalad and caudad from the injection site, the latter becomes an important determinant of dermatomes blocked. With mid- to high thoracic epidural blocks, local anesthetic molecules tend to diffuse in a caudal direction, whereas lower epidural blocks display a predominantly cephalad local anesthetic spread. Because the volume of the epidural space increases as one moves caudad, a greater local anesthetic dose is required to anesthetize the same number of dermatomes in the lumbar/caudal level compared to the thoracic level. Gravity, needle angulation, direction of needle aperture, and speed of injection confer negligible effects on the spread of epidural blocks.

3. **Patient factors.** The influence of pregnancy on the spread of epidural blockade is controversial. Interestingly, pregnant women are more sensitive to the effects of local anesthetics. In theory, increasing age, short stature, and obesity contribute to increase the spread of epidural blocks. However, the effect is small, and considerable interindividual variability exists.

CLINICAL PEARL The choice of local anesthetic dose remains highly subjective. One could use 15 mL as an average starting dose for lumbar epidural blocks. If clinical factors (i.e., extensive surgery, tall patient) suggest that a larger dose may be required, the operator could increase the injectate by 5 to 10 mL. Conversely, if factors (e.g., patient who is short, elderly, or obese) mandate a dose reduction, the operator could decrease the volume by 3 to 5 mL. For thoracic epidural blocks, one could start with 6 to 8 mL and use 2- to 4-mL increments or 1- to 2-mL decrements. The insertion of an epidural catheter will provide much clinical latitude, because it permits controlled titration of the epidural block.

CLINICAL PEARL If an epidural catheter traverses a vertebral foramen or lies anteriorly in the epidural space, local anesthetic spread may be asymmetric (i.e., unilateral) (4). Thus, the authors recommend not introducing the catheter more than 4 cm inside the epidural space. Malposition of epidural catheters may be particularly problematic in the setting of postoperative analgesia because low volumes of dilute local anesthetic agents are typically used.

III. Technique. Epidural blocks should be performed in a setting (e.g., induction room, operating room, or recovery room) with full monitoring capabilities (i.e., pulse oximetry, blood pressure, electrocardiogram) and ready access to an oxygen source as well as resuscitative equipment and drugs. The anesthesiologist should employ strict sterile precautions (i.e., cap, mask, and sterile gloves). The patient can be placed in the sitting or lateral decubitus position. Although the sitting position is preferred by beginners because it permits easier identification of the midline, the lateral

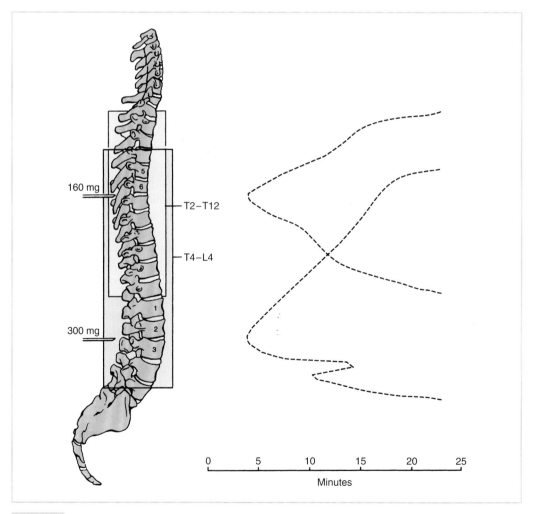

FIGURE 7.6 Diagram of spread of local anesthetic in the epidural space. The onset of epidural anesthesia is noted first in the segments nearest the site of injection, and spreads over the next 20 minutes both cephalad and caudad from this point.

TABLE 7.2   Factors affecting spread of epidural block

■ **Major factors**
Site of injection
Dose
■ **Minor factors**
Age
Height
Weight
Pregnancy
■ **Minimally relevant factors**
Speed of injection
Incremental injection
Direction of needle opening

decubitus position may improve patient comfort. If required, intravenous sedation (e.g., 2 mg of midazolam and 50 µg of fentanyl) can be administered, provided it does not hinder cooperation or verbal communication with the physician.

The appropriate level for the epidural block is selected based on cutaneous landmarks such as the scapular spine (T3 level), the inferior angle of the scapula (T8 level), and the intercristal line (L4–L5 intervertebral space) (*vide supra*). For abdominal and thoracic surgery, the anesthesiologist must provide analgesic coverage not only for somatic structures (i.e., skin and muscles) but also for the viscera (which receive innervation from the sympathetic chain). Somatic coverage can be easily inferred by the cutaneous incision itself. In terms of visceral coverage, the digestive tract (from the distal third of the esophagus to the splenic flexure of the colon) receives innervation from the T5 to T12 spinal levels, which give rise to the splanchnic nerves and the celiac plexus. Pelvic organs are supplied by the T10 to L2 spinal levels (hypogastric plexus), whereas the lung and heart receive innervation from the T1 to T4 levels (cardiac and pulmonary plexi).

Methods to identify the epidural space fall into three categories: LOR (tactile end point), negative-pressure recognition (visual end point) (5), and acoustic fall in tonal pitch (auditory end point). Despite the many devices aimed at detecting or augmenting negative pressure, few operators rely on the latter to identify the epidural space. Although preliminary works by Lechner et al (6) suggest that the fall in tonal pitch associated with needle transition from ligamentum flavum to epidural space can assist with catheter insertion, the sophisticated equipment required (pressure transducer, pressure amplifier, voltage-controlled oscillator, loudspeaker) limits its routine implementation. Thus, LOR, which was described in 1921, remains the most common method because of its simplicity (7).

LOR can be carried out with air or a liquid medium (i.e., normal saline) (8). Air runs the risk of creating a pneumocephalus if inadvertently injected into the subarachnoid space. Furthermore, excessive air administered inside the epidural space may result in a "patchy" block. On the other hand, LOR with saline could create confusion and hinder the diagnosis of a "wet tap" (i.e., accidental dural puncture). Despite these purported differences, studies comparing air and saline for LOR have not found major differences in terms of block efficacy.

The epidural space can be accessed using a midline or paramedian approach.

CLINICAL PEARL   If the operator favors the pneumatic feel of LOR to air but would like to avoid the occurrence of pneumocephalus or patchy blocks, a hybrid technique could be used: the LOR syringe could be filled with 3 mL of normal saline and 0.5 to 1 mL of air.

A. Midline approach

1. The skin is disinfected and draped in standard fashion. A chlorhexidine and alcohol solution is recommended for skin preparation. A transparent plastic drape will allow the operator to continuously visualize the cutaneous landmarks and surface anatomy of the back.

2. Using a 25-gauge needle, local anesthetic (e.g., lidocaine 1%) is used to infiltrate the skin and subcutaneous tissues.

3. The operator purposefully contacts the spinous process with the 25-gauge needle. This step serves to identify midline beyond a reasonable doubt. The operator should remember that, in patients with normal or low body mass indices, the spinous process is relatively shallow. If the 25-gauge needle contacts a deep bone, it has drifted away from the midline and contacted lamina.

4. The 25-gauge needle is angled slightly cephalad (or caudad), walked off the spinous process, and introduced into the interspinous ligament. Once the needle tip is inside the interspinous ligament, it feels well anchored and very stable to movement. This tactile sensation confirms midline puncture. The operator makes a mental note of the cephalad (or caudad) angle displayed by the 25-gauge needle.

5. A small amount of local anesthetic is injected and the 25-gauge needle removed.

6. The operator introduces the epidural needle into the interspinous ligament using the same cephalad (or caudad) angle as the one recorded for the 25-gauge needle. A glass or plastic syringe designed for LOR is attached to the epidural needle.

7. The epidural needle is slowly advanced forward while the operator applies pressure on the plunger of the LOR syringe.

8. When the epidural needle reaches the ligamentum flavum, resistance to advancement will increase. The operator slowly advances the epidural needle forward (while applying pressure on the plunger of the LOR syringe) until LOR occurs.

9. Using the markings present on the epidural needle, the operator determines the depth of the epidural space. An epidural catheter is introduced inside the needle and the latter is removed.

10. Three to four centimeters of catheter length is left inside the epidural space.

11. The catheter is secured to the skin using adhesive dressings.

12. After negative aspiration, a test dose (e.g., 3 mL of lidocaine 2% with epinephrine 5 µg/mL) is administered to rule out intravascular or intrathecal placement of the epidural catheter (9).

CLINICAL PEARL LOR can be easily identified with volumes as small as 0.2 to 0.3 mL of air or normal saline. In fact, the injection of "high" volumes (i.e., 2 mL) confers no additional tactile information compared to "micro" volumes (e.g., 0.2 mL). The authors strongly recommend not exceeding 0.5 mL to avoid patchy epidural blocks (if the LOR medium is air) or confusion with cerebrospinal fluid return (if the LOR medium is saline).

CLINICAL PEARL Different schools of thought exist on how to hold the epidural needle (one hand vs. two hands), how to advance the latter (intermittently vs. continuously), and how to apply pressure on the plunger of the LOR syringe (intermittently vs. continuously). No strong evidence exists to support any of these dogmas. The authors recommend that operators simply adopt a technique that feels natural and comfortable to them. Technically, the only important thing is that needle advancement be carried out in an incremental and controlled fashion.

CLINICAL PEARL If epidural catheter does not advance easily, the operator can rotate the bevel of the needle 180 degrees prior to a second attempt at catheter threading. However, during the rotation process, care should be taken not to inadvertently push the needle forward, because this could result in dural puncture.

B. Paramedian approach

1. The initial steps for the paramedian approach (i.e., skin disinfection, draping, local infiltration of skin and subcutaneous tissues) are identical to the ones used for the midline method.

2. The operator purposefully contacts the spinous process with the 25-gauge needle. This step serves to identify midline beyond a reasonable doubt.

3. The operator makes a mental note of the location of the spinous process. The 25-gauge needle is withdrawn from the skin. A second puncture site is made 2 cm lateral to the spinous process. The needle is advanced (while injecting local anesthetic) perpendicularly to the skin until bony contact. This step serves to identify the lamina beyond a reasonable doubt. The operator should remember that laminar bony contact must be reached at a greater depth than that of the spinous process. If the two bones are encountered at the same depth, the first bony contact was most likely lamina and not spinous process.

4. After contacting the lamina, the operator withdraws the 25-gauge needle and proceeds to anesthetize subcutaneous tissues in a cephalomedial direction (toward the midline). These are the tracks that will be used by the epidural needle to "triangulate" into the epidural space.

5. The 25-gauge needle is removed and the epidural needle is introduced perpendicularly to the skin until it contacts the lamina.

6. The operator then proceeds to redirect the epidural needle 15 degrees cephalad and 15 degrees medial so that laminar contact occurs at a second point slightly more cephalomedial to the first one. This process (triangulation) is repeated until the tip of the epidural needle is gently walked off the lamina.

7. A glass or plastic syringe designed for LOR is attached to the epidural needle.

8. The operator slowly advances the epidural needle forward (while applying pressure on the plunger of the LOR syringe) until LOR occurs.

9. The rest of the procedure is carried out in a similar fashion to the midline approach.

CLINICAL PEARL With the paramedian (lateral oblique) approach, during the triangulation process, care must be taken not to angle the epidural needle too medially to prevent the latter from walking off the spinous process instead of the lamina (Fig. 7.7). This would result in a nonepidural LOR.

CLINICAL PEARL A technical variant for the paramedian approach consists in using a puncture site just 1 cm lateral to the spinous process. The epidural needle is then walked off the lamina in a purely cephalad direction (without triangulation).

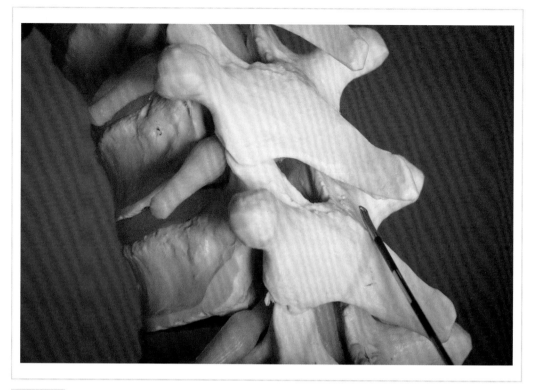

FIGURE 7.7 With the paramedian approach, an aggressive medial angulation results in the epidural needle walking off the spinous process instead of the lamina.

C. **Technical adjuncts.** Technical adjuncts for epidural blocks can be classified as navigational or confirmatory adjuncts.

1. **Navigational adjuncts.** Navigational adjuncts allow the operator to efficiently guide the epidural needle between adjacent spinous processes (midline approach) or laminae (paramedian approach). They include fluoroscopy and ultrasonography (US). Although fluoroscopy provides optimal versatility because it can also serve as a confirmatory adjunct (*vide infra*), the need for a lead-lined procedural room severely limits its widespread applicability in an operating room setting (10).

US can be used in two different ways. With *US guidance*, the operator advances the epidural needle toward the neuraxial space under real-time visualization. With *US assistance*, preprocedural US scanning is used to determine the optimal needle angulation and entry site. The epidural block is subsequently performed with a conventional "blind" technique. The prohibitive difficulty associated with US guidance lies in the need for an assistant, because a third hand is required to hold the US transducer while the operator advances the epidural needle and applies continuous (or intermittent) pressure on the plunger of the LOR syringe. Thus, at present time, only US assistance provides a modicum of user-friendliness. Ultrasound assistance has been investigated both for thoracic and lumbar (obstetric) epidural blocks. Randomized controlled trials reveal that, compared to their palpation-guided counterparts, US-assisted thoracic epidural blocks confer no additional benefits in terms of performance time and number of needle passes (11). In contrast, the available literature supports the use of US-assisted obstetric epidural blocks. Reported benefits include a decrease in performance time and number of needle passes as well as improved first-pass success (12). The technique for US-assisted lumbar epidural blocks is identical to the one used for US-assisted spinal blocks. The reader is referred to Chapter 6 (Spinal Anesthesia) for an in-depth description.

CLINICAL PEARL   At present time, the available evidence only supports the use of US assistance for lumbar (obstetric) epidural blocks.

CLINICAL PEARL   The acoustic window between contiguous spinous processes may be more difficult to find in elderly patients (with arthritic spines) than young parturients.

2. **Confirmatory adjuncts.** Despite its sensitivity, LOR lacks specificity, because cysts in interspinous ligaments, gaps in ligamenta flava, intermuscular planes, and thoracic paravertebral spaces can also yield a false-positive (i.e., nonepidural) LOR. Confirmatory adjuncts for LOR include a test dose, fluoroscopy, EWA, electrical stimulation [ES], and dural puncture.

a. **Epidural test dose.** Epidural test doses are frequently administered to rule out intravascular or intrathecal placement of catheters. Furthermore, a test dose can also confirm LOR (and correct positioning of the epidural catheter) by demonstrating the presence of a sensory block to ice (or pinprick). Unfortunately, the lack of "real-time" feedback limits its clinical usefulness. For instance, if sensory blockade were absent after 10 to 15 minutes, the operator would need to replace the faulty epidural catheter and wait an additional 10 minutes to confirm adequate placement of the latter. These cumulative delays would decrease operating room efficiency.

b. **Fluoroscopy.** Fluoroscopy (with contrast injection) enables confirmation of LOR obtained by the epidural needle as well as optimal placement of the catheter tip. Furthermore, fluoroscopy allows the operator to detect inadvertent catheter positioning in the intrathecal space and blood vessels. Unfortunately, in most centers, the additional equipment, manpower (i.e., radiology technologist), and radiation exposure often curtail its routine use in surgical and obstetric patients.

c. **Dural puncture.** When lumbar epidural catheters are inserted below the caudal end of the spinal cord (L1–L2), a 25- or 27-gauge spinal needle can be introduced through the epidural needle to carry out a "needle-through-needle" combined spinal–epidural (CSE) block. The spinal component of CSE decreases the onset of anesthesia/analgesia. However, "dry" dural puncture (without LA administration) can also be performed with the spinal needle: in this scenario, the small dural breach could facilitate LA translocation from the epidural space into the intrathecal space. More importantly, "dry" dural puncture provides LOR confirmation: if cerebrospinal fluid return is obtained through the spinal needle, the tip of the epidural needle is most likely positioned in the epidural space.

d. **Epidural waveform analysis.** EWA provides a simple confirmatory adjunct for LOR. When the needle (or catheter) is correctly positioned inside the epidural space, pressure measurement at its tip results in a pulsatile waveform synchronized with arterial pulsations. Waveform analysis can be carried out through the epidural needle or the catheter. The physics of waveform transmission reveals that a wave is less dampened by a short, rigid medium (i.e., epidural needle) than a long, flexible medium (i.e., epidural catheter). Thus, the sensitivity of EWA through the needle surpasses that of the catheter.

In recent observational trials (combined n = 241), EWA (through the needle) conferred 91% to 98% sensitivity, 84% to 100% specificity, 95% to 100% positive predictive value, and 50% to 74% negative predictive value for thoracic epidural blocks (13). Moreover, compared to traditional LOR, EWA-confirmed LOR led to a substantial decrease in the primary failure rate of thoracic epidural blocks (2% vs. 24%; $p = 0.002$) in two academic centers (14).

In clinical practice, EWA can be easily accomplished under 90 seconds. The operator first identifies LOR in the usual fashion. Subsequently, 5 mL of normal saline is injected through the epidural needle. The latter is then connected to a pressure transducer (leveled with the heart) via a sterile, rigid extension tubing (72″ male to female Luer Lock, Advance Medical Designs Inc., Marietta, GA, USA) (Fig. 7.8). A satisfactory end point is defined as the presence of waveforms synchronized with arterial pulsations (scale = 0 to 40 mm Hg). A video clip of EWA can be found on the authors' free access, educational website: www.regionalworks.ca.

CLINICAL PEARL   Because patients undergoing thoracotomy and laparotomy often require radial artery cannulation, the same pressurized normal saline bag and pressure transducer can be repurposed for EWA. Thus, for thoracic EWA, the only supplemental expense comes from the rigid extension tubing.

e. **Electrical stimulation.** ES for epidural catheters was pioneered by Tsui et al in 1998 (15). By priming the epidural catheter with normal saline, these authors were able to elicit myotomal contractions in 28 out of 39 patients using an average current of 3.78 mA (pulse width = 0.2 ms; frequency = 1 Hz). In subsequent studies, different investigators set out to assess the reliability of ES for the thoracic and lumbar epidural spaces. When compared to clinical response (sensory blockade/successful analgesia) or postoperative radiographic assessment of catheter placement, ES conferred 80% to 100% sensitivity, 83% to 100% specificity, 96% to 100% positive predictive value, and 16% to 100% negative predictive value.

In addition to LOR confirmation, ES provides additional benefits. For instance, placement of a catheter in the intrathecal and subdural spaces or alongside a nerve root will yield stimulation at a current less than 1 mA (pulse width = 0.2 ms). Intravascular placement can also be detected by the failure of LA to abolish myotomal contractions. More importantly, ES enables the operator to position the catheter tip at the desired spinal level, as evidenced by the contraction of corresponding myotomes.

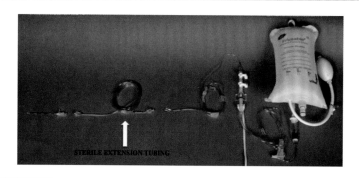

FIGURE 7.8   Setup for epidural waveform analysis through the needle. (Adapted from Leurcharusmee P, Arnuntasupakul V, Chora de le Garza D, et al. Reliability of waveform analysis as an adjunct to loss-of-resistance for thoracic epidural blocks. *Reg Anesth Pain Med* 2015;40(6):695.)

ES can be carried out with two different techniques. The epidural catheter could be primed with normal saline. Subsequently, an adaptor (Johans ECG Adaptor; Arrow International, Reading, PA, USA) enables the connection of the catheter to a nerve stimulator. With this method, the operator should ensure that there are no air bubbles in the system, because the presence of an "air lock" will dampen electrical conduction. Alternately, ES can be performed with an epidural catheter containing a removable stylet. The latter is connected to the neurostimulator via a two-headed alligator clip. A video clip of ES of the epidural space can be found on the authors' free access, educational website: www.regionalworks.ca.

CLINICAL PEARL   ES of the epidural space can be carried out with catheters designed for peripheral nerve blocks (StimuCath, Teleflex Medical, Research Triangle Park, NC, USA). Because these catheters connect directly to the neurostimulator, the two-headed alligator clip is no longer required. However, because they have not been officially approved for epidural blocks, their use should be considered off-label. Furthermore, because of the presence of metallic coils, they must be removed prior to magnetic resonance imaging (MRI).

CLINICAL PEARL   From an intellectual standpoint, the operator could conceptualize the technical performance of epidural blocks as a series of three distinct steps: (1) the search of a needle path between adjacent bones (spinous processes or laminae), (2) the search for LOR, and (3) confirmation of LOR. Most "difficult" epidural blocks originate from step 1 and could be remedied with US and, possibly, fluoroscopy. In contrast, most "failed" epidural blocks stem from the omission of step 3.

CLINICAL PEARL   For confirmation of LOR, the authors routinely use "dry" dural puncture for mid- to low lumbar epidural blocks. For thoracic and high lumbar epidural blocks, the authors employ waveform analysis through the epidural needle. ES of the catheter constitutes a possible alternative if the dedicated equipment (e.g., Johans ECG Adaptor, two-headed alligator clip, styletted epidural catheter, neurostimulator) is available.

IV. Combined spinal and epidural block. CSE blocks elegantly marry the quick onset time provided by spinal anesthesia with the prolonged postoperative analgesia conferred by the insertion of an epidural catheter. Furthermore, the ability to reload the latter intraoperatively enables the injection of a lower dose of local anesthetic for the initial spinal block. In turn, this curtails the occurrence and intensity of autonomic blockade and hypotension. Technically, two methods can be used to perform CSE blocks.

    A. Double puncture technique. The double puncture technique requires the performance of spinal and epidural blocks at different intervertebral spaces. Its main advantage stems from the ability to provide spinal anesthesia (carried out at the L3–L4 or L4–L5 level) when an epidural catheter is required above the L1–L2 level. The sequence in which the spinal and epidural blocks are performed depends on different clinical factors. If the operator plans to use a local anesthetic test dose to rule out intrathecal placement of the epidural catheter, the epidural block must be performed first because the test dose would be inconclusive in the presence of spinal anesthesia. In contrast, if the intrathecal and epidural blocks are performed at contiguous interspaces, the spinal block must be carried out first to avoid accidental puncture of a previously placed epidural catheter by the spinal needle.

B. Needle-through-needle technique. The needle-through-needle technique begins with the identification of LOR by the epidural needle. Subsequently, a (long) 25- or 27-gauge spinal needle is advanced through the latter in order to puncture the dura and arachnoid mater. The main advantage provided by the needle-through-needle technique lies in the fact that cerebrospinal fluid return (through the spinal needle) enables real-time confirmation that the tip of epidural needle is adequately positioned inside the epidural space (*vide supra*). Furthermore, the use of a single puncture site may increase efficiency and patient comfort.

There exist epidural needles with special ports designed to accommodate the spinal needle and to permit perpendicular dural puncture. Furthermore, some commercially available kits also allow the operator to mechanically secure the spinal needle inside its epidural counterpart prior to local anesthetic injection. However, conventional epidural and spinal needles can also be used with adequate efficacy.

CLINICAL PEARL For the needle-through-needle technique, the use of a fluid interface (normal saline) for LOR could interfere with the subsequent identification of dura/arachnoid puncture by the spinal needle, because saline flow back may mimic cerebrospinal fluid return. Thus, LOR to air may be preferable.

CLINICAL PEARL Irrespective of the technique selected for CSE blockade, the operator should remember that the level of the initial spinal block could be (intentionally or nonintentionally) increased by a loading dose through the epidural catheter. This phenomenon can be mechanically explained by the compression of the dural sac by the epidural bolus and the resultant rostral migration of local anesthetic molecules inside the intrathecal space.

V. Contraindications. Spinal and epidural blocks share a list of absolute and relative contraindications.

A. Absolute. Patient refusal, infection at the proposed puncture site, coagulopathy, allergy to local anesthetics and/or opioids, and intracranial hypertension.

B. Relative

1. **Neurologic.** The cost–benefit ratio of epidural blocks must be carefully analyzed in patients with known spinal stenosis. Despite historical concern, epidural blocks do not seem to exacerbate chronic back pain and demyelinating diseases (e.g., multiple sclerosis).

2. **Cardiovascular.** Patients with hypovolemia and fixed cardiac output pathology (e.g., aortic/mitral valve stenosis) may not be able to compensate for the sudden hypotension. Thus, epidural blocks should be carefully initiated with dilute boluses/infusions of local anesthetic agent and carefully titrated according to clinical response.

3. **Systemic infection.** If required, epidural (and spinal) blocks can be performed after the initiation of antibiotic therapy, provided there is an adequate response to treatment.

CLINICAL PEARL In trauma centers, anesthesiologists may be consulted to provide thoracic epidural analgesia for patients suffering from multiple rib fractures. Occasionally, some of these patients can also present concomitant head injury with intracranial hypertension. In this clinical scenario, the prudent anesthesiologist should refrain from carrying out epidural blocks, because accidental dural/arachnoid puncture (with a large bore epidural needle) could lead to brainstem herniation through the foramen magnum. Thoracic paravertebral blocks may provide a safer alternative.

CLINICAL PEARL   A history of spine surgery does not constitute a contraindication to epidural blocks *per se*. However, the latter may be technically challenging. In fact, because of extensive fibrosis, the epidural space may no longer be present. Furthermore, even if successful epidural catheter placement is achieved, the distribution of local anesthetic may be erratic and unpredictable.

VI. Complications. A detailed consideration of complications related to epidural block and their treatment can be found in Chapter 14.

    A. Failure. Epidural failure can be classified as primary (technical failure) or secondary (catheter dislodgement or inadequate pharmacologic regimen). In turn, technical failure can be ascribed to misidentification of the epidural space by the needle or misplacement of the epidural catheter. Using computed tomography scanning, Hogan has previously demonstrated that adequate epidural blockade could be obtained with various catheter tip positions: thus, misrecognition of the epidural space may explain most instances of technical failure.

        Technical failure is most problematic for thoracic epidural blocks performed in teaching centers. Its incidence can exceed 20%. In addition to the difficult anatomy of the thoracic spine and the unreliability of LOR, insufficient training may compound the problem, because pedagogical requirements are often inadequate and exposure during residency may be decreasing.

    B. Hypotension. Sympathetic blockade results in venous and, to a lesser degree, arterial vasodilatation. Venodilatation translates into decreased venous return (preload) and stroke volume. The clinical impact of these physiologic disturbances depends on the extent of sympathectomy as well as the patient's baseline cardiovascular status. The decrease in stroke volume is initially compensated by a reflexic increase in heart rate, which allows preservation of cardiac output and blood pressure. However, with mid to high thoracic epidural blocks, this compensatory reflex could be blunted and bradycardia may occur if the T1 to T4 levels (which give rise to the cardioaccelerator fibers) are anesthetized.

    C. Postdural (and arachnoid) puncture headache. Accidental dural (and arachnoid) puncture occurs in approximately 0.5% to 1% of cases. Female gender, young age, and large bore needle constitute risk factors to develop a spinal headache after inadvertent dural breach. Most measures used to prevent the occurrence of headache after proven dural puncture (e.g., bed rest, hydration, caffeine intake) are controversial at best. Treatment of postdural puncture headache can begin with conservative management (e.g., hydration, caffeine, as well as opioid and nonopioid analgesics). However, the most effective treatment remains an epidural autologous blood patch, a procedure whereby the patient's own blood (around 20 mL) is collected under sterile conditions and injected in the epidural space at a level contiguous to the one where dural puncture occurred.

    D. Total spinal anesthesia. Total spinal anesthesia usually occurs when an "epidural" dose of local anesthetic is administered in the intrathecal space following the accidental (and unrecognized) puncture of dural and arachnoid membranes. Manifestations include a denser sensorimotor block than expected, respiratory insufficiency, cardiovascular collapse, and loss of consciousness. The management of total spinal anesthesia requires control of the airway, mechanical ventilation, and hemodynamic support with vasopressors.

    E. Local anesthetic systemic toxicity. Local anesthetic systemic toxicity (LAST) usually results from the injection of local anesthetic inside an epidural vein. Test doses (i.e., 15 µg of epinephrine in 3 mL of local anesthetic) have contributed to decrease the occurrence of LAST. In addition to test doses, precautions such as aspiration and incremental local anesthetic injection should be used to minimize the occurrence of LAST. Management of LAST is covered in Chapter 14.

F. **Epidural hematoma.** Risk factors for epidural hematoma include female gender, advanced age, abnormal coagulation, spinal stenosis, and traumatic puncture. Total or partial recovery may be possible if decompression occurs within 8 to 12 hours of symptom onset. An epidural hematoma should be suspected when an epidural block lasts longer than usual, recurs after initial resolution, or involves myotomes/dermatomes inconsistent with the anticipated block level. Bladder or bowel dysfunction is usually a late finding. Urgent diagnostic imaging and surgical decompression are paramount. MRI differentiates soft tissues and identifies coexisting spinal canal pathology more effectively than computerized tomography (CT) scanning. However, in the absence of immediately available MRI, CT scans provide sufficient information for emergent surgical decompression.

G. **Neuraxial infection.** Epidural abscess and purulent meningitis have been reported after epidural blocks. Both may insidiously present several days after the initial block, with fever and back pain followed by rapid progression to neurologic impairment. Accurate diagnosis and treatment are paramount given the 15% mortality.

H. **Mechanical injury to the spinal cord and nerve roots.** Direct injury to the spinal cord or nerve roots by epidural needles or catheters can present with unilateral or bilateral symptoms, depending on the anatomic lesion. If the sole manifestation after suspected trauma is nonprogressive paresthesia, observant management suffices. However, widespread sensory and/or motor symptoms mandate urgent diagnostic imaging and neurologic consultation.

ACKNOWLEDGMENTS

The authors wish to acknowledge the contribution of Christopher M. Bernards, MD, who authored the chapter on epidural blocks in the previous edition.

REFERENCES

1. Pöpping DM, Elia N, Van Aken HK, et al. Impact of epidural analgesia on mortality and morbidity after surgery: systematic review and meta-analysis of randomized controlled trials. *Ann Surg* 2014;259:1056–1067.
2. Bromage PR. Identification of the epidural space. In: Bromage PR, ed. *Epidural Analgesia*. 1st ed. Philadelphia, PA: Saunders; 1978.
3. Tran DQH, Van Zundert TCRV, Aliste J, et al. Primary failure of thoracic epidural analgesia in training centers: the invisble elephant? *Reg Anesth Pain Med* 2016;41:309–313.
4. Hogan Q. Epidural anatomy catheter tip position and distribution of injectate evaluated by computed tomography. *Anesthesiology* 1999;90:964–970.
5. Todorov L, Vadeboncouer T. Etiology and use of the "hanging drop" technique: a review. *Pain Res Treat* 2014;2014:146750.
6. Lechner TJM, van Wijk MGF, Maas AJJ, et al. Thoracic epidural puncture guided by an acoustic signal: clinical results. *Eur J Anaesthesiol* 2004;21:694–699.
7. Tran DQH, González AP, Bernucci, F, et al. Confirmation of loss-of-resistance for epidural analgesia. *Reg Anesth Pain Med* 2015;40:166–173.
8. Antibas PL, do Nascimento Junior P, Braz LG, et al. Air versus saline in the loss of resistance technique for identification of the epidural space. *Cochrane Database Syst Rev* 2014;7:CD008938.
9. Larsson J, Gordh TE. Testing whether the epidural works: too time consuming? *Acta Anaesthesiol Scand* 2010;54:761–763.
10. Parra MC, Washburn K, Brown J, et al. Fluoroscopic guidance increases the incidence of thoracic epidural catheter placement within the epidural space: a randomized trial. *Reg Anesth Pain Med* 2017;42:17–24.
11. Auyong DB, Hostetter L, Yuan SC, et al. Evaluation of ultrasound-assisted thoracic epidural placement in patients undergoing upper abdominal and thoracic surgery. *Reg Anesth Pain Med* 2017;42:204–209.
12. Elgueta MF, Duong S, Finlayson RJ, et al. Ultrasonography for neuraxial blocks: a review of the evidence. *Minerva Anestesiol* 2017;83:512–523.

13. Leurcharusmee V, Arnuntasupakul A, Chora de la Garza D, et al. Reliability of waveform analysis as an adjunct to loss-of-resistance for thoracic épidural blocks. *Reg Anesth Pain Med* 2015;40:694–697.

14. Arnuntasupakul V, Van Zundert TCRV, Vijitpavan A, et al. A randomized comparison between conventional and waveform-confirmed loss-of-resistance for thoracic epidural blocks. *Reg Anesth Pain Med* 2016;41:368–373.

15. Tsui BCH, Sunil G, Finucane B. Confirmation of epidural catheter placement using nerve stimulation. *Can J Anesth* 1998;45:640–644.

8

Upper Extremity Blocks

De Q.H. Tran and Joseph M. Neal

I. Anatomy	**E.** Supplemental nerve blocks
II. Drugs	
III. Techniques	**IV.** Complications
A. Interscalene approach	**A.** Interscalene approach
B. Supraclavicular approach	**B.** Supraclavicular approach
C. Infraclavicular approach	**C.** Infraclavicular approach
D. Axillary approach	**D.** Axillary approach

KEY POINTS

1. For ambulatory surgery, compared to general anesthesia, brachial plexus blocks result in shorter discharge time, improved pain control, and fewer side effects (e.g., opioid-related nausea/vomiting, sore throat).

2. The combination of a long-lasting local anesthetic and proper adjuvant can provide analgesia for up to 24 hours. If acute postoperative pain is expected to exceed 24 hours, a continuous perineural catheter and local anesthetic infusion should be employed.

3. Knowledge of the brachial plexus anatomy and osseous innervation of the upper extremity will allow the operator to select the optimal approach for any type of surgical procedure.

4. The four main approaches to the brachial plexus are: interscalene, supraclavicular, infraclavicular, and axillary (1).

5. The interscalene or supraclavicular approaches should be used for shoulder and proximal humerus surgery.

6. The supraclavicular, infraclavicular, and axillary approaches can be used for elbow, forearm, and hand surgery. Selection between these three approaches depends on the patient's morphology (body mass index) and comorbidities (preexisting pulmonary compromise) as well as the operator's experience level.

7. Ultrasonography has supplanted neurostimulation as the preferred nerve localization technique for brachial plexus blocks (2).

8. Ultrasonography also allows the operator to selectively anesthetize individual nerves at distal locations (e.g., elbow, forearm, suprascapular fossa) in order to rescue failed brachial plexus blocks or to circumvent common side effects associated with traditional approaches (e.g., phrenic nerve block secondary to the interscalene approach).

I.   **Anatomy.** The anatomy of the brachial plexus (Fig. 8.1) may appear overwhelming. However, one need only remember some key facts:

    A.   **The brachial plexus can be divided into roots, trunks, divisions, cords, and terminal branches.** End branches can also originate from roots (dorsal scapular and long thoracic

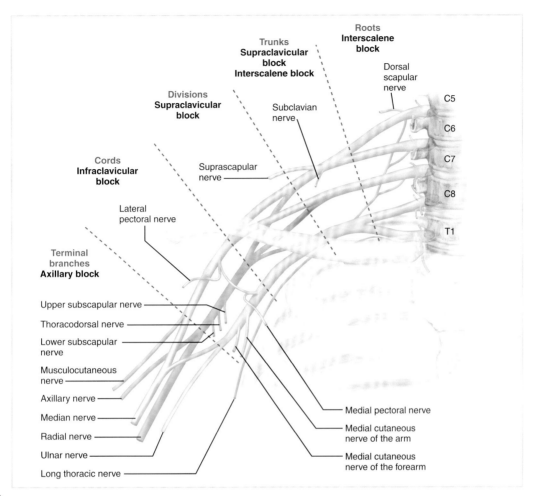

FIGURE 8.1   Anatomy of the brachial plexus. (Modified from Tank PW, Gest TR, Lippincott Williams & Wilkins Atlas of Anatomy, 2009.)

nerves), trunks (suprascapular and subclavian nerves), and cords (pectoral, subscapular, and thoracodorsal nerves).

B. **The interscalene, supraclavicular, infraclavicular, and axillary approaches anesthetize the brachial plexus at the level of its roots/trunks, trunks/divisions, cords, and terminal branches, respectively.**

C. **The suprascapular nerve originates from the superior trunk and supplies the posterior two-thirds of the shoulder joint as well as the acromioclavicular joint.** Thus, for shoulder surgery, it is important to block this nerve prior to its takeoff from the superior trunk. This is best achieved with an interscalene or supraclavicular approach.

D. **The subclavian nerve originates from the superior trunk and is responsible for most of the bony innervation of the clavicle.** Thus, for clavicular surgery, an interscalene or supraclavicular approach will anesthetize this nerve prior to its takeoff from the superior trunk.

E. **Cutaneous innervation of the shoulder and upper arm is separate from the brachial plexus and originates from the superficial plexus (supraclavicular nerves) and the intercostobrachial nerve.**

CLINICAL PEARL   In the literature, the term "approach" refers to the site where the brachial plexus is accessed (i.e., interscalene, supraclavicular, infraclavicular, or axillary). The term "technique" refers to the modality (e.g., neurostimulation, ultrasonography) or endpoints (e.g., single vs. multiple injections) used for a given approach.

3

CLINICAL PEARL   Although one can be tempted to select nerve blocks based on the cutaneous innervation of the surgical site, knowledge of its osseous innervation (Fig. 8.2) is far more important, because the most severe pain originates from periosteal trauma.

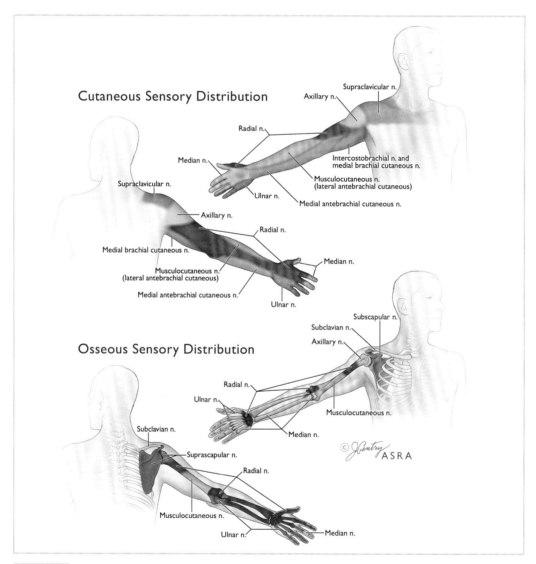

FIGURE 8.2   Osseous innervation of the upper limb. (Image Copyright 2017 American Society of Regional Anesthesia and Pain Medicine. Used with permission. All rights reserved.)

   II. Drugs. In order to select the optimal local anesthetic agent, the operator must decide whether the aim is postoperative analgesia (in the context of concomitant general anesthesia) or surgical anesthesia (Table 8.1).

TABLE 8.1   Recommended doses of local anesthetics and adjuvants

Purpose	Local anesthetic	Volume/Rate	Adjuvant
Postoperative analgesia (single-shot block)	Bupivacaine 0.25% *or* Ropivacaine 0.375% or 0.5%	Interscalene approach: 10–20 mL Supraclavicular, infraclavicular, or axillary approach: 30–35 mL	Epinephrine (2.5–5.0 µg/mL) ± Dexamethasone (4 mg)
Postoperative analgesia (continuous block)	Bupivacaine 0.125% *or* Ropivacaine 0.2%	6–10 mL/h *or* 6 mL/h with 4 mL each 30 min PRN	
Surgical anesthesia (single-shot block)	Lidocaine 1%–bupivacaine 0.25% (obtained by mixing equal parts of lidocaine 2% and bupivacaine 0.5%) *or* Mepivacaine 1.25%–1.5% *or* Bupivacaine 0.5% *or* Ropivacaine 0.75%	Interscalene approach: 10–20 mL Supraclavicular, infraclavicular, or axillary approach: 30–35 mL	Epinephrine (2.5–5.0 µg/mL) ± Dexamethasone (4 mg)
Surgical anesthesia (in the presence of a continuous perineural catheter)	Lidocaine 1.25%–1.5% *or* Mepivacaine 1.25%–1.5%	Interscalene approach: 10–20 mL Supraclavicular, infraclavicular, or axillary approach: 30–35 mL	Epinephrine (2.5–5.0 µg/mL)

Independently of the local anesthetic selected, maximal recommended doses should be respected (cf Chapter 5).

If the goal is to maximize postoperative analgesia, block duration should be the overriding concern. Thus, long-acting agents (such as bupivacaine or ropivacaine) should be selected. Moreover, adjuvants can prolong the duration of brachial plexus blocks. Epinephrine is useful as an intravascular injection marker and for increasing the duration of action of intermediate local anesthetic agents. Clonidine provides similar intermediate prolongation as epinephrine, but is associated with increased costs and potential side effects (hypotension, sedation) (3). Dexmedetomidine is effective with long-acting agents, but can be prohibitively expensive. Despite dexamethasone's popularity, the optimal administration route (intravenous vs. perineural) remains controversial (4,5). Perineural dexamethasone has not received official FDA approval, and its use remains off-label for now. Moreover, dexamethasone may have a potential for neural toxicity in diabetic patients. In-depth discussion of adjuvants can be found in Chapter 5.

If the operator wishes to achieve surgical anesthesia, three options exist. Firstly, the brachial plexus block is performed with bupivacaine 0.5% or ropivacaine 0.75% at least 45 to 60 minutes before surgery to provide sufficient "soak time." This strategy requires an induction room and efficient planning. Secondly, the brachial plexus block is performed with lidocaine or mepivacaine (1.25% to 1.5%), thereby ensuring a swift onset, and a perineural catheter is inserted. Postoperatively, the latter is injected with bupivacaine/ropivacaine prior to removal (if additional analgesia is required) or transitioned to a continuous local anesthetic infusion. Albeit the most versatile, this strategy requires increased technical skills, performance time, and equipment costs. Finally, a mix of lidocaine and bupivacaine/ropivacaine is employed. Although the mix may not have the swift onset of pure lidocaine or the long duration of bupivacaine/ropivacaine, its simplicity makes it attractive.

2   **CLINICAL PEARL**   **The combination of a long-lasting local anesthetic and proper adjuvant can provide analgesia for up to 24 hours.** If acute postoperative pain is expected to exceed 24 hours, the operator should consider using a continuous perineural catheter and local anesthetic infusion.

CLINICAL PEARL   Orthopedists may need to confirm neural integrity after certain surgical procedures (e.g., axillary nerve after shoulder surgery, radial nerve after proximal humerus surgery, radial nerve after distal bicipital tendon repair, ulnar nerve after elbow surgery). In such instances, consideration should be given to performing the brachial plexus block after the postoperative sensorimotor exam. Alternately, a perineural catheter can be inserted preoperatively, but not bolused until after postoperative neurologic assessment.

III. Techniques

    A. Interscalene approach

        1. Indication

           a. Shoulder and proximal humerus surgery

        2. Contraindications

           a. Usual contraindications to peripheral nerve blocks (i.e., lack of consent, local infection at the injection site, allergy to local anesthetic agent).

           b. Patients with preexisting obstructive or restrictive pulmonary pathology who are unable to withstand up to 30% reduction in pulmonary function consequent to ipsilateral phrenic nerve block/hemidiaphragmatic paralysis. In general, such patients have severe chronic obstructive pulmonary disease (COPD) and may be on home oxygen therapy.

CLINICAL PEARL   With ultrasound guidance, coagulopathy no longer constitutes an absolute contraindication to brachial plexus blocks. Nonetheless, the prudent operator should select approaches with easily discernible and compressible vascular structures (e.g., interscalene or axillary approaches).

CLINICAL PEARL   Various maneuvers have been tried to prevent hemidiaphragmatic paralysis with interscalene blocks: proximal digital pressure (to minimize cephalad spread of local anesthetic), low injectate volume (5 mL), injection of the local anesthetic in the middle scalene muscle away from the brachial plexus. To date, no strategy can reliably circumvent the occurrence of phrenic nerve block.

        3. Single injection technique. The patient is placed in a supine or semi-sitting position with the head turned toward the contralateral side. An ultrasound-guided traceback technique (starting from the supraclavicular fossa) is commonly used. The supraclavicular area is first scanned to locate the subclavian artery. The brachial plexus (cluster of trunks and divisions) can be found superolateral to the artery. Subsequently, the plexus is traced cephalad toward the cricoid cartilage until it becomes a column of hypoechoic nodules (roots/trunks) (Figs. 8.3 and 8.4). Using an in-plane technique and a lateral-to-medial direction, the subcutaneous tissues are infiltrated with local anesthesia. A 5-cm, short-beveled block needle is then inserted. The target for this block is situated under the paraneurium, between the first and second hypoechoic nodules. Alternately, the operator can elect to deposit local anesthetic outside the paraneurium, between the middle scalene muscle and the brachial plexus. Extraparaneural injection will not affect the success rate, but the block will have a slightly shorter duration (6). A volume of 10 to 20 mL of local anesthetic is commonly used.

The operator should refrain from injecting local anesthetic between the second and third hypoechoic nodules. In many instances, the latter do not represent middle/inferior trunks or C6/C7 roots but two divisions of the same C6 nerve root. Thus, deposition of local anesthetic between them may equate to intraneural injection, which could lead to neural injury and/or promote local anesthetic spread toward the neuraxis (7).

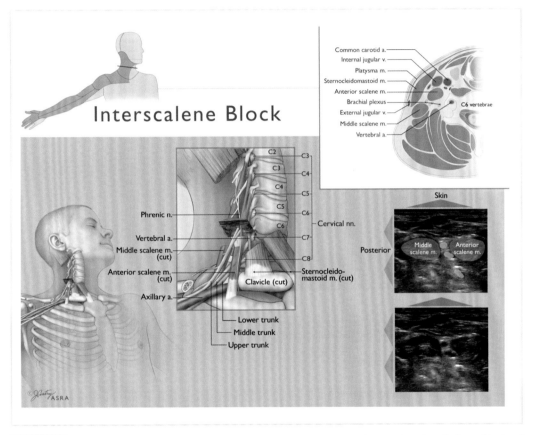

FIGURE 8.3 Overview of the interscalene brachial plexus block. (Image Copyright 2017 American Society of Regional Anesthesia and Pain Medicine. Used with permission. All rights reserved.)

4. **Continuous technique.** The sonographic target for continuous interscalene block is identical to the one used for its single-shot counterpart. As a general rule, advancement of any perineural catheter beyond the needle tip should be followed in real time with ultrasonography. An assistant may be required, because a third hand is required to stabilize the transducer while the operator feeds the catheter through the needle. The final position of the catheter tip should be confirmed sonographically with the injection of a 1 to 2 mL of local anesthetic, normal saline, or air. In-depth discussion of perineural catheters can be found in Chapter 2.

CLINICAL PEARL   The optimal length of catheter that needs to be advanced beyond the needle tip remains controversial. On the one hand, a short distance (1 cm) ensures almost identical positions of the needle and catheter tips next to the nerve, but may predispose to premature catheter dislodgement. On the other hand, a greater distance (4 to 5 cm) ensures stability by coiling and anchoring the catheter next to the nerve. However, one runs the risk of "overthreading" the catheter tip away from the sonographic target. Regardless of the length of catheter inserted beyond the needle tip, the final position of the catheter tip should always be verified by ultrasound to ensure continued nerve–catheter proximity.

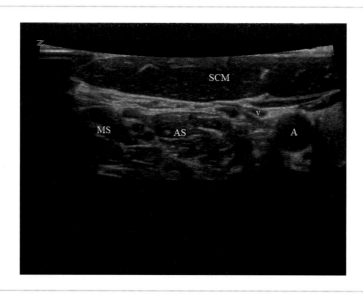

FIGURE 8.4   Sonographic appearance of the interscalene brachial plexus. A, carotid artery; AS, anterior scalene muscle; MS, middle scalene muscle; SCM, sternocleidomastoid muscle; V, internal jugular vein. (Reproduced from Kaye AD, Urman RD, Vadivelu N, eds. *Essentials of Regional Anesthesia.* 1st ed, "Upper Extremity Nerve Blocks." New York: Springer; 2012:346; with permission of Springer.)

B. **Supraclavicular approach**

5
1. **Indication**
   a. The supraclavicular approach is extremely versatile and can be used for surgery of the entire upper limb.

6
2. **Contraindications**
   a. Usual contraindications to peripheral nerve blocks (*vide supra*).
   b. Patients with preexisting obstructive or restrictive pulmonary pathology who are unable to withstand up to 30% reduction in pulmonary function consequent to ipsilateral phrenic nerve block/hemidiaphragmatic paralysis. In general, such patients have severe COPD and may be on home oxygen therapy.
      Compared to their interscalene counterparts, supraclavicular blocks are less prone to incidental phrenic nerve block, but the risk remains significant, particularly when higher volumes are used.

3. **Single injection technique.** The patient is positioned in a supine or semi-sitting position with the head turned toward the contralateral side. Using a high-frequency transducer, the supraclavicular area is scanned to identify a short-axis view of the subclavian artery. It is

crucial to visualize the first rib underneath the subclavian artery: it serves as a backstop and prevents pleural breach. The first rib is identified by the acoustic drop-out consequent to dense bone; in contrast, the pleura, which is less dense, results in a hyperechoic shimmering image. Superolateral to the artery, collections of neural clusters (trunks/divisions) can be seen.

A "targeted intracluster injection" technique can be used (8). The operator identifies the main (largest) cluster. The latter is usually flanked by two to three satellite (smaller) clusters (Figs. 8.5 and 8.6). The subcutaneous tissues are infiltrated with local anesthesia. Using an in-plane technique and a lateral-to-medial direction, a 5-cm, short-beveled block needle is first directed toward the main cluster. Half the volume of local anesthetic is injected in this location. The remaining half is divided in equal aliquots and injected inside each satellite cluster. A total volume of 30 to 35 mL of local anesthetic is commonly used.

Because of its multiple targets, the "targeted intracluster injection" method constitutes an advanced technique. Less experienced operators may prefer a simplified version whereby half the volume of local anesthetic is injected inside the main (largest) neural cluster and the remaining half deposited at the "corner pocket" (i.e., intersection of the first rib and subclavian artery). Because the satellite neural clusters are not directly targeted, the onset time will be somewhat slower.

CLINICAL PEARL   Needle penetration of neural clusters can be controversial. Although some authors equate it to transfixing epineurium, recent evidence suggests that a paraneural sheath surrounds the neural clusters. Thus, intracluster (i.e., subparaneural) and intraneural (i.e., subepineural) injections are not necessarily synonymous.

CLINICAL PEARL   If shoulder or clavicle surgery is carried out solely with interscalene or supraclavicular nerve blocks, brachial plexus blocks should be combined with superficial (or intermediate) cervical plexus blocks to anesthetize the supraclavicular nerves (C3–C4) that innervate the skin overlying the "cape" region of the shoulder. Superficial and intermediate cervical plexus blocks provide coverage for skin incision/closure and are easily performed with ultrasound guidance or simple subcutaneous infiltration along the posterior border of the sternocleidomastoid muscle between the mastoid and the clavicle (Chapter 13).

4. **Continuous technique.** The sonographic target for continuous supraclavicular block is the "corner pocket." Standard steps for perineural catheter insertion should be used (*vide supra*). In-depth discussion of perineural catheters can be found in Chapter 2.

C. **Infraclavicular approach**

1. **Indication**
   a. Elbow, forearm, and hand surgery

2. **Contraindications**
   a. Usual contraindications to peripheral nerve blocks (*vide supra*).

3. **Single injection technique.** The patient is positioned supine. The arm is flexed so that the forearm and hand can rest comfortably on the torso. A high-frequency ultrasound transducer is placed in the infraclavicular fossa, medial to the coracoid process, to obtain a short-axis view of the axillary vessels. The second part of the axillary artery and axillary vein can be found under the pectoralis major and minor muscles. The pleura can sometimes be seen under the vessels: when observed, the transducer should be moved lateral to avoid

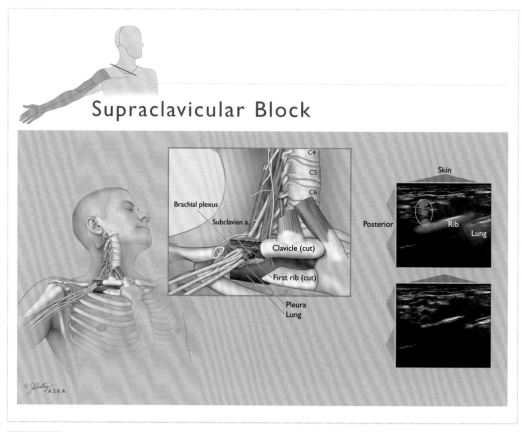

FIGURE 8.5 Overview of the supraclavicular brachial plexus block. (Image Copyright 2017 American Society of Regional Anesthesia and Pain Medicine. Used with permission. All rights reserved.)

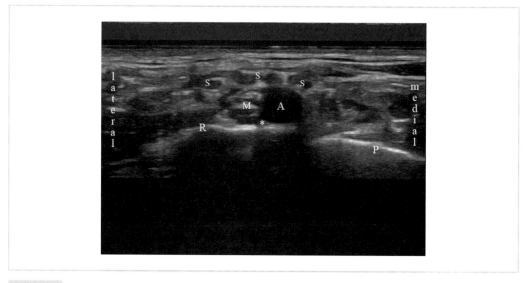

FIGURE 8.6 Sonographic appearance of the supraclavicular brachial plexus. A, subclavian artery; M, main neural cluster; R, first rib; P, pleura; S, satellite neural cluster; *, "corner pocket." (Adapted from Kaye AD, Urman RD, Vadivelu N, eds. *Essentials of Regional Anesthesia*. 1st ed, "Upper Extremity Nerve Blocks." New York: Springer; 2012:351; with permission of Springer.)

it (Figs. 8.7 and 8.8). The subcutaneous tissues are infiltrated with local anesthesia. Using an in-plane technique and a cephalad-to-caudad direction, a 10-cm, short-beveled block needle is advanced until the tip lies just dorsal to the artery (6 o'clock position) (9). Usually, a pop can be felt just before the needle assumes the correct position. Thirty to thirty-five milliliters of local anesthetic agent is administered. With local anesthetic injection, the artery will be gently pushed ventrally. If the artery fails to rise, the needle tip may be too dorsal in relation to the artery; thus, it should be repositioned to lie immediately adjacent to the latter.

CLINICAL PEARL   Occasionally, two arteries can be identified side by side. In such a situation, another approach should be selected to ensure singularity of the target and to avoid vascular puncture.

CLINICAL PEARL   In patients with elevated body mass indices, shoulder abduction (or raising the arm above the shoulder) will decrease the depth of the axillary artery and facilitate the performance of the infraclavicular block.

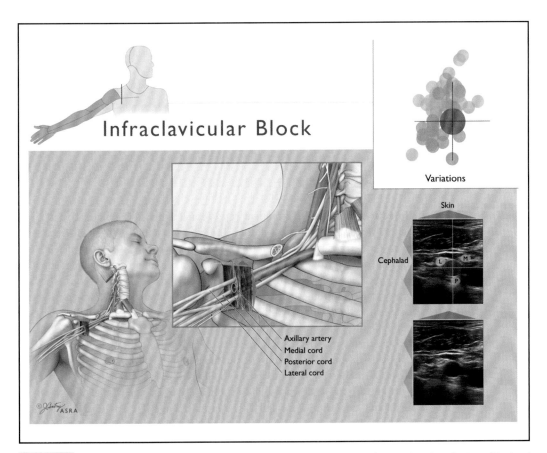

FIGURE 8.7   Overview of the infraclavicular brachial plexus block. (Image Copyright 2017 American Society of Regional Anesthesia and Pain Medicine. Used with permission. All rights reserved.)

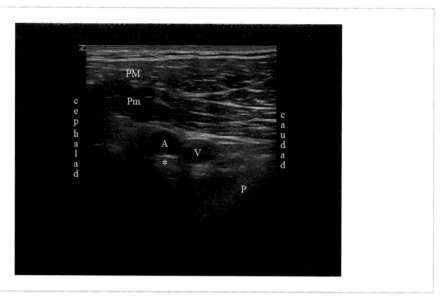

FIGURE 8.8 Sonographic appearance of the infraclavicular brachial plexus. A, axillary artery; P, pleura; PM, pectoralis major muscle; Pm, pectoralis minor muscle; V, axillary vein; *, target. (Reproduced from Kaye AD, Urman RD, Vadivelu N, eds. *Essentials of Regional Anesthesia.* 1st ed, "Upper Extremity Nerve Blocks." New York: Springer; 2012:354; with permission of Springer.)

4. **Continuous technique.** The sonographic target for continuous infraclavicular block is the 6 o'clock position of the axillary artery. Standard steps for perineural catheter insertion should be used (*vide supra*). In-depth discussion of perineural catheters can be found in Chapter 2.

D. **Axillary approach**

1. **Indication**
   a. Forearm and hand surgery

2. **Contraindications**
   a. Usual contraindications to peripheral nerve blocks (*vide supra*)

3. **Single injection technique.** The patient is positioned with the shoulder abducted (no more than 90 degrees) and the elbow flexed. The axilla is scanned with a high-frequency, linear ultrasound transducer to identify a short-axis view of the axillary artery. The musculocutaneous nerve, a hyperechoic structure, can be found anterior and lateral to the artery (Figs. 8.9 and 8.10). Using an in-plane technique, the subcutaneous tissues are infiltrated with local anesthesia. A 5-cm, short-beveled block needle is then inserted. The needle is first directed toward the musculocutaneous nerve. Six milliliters of local anesthetic is deposited near the nerve (within the fascial plane between the biceps and the coracobrachialis muscles). Subsequently, the needle is redirected toward the six o'clock position of the axillary artery. If the needle tip is correctly positioned inside the neurovascular sheath, injection of a few milliliters will result in a "silhouette sign" (blurring of the arterial wall because of the contiguity of anechoic blood and anechoic local anesthetic). If a "silhouette sign" fails to form, the needle tip may be too dorsal in relation to the vessel (i.e., deep to the conjoint tendon); thus, it should be repositioned to lie immediately adjacent to the axillary artery. Twenty-four milliliters of local anesthetic is then injected. This typically results in the axillary artery being surrounded by local anesthetic (donut sign).

CLINICAL PEARL   Although some authors prefer a "perineural" technique (whereby the musculocutaneous, median, radial, and ulnar nerves are painstakingly identified and individually injected with local anesthetic), the latter offers no real benefits compared to the previously described "perivascular" technique for axillary blocks (10).

CLINICAL PEARL   In some patients, the musculocutaneous nerve cannot be visualized in its usual position, because it travels together with the median/radial/ulnar nerves inside the neurovascular bundle. In such cases, the entire volume of local anesthetic (30 mL) is injected at the 6 o'clock position of the axillary artery after obtaining a "silhouette sign."

4. **Continuous technique.** The sonographic target for continuous axillary block is the 6 o'clock position of the axillary artery. Standard steps for perineural catheter insertion should be used (*vide supra*). In-depth discussion of perineural catheters can be found in Chapter 2.

CLINICAL PEARL   Because of the increased risk of dislodgement (as a result of sweating and hair), axillary perineural catheters are seldom used. Supraclavicular or infraclavicular catheters provide similar efficacy coupled with increased stability.

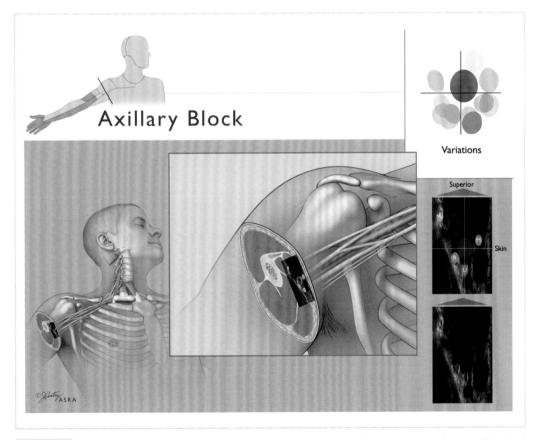

FIGURE 8.9   Overview of the axillary brachial plexus block. (Image Copyright 2017 American Society of Regional Anesthesia and Pain Medicine. Used with permission. All rights reserved.)

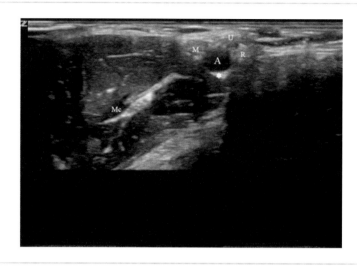

FIGURE 8.10 Sonographic appearance of the axillary brachial plexus. A, axillary artery; M, median nerve; Mc, musculocutaneous nerve; R, radial nerve; U, ulnar nerve; *, target for perivascular injection. (Adapted from Kaye AD, Urman RD, Vadivelu N, eds. *Essentials of Regional Anesthesia.* 1st ed, "Upper Extremity Nerve Blocks." New York: Springer; 2012:357; with permission of Springer.)

E. Supplemental nerve blocks

1. **Suprascapular nerve block.** The patient is positioned in the lateral decubitus position, with the side to be blocked uppermost. Using a high-frequency, linear ultrasound transducer, the area cephalad to the scapular spine is scanned to identify the suprascapular fossa (Fig. 8.11). The subcutaneous tissues are infiltrated with local anesthesia. Using an out-of-plane technique, a 10-cm, short-beveled block needle is advanced toward the suprascapular fossa. After bony contact, a volume of 10 mL of local anesthetics is deposited in the latter.

> **CLINICAL PEARL** Patients afflicted with severe pulmonary pathology and requiring shoulder surgery constitute a classic regional anesthesia dilemma. Parenteral opioids interfere with breathing. Subacromial local anesthetic injection provides limited pain control and is associated with local anesthetic-induced chondrolysis. Two strategies can be used to circumvent interscalene block. Targeted axillary *nerve* blocks and suprascapular nerve blocks can be combined to anesthetize the anterior and posterior shoulder, respectively (11). Unfortunately, this strategy does not allow the insertion of perineural catheters. Furthermore, surgical procedures like rotator cuff repair and proximal humeral fracture repair also involve territories innervated by the subscapular and radial nerves, respectively. Expectedly, these nerves will not be anesthetized with axillary–suprascapular nerve blocks. Alternately, suprascapular nerve blocks can be combined with the infraclavicular approach. The latter enables perineural catheter insertion. More importantly, it anesthetizes the posterior cord, thus providing coverage for both axillary and radial nerves (Fig. 8.1).

2. **Radial and median nerve at the elbow.** The patient is positioned supine with the upper extremity abducted. At the level of the elbow crease, a high-frequency, linear ultrasound transducer is used. The radial nerve appears as a hyperechoic crescent (Fig. 8.12). The median nerve is located medial to the brachial artery (Fig. 8.13). Using an in-plane technique, a 5-cm, short-beveled block needle is advanced toward the two nerves. A volume of 5 to 7 mL of local anesthetic is deposited around each nerve. If the median nerve cannot be visualized, a perivascular injection can be carried out medial to the brachial artery.

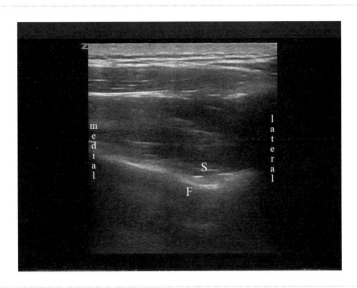

FIGURE 8.11 Suprascapular nerve in the suprascapular fossa. F, suprascapular fossa; S, fascia of the supraspinatus muscle. (Reproduced from Kaye AD, Urman RD, Vadivelu N, eds. *Essentials of Regional Anesthesia*. 1st ed, "Upper Extremity Nerve Blocks." New York: Springer; 2012:362; with permission of Springer.)

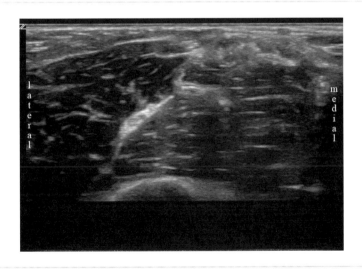

FIGURE 8.12 Sonographic appearance of the radial nerve at the elbow. (Reproduced from Kaye AD, Urman RD, Vadivelu N, eds. *Essentials of Regional Anesthesia*. 1st ed, "Upper Extremity Nerve Blocks." New York: Springer; 2012:365; with permission of Springer.)

3. **Ulnar nerve.** The patient is positioned supine. The elbow is flexed and the forearm internally rotated so that its radial aspect rests comfortably on the torso. A high-frequency, linear ultrasound transducer is used to scan the proximal forearm. The ulnar nerve appears as a hyperechoic structure (Fig. 8.14). Using an in-plane technique, a 5-cm, short-beveled block needle is advanced toward the nerve. A volume of 5 to 7 mL of local anesthetic is deposited around the nerve.

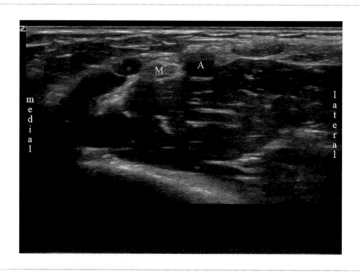

FIGURE 8.13 Sonographic appearance of the median nerve at the elbow. A, brachial artery; M, median nerve. (Reproduced from Kaye AD, Urman RD, Vadivelu N, eds. *Essentials of Regional Anesthesia.* 1st ed, "Upper Extremity Nerve Blocks." New York: Springer; 2012:366; with permission of Springer.)

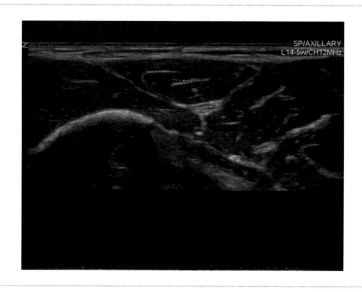

FIGURE 8.14 Sonographic appearance of the ulnar nerve at the elbow. (Reproduced from Kaye AD, Urman RD, Vadivelu N, eds. *Essentials of Regional Anesthesia.* 1st ed, "Upper Extremity Nerve Blocks." New York: Springer; 2012:367; with permission of Springer.)

CLINICAL PEARL   The median, radial, and ulnar can also be anesthetized in the distal forearm. However, the presence of a cast often limits access to this location. Furthermore, this approach does not provide anesthesia for upper arm or forearm tourniquets.

CLINICAL PEARL   Although most textbooks advocate supplemental intercostobrachial nerve block to ensure tourniquet tolerance, this step is seldom necessary. The intercostobrachial nerve provides cutaneous innervation to the medial aspect of the arm. However, tourniquet pain stems from muscular and not skin compression. The biceps and triceps muscles are innervated by the musculocutaneous and radial nerve, respectively, and can be readily anesthetized with all four approaches to the brachial plexus.

CLINICAL PEARL   For superficial surgical procedures of the forearm (e.g., creation of arteriovenous fistula), anesthesia can be achieved with combined lateral and medial antebrachial cutaneous nerve blocks. This strategy would avoid the inherent motor block associated with supraclavicular, infraclavicular, or axillary approaches to the brachial plexus.

IV. Complications. A detailed consideration of block complications can be found in Chapter 14. Complications specific to brachial plexus blocks are listed below.

   A. **Interscalene approach.** Vascular puncture, neuraxial injection, recurrent laryngeal nerve paralysis, and Horner syndrome can occur after interscalene blocks. Inadvertent local anesthetic injection into the carotid (or vertebral) artery will result in central nervous system toxicity with a very low volume. Because of the risk of phrenic nerve block, the interscalene approach should be avoided in patients with pulmonary compromise who cannot withstand a potential 30% reduction in vital capacity and/or forced expiratory volume over 1 second (FEV_1).

   B. **Supraclavicular approach.** Vascular puncture, pneumothorax, recurrent laryngeal nerve paralysis, and Horner syndrome can occur after supraclavicular blocks. Because of the risk of phrenic nerve block, the supraclavicular approach should be avoided in patients with pulmonary compromise who cannot withstand a potential 30% reduction in vital capacity and/or FEV_1.

   C. **Infraclavicular approach.** Vascular puncture can occur. Phrenic paralysis occurs in a minority of patients. There have been anecdotal reports of Horner syndrome and pneumothorax associated with infraclavicular blocks.

   D. **Axillary approach.** Vascular puncture, intravascular injection, bruising, and soreness at the injection site have been reported, but the overall safety margin is very high.

ACKNOWLEDGMENTS

The authors wish to acknowledge the contributions of Susan B. McDonald, MD, who authored the upper extremity block chapters in the previous edition.

REFERENCES

1. Neal JM, Gerancher JC, Hebl JR, et al. Upper extremity regional anesthesia: essentials of our current understanding, 2008. *Reg Anesth Pain Med* 2009;34:134–170.
2. Neal JM, Brull R, Horn JL, et al. The second American Society of Regional Anesthesia and Pain Medicine evidence-based medicine assessment of ultrasound-guided regional anesthesia: executive summary. *Reg Anesth Pain Med* 2016;41:181–194.
3. Popping DM, Ella N, Marret E, et al. Clonidine as an adjuvant to local anesthetics for peripheral nerve and plexus blocks: a meta-analysis of randomized trials. *Anesthesiology* 2009;111:406–415.

4. Albrecht E, Kern C, Kirkham KR. A systematic review and meta-analysis of dexamethasone for peripheral nerve blocks. *Anaesth* 2015;70:71–83.

5. Leurcharusmee P, Aliste J, Van Zundert TCRV, et al. A multicenter randomized comparison between intravenous and perineural dexamethasone for ultrasound-guided infraclavicular block. *Reg Anesth Pain Med* 2016;41:328–333.

6. Spence BC, Beach ML, Gallagher JD, et al. Ultrasound-guided interscalene blocks: understanding where to inject the local anesthetic. *Anaesth* 2011;66:509–514.

7. Franco CD, Williams JM. Ultrasound-guided interscalene block. Reevaluation of the "stoplight" sign and clinical implications. *Reg Anesth Pain Med* 2016;41:452–459.

8. Techasuk W, González AP, Bernucci F, et al. A randomized comparison between double-injection and targeted intracluster-injection for ultrasound-guided supraclavicular brachial plexus block. *Anesth Analg* 2014;118:1363–1369.

9. Desgagnés MC, Levesque S, Dion S, et al. A comparison of a single or triple injection technique for ultrasound-guided infraclavicular block: a prospective randomized controlled study. *Anesth Analg* 2009;109:668–672.

10. Bernucci F, González F, Finlayson RJ, et al. A prospective randomized comparison between perivascular and perineural ultrasound-guided axillary brachial plexus block. *Reg Anesth Pain Med* 2012;37:473–477.

11. Price DJ. The shoulder block: a new alternative to interscalene brachial plexus blockade for the control of postoperative shoulder pain. *Anaesth Intens Care* 2007;35:575–581.

9 Intravenous Regional Anesthesia

Joseph M. Neal and Susan B. McDonald

I. Anatomy
 A. Venous plexi of the extremities
 B. Mechanism of action
II. Drugs
 A. Local anesthetics
 B. Additives
III. Technique
 A. Indications
 B. Contraindications

C. Preparation for block
D. Cuff inflation
E. Injection of local anesthetic solution
F. Cuff deflation
IV. Complications
 A. LAST is the major risk of IVRA
 B. Other side effects of IVRA

KEY POINTS

1. The use of IVRA has lessened as anesthesiologists have become more proficient with peripheral nerve blocks, which provide denser anesthesia and the potential for prolonged analgesia.

2. Lidocaine 0.5% is used most commonly for IVRA and has distinct safety advantages over other local anesthetics.

3. Ketorolac is the most effective adjuvant drug in terms of improved anesthesia, prolonged analgesia, tourniquet tolerance, and cost.

4. Intravenous regional anesthesia (IVRA) is a simple technique for quick operations that involve the distal upper or lower extremity.

5. Single- and double-cuff pneumatic tourniquets have specific roles in IVRA. In select cases, forearm or ankle/calf tourniquets are advantageous.

6. Careful attention to tourniquet integrity, slow injection of local anesthetic into a distal vein, and immediate availability of resuscitation equipment lessen the risk of local anesthetic systemic toxicity.

1 **INTRAVENOUS REGIONAL ANESTHESIA (IVRA)** of the extremities is one of the simplest and oldest regional anesthetic techniques available, but requires understanding of peripheral venous anatomy, local anesthetic pharmacology, and physiology to ensure safe and effective anesthesia. Introduced in 1908 by August Bier, the eponymous *Bier block* was initially a surgical technique that required exposure of the veins. Subsequent development of the intravenous cannula and pneumatic tourniquet enabled modern IVRA techniques, which for years were the mainstay of extremity regional anesthesia in many operating suites. The growth of ultrasound-guided regional anesthesia and peripheral nerve blocks has lessened the role of IVRA in contemporary anesthetic practice.

I. Anatomy

A. **Venous plexi of the extremities.** The peripheral nerves of the extremities are nourished by small arteries, the vasa nervorum. Metabolic by-products are cleared via venules, which flow into the extremity's venous plexus. Injection of sufficient volume of local anesthetic into the venous plexus leads to retrograde diffusion of drug into the nerve's microcirculation and thereby produces anesthesia. Sufficient volume is attained by using a proximal pneumatic tourniquet to prevent egress of local anesthetic into the systemic circulation.

B. **Mechanism of action. Surgical anesthesia is produced by several complimentary mechanisms.** Diffusion of local anesthetic to small peripheral nerves throughout the extremity constitutes the initial effect of IVRA. The main anesthetic effect results from conduction blockade of larger nerves at more proximal sites. Tourniquet-induced ischemia and direct nerve compression further impede nerve conduction (1).

II. Drugs

A. Local anesthetics

1. **Lidocaine** is the most commonly used drug and has a long safety record. Because large volumes are necessary to distend the venous plexus, lidocaine 0.5% is used in volumes of 50 mL for the upper extremity or 100 mL for the lower extremity. These volumes can be reduced to 30 mL or 50 mL when forearm or calf tourniquets, respectively, are used. In children or small adults, volumes should be reduced on the basis of a dose of 3 mg/kg lidocaine. A separate priming dose of intravenous lidocaine 1 mg/kg administered minutes before IVRA institution reduces tourniquet pain (2).

2. **Bupivacaine** has been used for IVRA, but is not recommended because of significant concern for local anesthetic systemic toxicity (LAST) in the event of tourniquet failure or early release. Although ropivacaine has also been used (3), similar concerns remain for those patients at higher risk for LAST. Such patients include those at the extremes of age, with small muscle mass, or with cardiac disease (4).

3. Despite rapid clearance, 2-chloroprocaine has been associated with LAST and phlebitis (5).

B. Additives

1. Numerous studies have evaluated local anesthetic additives to improve IVRA anesthesia, analgesia, and tourniquet tolerance. Evidence supports nonsteroidal anti-inflammatory drugs (NSAIDs), clonidine, and dexmedetomidine. Other additives, including opioids, muscle relaxants, magnesium, neostigmine, dexamethasone, and tramadol, have relatively limited clinical benefit and/or are associated with unwanted side effects (6).

2. **Nonsteroidal anti-inflammatory drugs**
   a. Presumably through a peripheral site mechanism of action, NSAIDs mixed with local anesthetic for IVRA improve block quality and tourniquet tolerance.
   b. **Ketorolac 20 mg** added to lidocaine for upper extremity surgery reduces the need for rescue analgesics in the post-anesthesia recovery unit (6).

3. **α_2-Agonists**
   a. **Clonidine 1 μg/kg** improves postoperative analgesia and prolongs tourniquet tolerance (7).
   b. **Dexmedetomidine 0.5 μg/kg** improves the quality of perioperative analgesia when added to lidocaine, with minimal side effects (8).
   c. Both α_2-agonists are more expensive than ketorolac.

4. **Muscle relaxants**
   a. Nondepolarizing agents can provide muscle relaxation that can assist with fracture reduction, but may risk airway compromise in the case of tourniquet failure or residual systemic effects (6).

III. **Technique**

A. **Indications**

1. The primary advantages of IVRA are its simplicity and reliability. It is **the easiest and most effective block of the distal upper extremity for simple,** quick procedures, and it is therefore well suited for novices and for ambulatory surgery.

2. IVRA is suitable for many operations on the distal extremities when **a proximal occlusive tourniquet** can be applied safely.

   a. The block is used primarily in the arm. An upper-arm single- or double-cuff pneumatic tourniquet is used commonly. A forearm tourniquet allows reduction of local anesthetic dose and is advocated for rescue when upper-arm tourniquet pain ensues.

   b. In the leg, larger volumes of local anesthetic are required and adequate occlusion of vessels is harder to attain because of thicker muscles and the thigh's irregular shape. Alternatively, a calf or ankle tourniquet facilitates reduction of local anesthetic dose. Compared with the arm, the leg's large-capacity intraosseous channels lead to concern regarding local anesthetic leakage into the systemic circulation and consequent risk for LAST.

3. **A variety of minor surgical procedures are amenable to IVRA, including foreign body extraction, laceration repair, and tendon, nerve, or ligament procedures**.

4. Although periosteal anesthesia is not as dense as that achieved with peripheral nerve blocks, IVRA is used successfully for bunionectomy or simple fracture reduction.

5. Rapid functional recovery of the extremity is an advantage.

B. **Contraindications**

1. Ischemic vascular disease, which contraindicates vascular occlusion with a tourniquet

2. Pneumatic tourniquet use in sickle cell anemia may induce localized stasis of blood flow, hypoxemia, and acidosis and induce formation of sickle cells in the involved extremity.

3. Some surgeons may be dissatisfied with the amount of fluid exuded into the surgical field (especially if performing microscopic procedures).

4. **Surgical length must reliably fit within a relatively short duration of approximately 20 to 60 minutes**.

5. Because **postoperative analgesia is limited** when using IVRA, other regional block techniques are recommended for extended analgesia.

C. **Preparation for block**

1. The patient is placed in the supine position, and standard American Society of Anesthesiologists (ASA) monitors are placed. The systolic blood pressure obtained in the contralateral arm will guide **pneumatic tourniquet settings**. Intravenous (IV) access is established in another extremity.

2. A **small-gauge IV catheter** is inserted distally in the hand or foot to be operated on in a position where it will not be dislodged by the Esmarch bandage used for exsanguination.

Distal IV catheter placement, rather than in the antecubital fossa, is associated with less local anesthetic leakage under the cuff (9). The catheter is taped loosely in place and a small syringe or injection cap is fitted over it after a dilute heparin or saline flush is used to clear the lumen.

D. Cuff inflation

1. The pneumatic tourniquet is placed securely on the proximal part of the extremity to be operated on.

   a. **The extremity is elevated to promote venous drainage and is then exsanguinated with an Esmarch bandage** wrapped from the distal end up to the tourniquet itself (Fig. 9.1).

   b. **The tourniquet is inflated to a pressure of 100 mm Hg above the systolic blood pressure, not to exceed 300 mm Hg**. Tourniquet inflation is checked by balloting the cuff and observing oscillation of the pressure gauge.

   c. After tourniquet inflation and removal of the Esmarch wrap, adequate occlusion is confirmed by the absence of the radial or posterior tibial pulse.

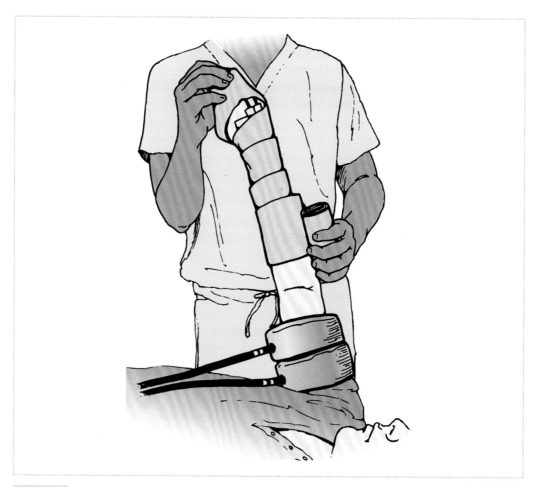

FIGURE 9.1   Technique for intravenous regional anesthesia. A small intravenous catheter is placed in the hand and the tourniquet is applied to the upper arm. A single tourniquet may be used for shorter operations and may provide more reliable compression of the venous system than the double-tourniquet system shown. Exsanguination of the arm is attained by elevation and wrapping with the Esmarch elastic bandage. The tourniquet is then inflated and the local anesthetic injected.

2. A constant pressure gas source must be used to maintain inflation of the cuff. All cuffs have some degree of volume leak—a standard blood pressure cuff will gradually lose cuff pressure and allow leakage of local anesthetic with potentially catastrophic results. The cuffs should be checked before injection and frequently during the procedure.

3. **Tourniquet selection**

   a. **Single cuff versus double cuff.** The "double cuff" was used traditionally to reduce pressure pain of the unanesthetized skin under the cuff, which worsens progressively during operations.

      (1) **Caution regarding the "double cuff."** The presence of two cuffs requires that they both be narrower (5 to 7 cm) than the standard blood pressure arm cuff (12 to 14 cm). Narrower cuffs do not effectively transmit the indicated gauge pressure to deep tissues, and therefore venous occlusion pressures are less than presumed (9). The use of a standard, wide, single cuff may be more desirable if the procedure lasts less than an hour (about the time for pressure discomfort/tourniquet pain to develop).

      (2) If the procedure exceeds 45 minutes, the double cuff may be preferable. In this situation, the proximal cuff is inflated for the first 45 minutes of anesthesia. The distal cuff is then inflated over anesthetized tissue. The proximal cuff (overlying unanesthetized skin) is then deflated. The adequacy of distal cuff inflation must be checked before the proximal cuff is deflated. Although this technique reportedly reduces patient discomfort at the area of the tourniquet, the complex procedure of shifting between inflated cuffs adds the risk of unintentional deflation.

   b. **Forearm cuff.** The use of a forearm cuff has some advantages over either a single or double upper-arm cuff. Because it is placed more distally, the forearm cuff allows a smaller volume of local anesthetic (10). A forearm cuff may also play a role in rescue from tourniquet pain. In this scenario, placement and inflation of a forearm cuff before deflation of the arm tourniquet is better tolerated than use of a double-cuff tourniquet (11).

CLINICAL PEARL The type of tourniquet selected depends on anticipated surgical time and if the surgery site is distal enough to accommodate the use of a forearm tourniquet.

E. **Injection of local anesthetic solution**

   1. After exsanguination, the limb is returned to the neutral position and the local anesthetic drug is injected through the previously placed IV catheter. The **injection is performed slowly (90 seconds or more) to avoid peak venous pressure from exceeding the tourniquet-occluding pressure** (9). If the tourniquet is functioning properly, the extremity will appear pale and mottled.

   2. The IV catheter is removed if the planned surgical procedure is expected to last less than an hour, and pressure is placed over the entry site until it seals. Adequate sensory anesthesia will ensue in 5 minutes.

   3. **If more than 45 minutes have elapsed after injection**, anesthesia may begin to diminish. If the surgeon requires more time, the intravenous catheter may be reinjected with local anesthetic solution after 60 to 90 minutes. This is disruptive to the surgery and potentially to the sterile field, and, because of this, for longer procedures, peripheral nerve blocks are a more appropriate plan.

F. Cuff deflation

1. Because local anesthetic binds to tissues, deflation of the tourniquet can be performed after 45 minutes with minimal risk of LAST (12).

2. **If less than 45 minutes have elapsed**, a two-stage release is recommended, where the cuff is deflated for 10 seconds and reinflated for a minute before final release. This allows a gradual washout of anesthetic. Cycling the cuff three times in this manner will delay the onset of peak blood levels, although it does not significantly reduce the level attained with a single deflation (13).

3. Under no circumstances is the cuff deflated in the first 20 minutes after injection. If less than 20 minutes have elapsed, the patient should be simply monitored until the 20-minute interval has passed and a two-stage release can be performed. These steps do not guarantee the absence of LAST (Fig. 9.2).

CLINICAL PEARL Safe IVRA is enhanced by injecting local anesthetic solution slowly at a site distal to the tourniquet and by extreme vigilance during tourniquet deflation sequences.

IV. Complications (14)

A. LAST is the major risk of IVRA

1. The greatest danger is from an inadequate venous occlusion or tourniquet failure early in the procedure when the intravenous volume is large.

2. Even with adequate inflation, the narrow cuffs (5 to 7 cm width) used for the double-tourniquet system sometimes allow leakage. The use of a standard-width adult cuff (12 to 14 cm) or a forearm cuff provides more reliable venous compression. This is especially true for leg tourniquets.

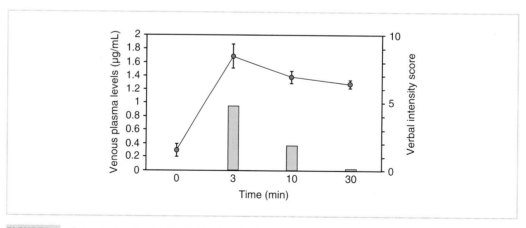

FIGURE 9.2 Systemic blood levels of 0.5% lidocaine after intravenous regional blockade. After release of the tourniquet, blood levels of local anesthetic increase rapidly, but are also rapidly cleared. After 72 ± 22 minutes of total tourniquet inflation time, the *colored circles* indicate blood levels following injection of 40 mL of 0.5% lidocaine (range to 2 µg/mL). The *solid bars* indicate the verbal numerical intensity score (on scale of 0 to 10) of central nervous system symptoms of light-headedness, dizziness, and tinnitus at 3, 10, and 30 minutes after deflation. (Adapted from Atanassoff PG, Hartmannsgruber MWB. Central nervous system side effects are less important afteriv regional anesthesia with ropivacaine 0.2% compared to lidocaine 0.5% in volunteers. *Can J Anaesth* 2002;49(2):169–172; with permission of Springer).

3. Leakage is more likely if the injection is made rapidly under high pressure into a proximal vein near the cuff.

4. The least leakage occurs when injection is made into a distal vein over more than 90 seconds.

5. Tourniquet release inevitably washes drug into the systemic circulation because some local anesthetic remains in the veins. With lidocaine, plasma levels are subtoxic after 45 minutes, but may reach toxic levels within the first 20 minutes after injection (12).

6. Because safety cannot be guaranteed, all IVRA patients must be monitored closely for LAST. Immediate access to resuscitation equipment and IV access in another extremity (typically the contralateral upper extremity) is indicated.

B. **Other side effects of IVRA include phlebitis and tourniquet-related discomfort and rare case reports of compartment syndrome.**

REFERENCES

1. Rosenberg PH. Intravenous regional anesthesia: nerve block by multiple mechanisms. *Reg Anesth* 1993;18:1–5.
2. Estebe JP, Gentilli ME, Langlois G, et al. Lidocaine priming reduces tourniquet pain during intravenous regional anesthesia: a preliminary study. *Reg Anesth Pain Med* 2003;28:120–123.
3. Atanassoff PG, Ocampo CA, Bande MC, et al. Ropivacaine 0.2% and lidocaine 0.5% for intravenous regional anesthesia in outpatient surgery. *Anesthesiology* 2001;95:627–631.
4. Neal JM, Bernards CM, Butterworth JF, et al. ASRA practice advisory on local anesthetic systemic toxicity. *Reg Anesth Pain Med* 2010;35:152–161.
5. Marsch SC, Sluga M, Studer W, et al. 0.5% versus 1.0% 2-chloroprocaine for intravenous regional anesthesia: a prospective, randomized, double-blind trial. *Anesth Analg* 2004;98:1789–1793.
6. Choyce A, Peng P. A systematic review of adjuvants for intravenous regional anesthesia for surgical procedures. *Can J Anaesth* 2002;49:32–45.
7. Reuben SS, Steinberg RB, Klatt J, et al. Intravenous regional anesthesia using lidocaine and clonidine. *Anesthesiology* 1999;91:654–658.
8. Memis D, Turan A, Karamanlioglu B, et al. Adding dexmedetomidine to lidocaine for intravenous regional anesthesia. *Anesth Analg* 2004;98:835–840.
9. Grice SC, Morell RC, Balestrieri FJ, et al. Intravenous regional anesthesia: evaluation and prevention of leakage under the tourniquet. *Anesthesiology* 1986;65:316–320.
10. Coleman MM, Peng PW, Regan JM, et al. Quantitative comparison of leakage under the tourniquet in forearm versus conventional intravenous regional anesthesia. *Anesth Analg* 1999;89:1482–1486.
11. Perlas A, Peng PW, Plaza MB, et al. Forearm rescue cuff improves tourniquet tolerance during intravenous regional anesthesia. *Reg Anesth Pain Med* 2003;28:98–102.
12. Tucker GT, Boas RA. Pharmacokinetic aspects of intravenous regional anesthesia. *Anesthesiology* 1971;34:538–549.
13. Sukhani R, Garcia CJ, Munhal RJ, et al. Lidocaine disposition following intravenous regional anesthesia with different tourniquet deflation techniques. *Anesth Analg* 1965;68:633.
14. Guay J. Adverse events associated with intravenous regional anesthesia (Bier block): a systematic review of complications. *J Clin Anesth* 2009;21:585–594.

Lower Extremity-Blocks of the Lumbar Plexus and Lumbar Plexus Peripheral Nerves

Francis V. Salinas

KEY POINTS

1. Detailed knowledge of the lumbar plexus, and the osseous and articular innervation of the joints of the lower extremity, will allow the operator to select the optimal approach based on the surgical procedure.

2. Ultrasonography has become the predominant technique for localization of the lumbar plexus and its peripheral nerve branches.

3. Successful ultrasound-guided nerve block of the lumbar plexus and lower extremity peripheral nerves relies on visualization and identification of both the neural structures and the fascial compartments that contain the target nerves.

4. The lumbar plexus approach (psoas compartment) blocks all three peripheral nerve branches (femoral, obturator, and lateral femoral cutaneous) within the substance of the psoas muscle.

5. Successful femoral nerve block relies on placement of the local anesthetic deep to the fascia iliaca. Femoral nerve block provides effective postoperative analgesia after major knee surgery and provides effective preoperative analgesia for hip fractures.

6. Ultrasound-guided subsartorial femoral triangle block is a relatively new technique, but has gained widespread adoption for total knee arthroplasty because of its analgesic efficacy and minimum effect on quadriceps motor function. It has been has referred to as adductor canal block, but the correct anatomic location for block placement is within the subsartorial apex of the femoral triangle

1

I. Anatomy

CLINICAL PEARL The clinically relevant branches of the lumbosacral plexus for lower extremity block are derived from the ventral rami of the L2–S4 spinal nerves. Anatomically, the lumbar and sacral plexus are connected through L4 as it bifurcates to join with L5 and form the lumbosacral trunk (Fig. 10.1). In contrast to the brachial plexus, there is no technique that allows the entire lumbosacral plexus to be anesthetized with a single injection. Therefore, for functional purposes, the lumbar and sacral plexus are distinct entities and must be blocked separately to provide complete unilateral lower extremity anesthesia and/or analgesia.

A. Lumbar plexus

    1. The clinically relevant motor and sensory innervation of the lumbar plexus arises from the ventral rami of the L2–L4 spinal nerve roots, which give rise to the lateral femoral cutaneous nerve (**LFCN**), femoral nerve (**FN**), and obturator nerve (**ON**). Shortly after exiting from their respective intervertebral foramina, the L2–L4 nerve roots lie within a fascial plane within the posterior aspect of the psoas major muscle (**PMM**) (Fig. 10.1).

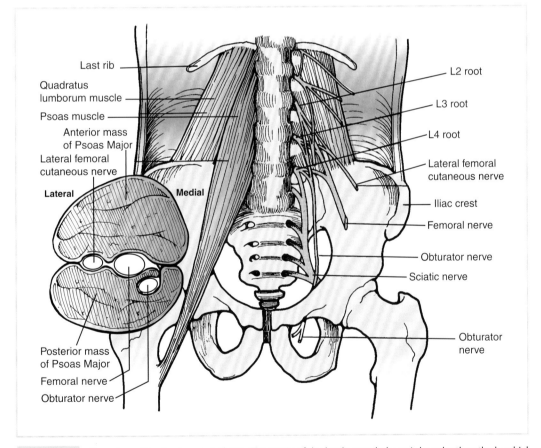

FIGURE 10.1 Overview of the lumbosacral plexus. The origin of the lumbosacral plexus is broader than the brachial plexus in the cervical region. The ventral rami of the L2–L4 spinal nerve roots emerge from their respective intervertebral foramina and travel within a fascial plane located between the posterior third and anterior two-thirds of the psoas major muscle (PMM). Within the substance of the PMM, the ventral rami form the peripheral nerves of the lumbar plexus. From a medial to lateral orientation, the obturator nerve is located most medial, the lateral femoral cutaneous nerve most lateral, and the femoral nerve located in between (see inset). The sacral spinal nerve roots (S1–S4) give rise to the sacral plexus and sciatic nerve, and require a separate injection.

2. The origins of the larger anterior PMM include the lateral surfaces of the lumbar vertebral bodies and their associated intervertebral discs, whereas the origins of the smaller posterior PMM are the ventral and lower surfaces of the respective transverse processes. The intervertebral foramina lie anterior to the transverse processes and posterior to the anterior muscular attachments to the vertebral bodies. Therefore, the nerve roots enter the PMM between their respective anterior and posterior segments.

3. Within the PMM, the ventral rami divide into anterior and posterior branches, which reunite to give rise to the individual peripheral nerves of the lumbar plexus. The lumbar plexus descends vertically within the substance of the psoas, and at the L4 and L5 levels, the terminal nerves have been formed.

4. Based on anatomic dissections and computed tomography imaging, the terminal nerves are arranged in a medial to lateral topographic arrangement, with the ON most medial, the LFCN most lateral, and the FN located in between[1,2] (Fig. 10.1). Although all the three terminal nerves are located within the PMM, anatomic studies have demonstrated that the ON may be separated from the FN and LFCN by a muscular fold more than 50% to 60% of the time, which may potentially lead to incomplete blockade of the lumbar plexus.[1,2]

B. Femoral nerve

1. **The FN** is derived from dorsal divisions of the ventral rami of the L2–L4 spinal nerve roots. It is the largest and most commonly blocked peripheral nerve branch of the lumbar plexus. Within the pelvis, the FN supplies muscular branches to the iliacus muscle and pectineus muscle (PM), as well as an articular branch to the hip joint.[3] The FN continues distally to enter the base of the femoral triangle (**FT**) in the proximal aspect of the anterior thigh by passing deep to the inguinal ligament (Fig. 10.2). The borders of the FT include the inguinal ligament (base), the sartorius muscle (lateral), and adductor longus muscle (AL) (medial). The iliacus muscle and PMM form the floor of the FT laterally and the PL and AL medially, while the roof is the overlying fascia lata. The apex of the FT is the intersection of the medial borders of the sartorius muscle and AL. In contrast, the medial border of the sartorius muscle, but the lateral border of the AL corresponds to the apex of the iliopectineal fossa (**IPF**), which is a proximal subset of the FT.[4]

2. The FN and femoral vessels continue distally from the base to the apex of the IPF. At the level of the inguinal ligament, the FN is within the IPF and is located 1 to 2 cm lateral to the femoral artery (**FA**), with the femoral vein (**FV**) located immediately medial to the FA (Fig. 10.2). As the FN continues further distally to the level of the inguinal crease, it is just lateral or posterolateral to the **FA**. Within the FT, the FN is located deep to both the fascia lata and fascia iliaca. In contrast, the femoral vessels (enveloped by the femoral sheath) are located deep to the fascia lata, but are superficial to the fascia iliaca. Thus, the fascia iliaca physically separates the FN (located within the muscular fascia iliaca compartment) from the femoral vessels (located within the vascular fascial compartment of the femoral sheath) (Fig. 10.3).

3. The topography of the FN demonstrates a relatively flat cross-sectional diameter with a mean medial to lateral width of 9 to 11 mm and a mean anterior to posterior height of 1.3 to 2.3 mm.[5] The FN is composed of multiple fascicles supplying muscular and cutaneous branches to the anterior compartment of the thigh, articular branches to the hip and knee joints, and cutaneous branches to the medial aspect of the lower leg (Fig. 10.4). Fascicular branches innervating the vastus medialis muscle (**VMM**), vastus intermedius muscle, and vastus lateralis muscle are positioned in the central and dorsal portion of the FN. The fascicular branches innervating the rectus femoris (laterally located), PMs (medially located), and the cutaneous nerves to the anterior and medial thigh are located on the peripheral aspects of the FN. The fascicular branch supplying the sartorius muscle is typically located

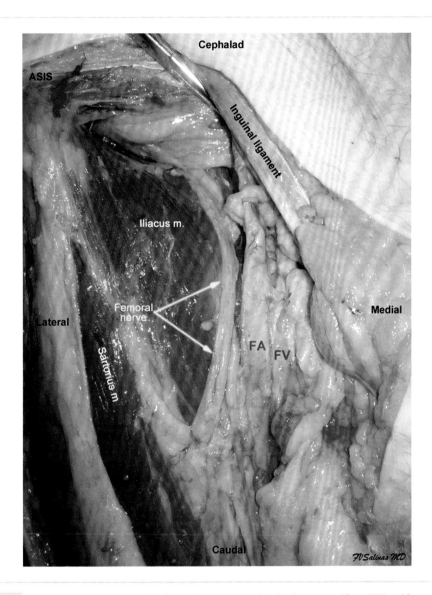

FIGURE 10.2 Fresh cadaver dissection of the femoral nerve (FN) within the iliopectineal fossa (IPF) and femoral triangle (FT). The inguinal ligament is retracted cephalad to show the course of the FN in the base of the FT. Several centimeters caudad to the inguinal ligament, the FN assumes a more superficial location within the FT. At the level of the inguinal crease, note that the FN lays just anterior to the iliacus muscle and just lateral to the femoral artery. The FN has a flattened appearance grossly and has a wider medial to lateral dimension compared to its anterior to posterior dimensions.

on the ventral aspect of the FN, but may be in a lateral, medial, or central position within the FN.[5] The saphenous nerve (**SN**) is consistently medial to the nerve branch to vastus medialis muscle (**N-VMM**) and together, they continue distally with the FA and FV (as a neurovascular bundle) toward the apex of the FT[4] (Fig. 10.5).

4. In the distal part of the FT, the N-VMM lies between the sartorius muscle and **VMM**. The posterior branch of the medial femoral cutaneous lies along the posterior side of the sartorius muscle and communicates with the SN and anterior branch of the ON forming the subsartorial plexus superficial to the vasoadductor membrane (**VAM**). These three

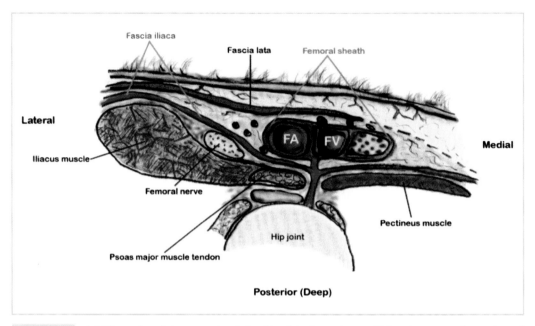

FIGURE 10.3 Axial illustration of the anatomic relationship of the femoral nerve (FN) to the surrounding perineural structures within the iliopectineal fossa (IPF). The FN lays directly anterior to the iliacus muscle and just posterior (deep) to the fascia iliaca. The FN is contained within the fascia iliaca compartment, just lateral to the femoral artery (FA). The FA (contained within the femoral sheath) is deep to the fascia lata but superficial to the fascia iliaca and is in a separate fascial compartment from the FN. This illustration most closely represents the ideal two-dimensional ultrasound short-axis image of the FN–FA anatomic relationship observed at the inguinal crease.

nerves lie deep to the sartorius muscle and lateral to the **FA** within the subsartorial apex (Scarpa) of the **FT**.

5. At the apex of the FT, the neurovascular bundle dives deep to the sartorius muscle into the groove of the FT. The SN and N-VMM exit the apex of the FT, but only the saphenous enters the adductor canal (**AC**) in conjunction with the superficial femoral artery (**SFA**) and superficial femoral vein (**SFV**). The AC is the neurovascular pathway from the apex of the FT to the adductor hiatus. The SFA exits the adductor hiatus and dives posterior in to the popliteal fossa to become the popliteal artery. Within the AC, the neurovascular bundle is sandwiched between the AI and AM posteromedially, the VMM anterolaterally, and the **VAM** anteromedially.[4,6] Within the AC, the SN is initially located lateral to the SFA, but as it continues distally, the SN assumes a position anterior and then medially located to the SFA within the distal AC.

6. Although the anatomic data is conflicting (because of differences in dissection technique),[4,6,7] the **N-VMM** is consistently located in a separate myofascial tunnel running alongside, but superficial to the AC. It gives rise to muscular branches that supply both the VMM and then continues further distally to supply the anterior and medial capsule of the knee joint and the medial retinaculum[4,6] (Fig. 10.6).

7. Both the SN and muscular branches from N-VMM give rise to branches that form a deep plexus lying between the SFA and femur. This deep plexus gives rise to anterior and medial genicular nerves that supply the deep anteromedial aspect of the knee joint.[4,6]

8. At the distal end of the AC, the SN pierces the VAM and emerges subcutaneously between the sartorius and gracilis muscles. As the SN continues further distally toward the joint line of the knee, it further divides into infrapatellar and sartorial branches. The infrapatellar branch provides cutaneous sensory innervation around the anterior aspect of the knee and an articular branch to the medial aspect of the knee joint. The sartorial branch continues

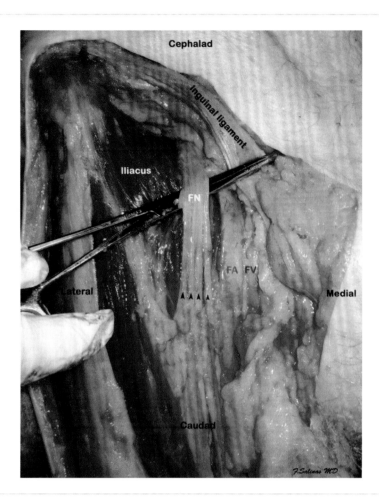

FIGURE 10.4   The tip of the clamp is over the inguinal ligament, whereas the middle of the clamp is under the proximal femoral nerve (FN). Distally, at least four individual fascicular components (branches) of the FN (*black arrowheads*) are visible. At this level, the branches of the femoral nerve will likely have arborized to supply their respective muscles of the quadriceps muscle group.

distally in the subcutaneous tissue of the lower leg, and continues further distally passing anteromedial to the medial malleolus to provide cutaneous innervation to the anteromedial lower leg and medial aspect of the foot. The sartorial branch also provides articular branches to the medial ankle and talocalcaneonavicular joint.[8]

C. Obturator nerve

1. The **ON** is formed within the substance of the PMM from the anterior divisions (ADs) of the ventral rami of the L2–L4 spinal nerves. The ON is the most medial branch of the lumbar plexus within the PMM. It emerges from the posterior border of the PMM and descends along the lateral wall of the pelvis toward the superior part of the obturator foramen (Fig. 10.1). The ON then enters the adductor compartment of the proximal thigh by passing through the obturator foramen. After emerging through the obturator foramen and just inferior to the superior pubic ramus, the ON continues distally in an interfascial plane anterior to the obturator externus muscle (OE) and deep to the PMs[9] (Fig. 10.7 A, B).

2. The ON has AD and posterior division (PD) that provide muscular branches to the adductor muscles of the thigh, articular branches to the hip and knee joints, and variable cutaneous sensory

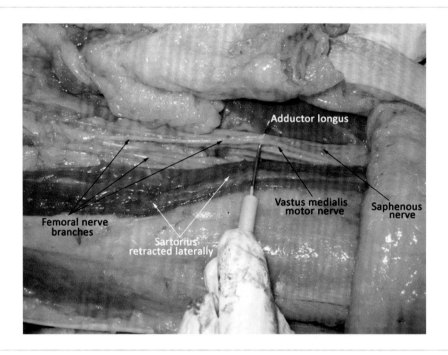

FIGURE 10.5 The course of the individual fascicular components of the femoral nerve is illustrated. The arrows indicate muscular branches to the vastus muscles. Note the two more medially located fascicular components (under the tip of the dissecting needle), accompanied by the femoral artery coursing caudad to the apex of the femoral triangle. The sartorius muscle has been retracted laterally.

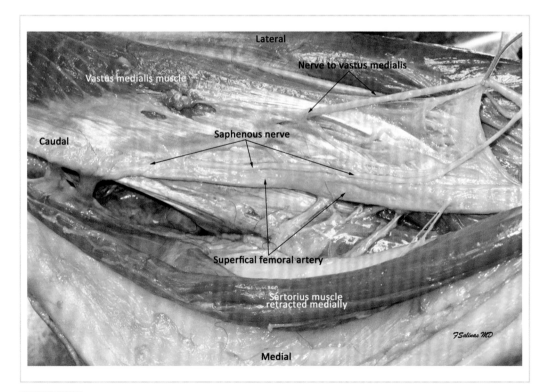

FIGURE 10.6 The contents of the adductor canal (AC). The sartorius muscle has been retracted medially. The nerve branch to the vastus medialis muscle (V-MMN) continues alongside and superficial to the AC then provides muscular branches to VMM. The saphenous nerve (SN) continues distally within the AC, initially lateral to the superficial femoral artery, courses anteriorly and then medially prior to exiting through the adductor hiatus.

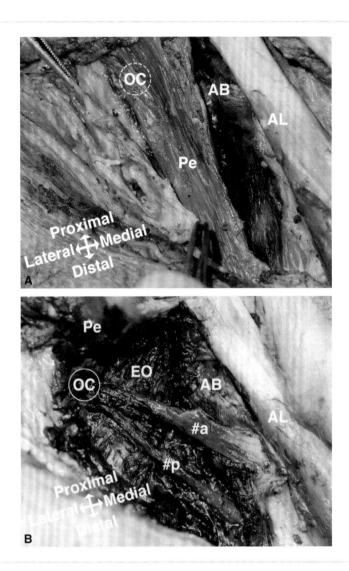

FIGURE 10.7 **A:** Cadaver dissection demonstrating the anatomy of the obturator nerve. Exposure of the structures before transection and reflection of the pectineus muscle from the superior pubic ramus. An ultrasound-guided injection into the fascial between the pectineus and obturator externus muscles was performed with 15 mL of methylene blue prior to transection. OC indicates the orifice of the obturator canal (depiction of the deeper position). **B:** After reflection of the PM, the anterior (#a) and posterior (#p) divisions of the obturator nerve exiting the OC, and are visibly stained in their extrapelvic trajectory anterior to the obturator externus muscle (OE). Note that the deep surface of the PM and the superficial surface of the OE are stained by methylene blue. AB, adductor brevis muscle; AL, adductor longus muscle; PM, pectineus muscle. (From Nielsen TD, et al. A cadaveric study of ultrasound-guided subpectineal injected spread around the obturator nerve and its articular branches. *Reg Anesth Pain Med.* 2017;42(3):357–361.)

branches to the posteromedial distal thigh. Anatomic studies have demonstrated a considerable degree of variability in the anatomy of the ON. It may divide into its respective AD and PD within the pelvis (23%) as it enters the obturator foramen, within the obturator foramen (52%), or may emerge united from the obturator foramen and divide in the proximal medial thigh (25%).[9] One to three articular branches innervate the hip joint: they typically arise from the proximal ON. However, the hip joint may also be supplied directly from both the AD and PD.[9,10]

3. The AD courses between the AL and the adductor brevis (AB), whereas the PD courses between the AB and adductor magnus (AM). Most commonly, the AD provides 2 to 3

branches (95%) to the AL, AB, and gracilis muscle. Less commonly, the AD may provide a fourth branch (5%) to the PM.[9] The AD provides a variable degree of cutaneous sensory distribution to the distal medial thigh.[11] At the lower border of the AL, the distal continuation of the AD occasionally communicates with the medial cutaneous and saphenous branches of the FN to form a subsartorial plexus that supplies the skin on the medial side of the thigh.

4. The PD commonly separates into two muscular branches providing innervation to the AB and AM. Less commonly, the PD may provide additional branches that supply the OE and AL. The posterior branch descends between the AB and AM and perforates the AM distally at its opening. It then enters the distal aspect of the AC and courses with the SFA through the adductor hiatus to enter the popliteal fossa. Within the popliteal fossa, the posterior branch anastomoses with branches of the tibial nerve to supply the posterior aspect of the knee joint.[4,6]

5. An accessory obturator nerve (**AON**) may be present in 10% to 30% of patients and is derived from the ventral rami of the L3 and L4 spinal nerves or directly from the ON.[12] The AON courses along the posterior aspect of the external iliac artery and descends caudally over the superior pubic ramus giving off branches to the pectineus and hip joint. The presence of an AON may have clinical consequences for hip surgery. Consequently, achievement of complete ON block, especially to the hip joint, may require an approach that consistently blocks the AON, when present.

D. **Lateral femoral cutaneous nerve**

1. The **LFCN** is a purely sensory nerve formed from the PDs of the ventral rami of the L2 and L3 spinal nerves (Fig. 10.8A). It emerges from the lateral border of the PMM coursing obliquely across the iliacus muscle (deep to the fascia iliaca) toward the anterior superior iliac spine (**ASIS**) (Fig. 10.8A). The LFCN continues distally, most commonly, deep to the inguinal ligament. However, it may also pass through a split in the inguinal ligament, and in cases of nerve entrapment, through an iliac bone canaliculus.[13]

2. The course of the LFCN as it enters the thigh, particularly in relation to the inguinal ligament and ASIS demonstrates considerable variability.[13,14] It is typically located within 2 to 3 cm medial to the ASIS, although it may be located up to 7 cm medial, or even lateral to ASIS. The LFCN most commonly enters the thigh as a single branch (72% of cases), although it can divide into 2 to 5 branches proximal to the inguinal ligament. As the LFCN enters the thigh, it is most commonly located superficial to the sartorius muscle and deep to the fascia iliaca. It may also pass through the muscle (in up to 22% of cases), and rarely it may even pass superficial to the fascia lata.

3. The LFCN provides cutaneous sensory innervation of the lateral thigh from the area of the greater trochanter as far distal as the lateral aspect of the knee, but may also extend to the medial aspect of the thigh and distally to the patella (Fig. 10.8B).[14,15]

II. **Drugs.** To select the optimal local anesthetic agent, the operator must decide whether the aim is postoperative analgesia (in the context of concomitant general anesthesia or spinal anesthesia, as well as the presence of continuous perineural catheter) or surgical anesthesia. Tables 10.1 and 10.2 provide suggested duration(s) of anesthesia and analgesia, but may vary significantly with type and dose of local anesthetic, local anesthetic adjuvants (e.g., epinephrine or dexamethasone) interindividual patient variability, and block location. Surgical anesthesia for lower extremity surgery will require additional neural blockade (sciatic nerve) based on the surgical considerations (i.e., location of surgery and tourniquet requirements). ON or LFCN blocks are rarely indicated for surgical anesthesia.

TABLE 10.1   Local anesthetic choices for posterior lumbar plexus (psoas compartment) block

Local anesthetic (%)	Duration of anesthesia (h)	Duration of analgesia (h)
Lidocaine 1.5–2	2–4	4–8
Mepivacaine 1.5–2	3–5	5–8
Ropivacaine 0.5–0.75	4–6	6–12
Bupivacaine 0.5	4–6	6–12

TABLE 10.2   Local anesthetic choices for femoral nerve block

Local anesthetic (%)	Duration of anesthesia (h)	Duration of analgesia (h)
Lidocaine 1.5–2	2–3	4–6
Mepivacaine 1.5–2	3–4	5–8
Ropivacaine 0.5–0.75	4–6	6–12
Bupivacaine 0.25–0.5	6–8	8–24

III. Approaches and techniques

CLINICAL PEARL   The term *"approach"* refers to the anatomic location where the lumbar plexus or its peripheral nerve branches are targeted (e.g., posterior paravertebral for psoas compartment vs. inguinal perivascular for FN). The term *"technique"* refers to the modality for nerve localization (e.g., ultrasound guidance [USG], peripheral nerve stimulation [PNS], loss of resistance, or a combined technique) utilized for a given approach.

In addition, continuous lumbar plexus and lower extremity perineural catheter techniques provide superior postoperative analgesia compared to traditional systemic opioid-based therapy and comparable postoperative analgesia to lumbar epidural infusions after major lower extremity surgery.[16]

2   USG has become the predominant technique for lower extremity peripheral nerve localization. USG has not only been shown to increase the onset of complete sensory block but also decreases block performance time, block onset time, and local anesthetic requirements compared to **PNS**.[17] There is no evidence to support the routine use of concurrent PNS to supplement a primary USG (*"dual-guidance"*) technique, especially when the target nerve is well visualized.

However, dual guidance may be useful in two specific circumstances: (1) when target nerve visualization is difficult in specific circumstances, such as increased body habitus, deep nerve location (lumbar plexus–psoas compartment approach), or anatomic variation and (2) evoked motor responses at current output ≤0.2 mA is highly suggestive of intraneural needle placement, and should prompt slight withdrawal or repositioning of the needle tip prior to local anesthetic injection; however, stimulatory thresholds >0.2 mA do not offer a fail-safe guarantee that the needle tip is extraneural.

4   **A. Lumbar plexus (psoas compartment approach) block**

CLINICAL PEARL   The lumbar plexus approach (psoas compartment block) anesthetizes all three peripheral nerve branches of the lumbar plexus within the PMM. Lumbar plexus block (LBP) may be successfully performed with a variety of surface landmark-based techniques in combination with PNS. However, it is an advanced regional anesthetic technique because of a combination of the depth of the target nerves and inconsistent surface landmarks. Owing to the deep anatomic location (and variation in depth based on gender and body mass index) of the lumbar plexus, small errors in surface landmark estimations combined with angle miscalculations can lead to inaccurate needle tip placement. Advances in the technology and application of US imaging facilitates preprocedural mapping of the location and depth of key anatomic landmarks, and intraprocedural imaging facilitates real-time assessment of needle trajectory and local anesthetic spread.

1. **Indications.** In combination with a sacral plexus block, LPB provides operative anesthesia-postoperative analgesia for hip surgery (total hip arthroplasty [THA], hip and femoral shaft fracture repair, acetabular reconstruction/osteotomy). In combination with a sciatic nerve block, operative anesthesia-postoperative analgesia for surgical procedures from the femoral shaft to the foot. Postoperative analgesia for THA, hip and femoral shaft fracture repair, acetabular reconstruction/osteotomy, total knee arthroplasty (TKA).

2. **Contraindications.** Usual contraindications to peripheral nerve blocks (i.e., lack of consent, infection at the injection site, allergy to local anesthetics). Preexisting neural compromise is considered a relative contraindication; a careful discussion regarding the potential risks and benefits of performing peripheral nerve blocks in patients with preexisting neural compromise is strongly recommended.[18] For the posterior paravertebral approach to the lumbar plexus, follow current American Society of Regional Anesthesia recommendations for neuraxial techniques in the anticoagulated patient.[19]

3. **Single-injection technique**

   a. **Patient position.** The patient is placed in the lateral decubitus position with a slight forward tilt, hips flexed with the operative side uppermost.

CLINICAL PEARL The operator should be positioned behind the patient so that evoked motor responses of the quadriceps muscle and patella may be easily seen or palpated when concurrent PNS is utilized. First, mark a line (intercristal line) connecting the iliac crests, which provides an approximation of the L4 vertebral body or the L4 and L5 intervertebral space. Second, draw a line connecting adjacent spinous processes to identify the midline. These two lines will provide a reference point for the initial US scanning-surface mapping of the key sonographic landmark, the transverse process of the L4 vertebral body (Fig. 10.9).

   b. **Ultrasound transducer selection-scanning technique**

CLINICAL PEARL Owing to the depth of the transverse processes and the required wide field of view, a low-frequency (2 to 5 MHz) curved array transducer should be utilized.

   (1) The US scanning technique consists of two phases:
       (a) **Preprocedural surface mapping of the lumbar transverse processes to confirm depth of the transverse process and needle insertion location.**
       (b) **Real-time US imaging of the needle advancement.**
   (2) **A standard stepwise process requiring two transducer locations is recommended as follows:**
       (a) Initially, place the transducer in a parasagittal (PS; just lateral to the midline) orientation over the proximal sacrum of the patient (Fig. 10.10A). Sonographically, the sacrum is recognizable as a continuous hyperechoic line with posterior acoustic shadowing beneath (Fig. 10.10B). The transducer is slid in a cephalad direction to obtain a PS view of the L5 and S1 articular process, followed then

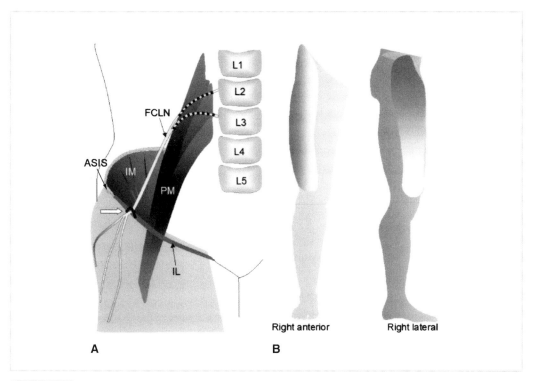

FIGURE 10.8   Illustration showing the formation of the right lateral femoral cutaneous nerve (LFCN). The LFCN exits from the posterolateral border of the psoas major muscle traveling obliquely over the iliac muscle toward the anterior superior iliac spine and deep to the inguinal ligament. The gray-coded signed area shows the sensory cutaneous distribution along the anterolateral thigh. (From Bodner G, et al. Ultrasound of the lateral femoral cutaneous nerve: normal findings in a cadaver and in volunteers. *Reg Anesth Pain Med.* 2009;34:265–268, p. 266).

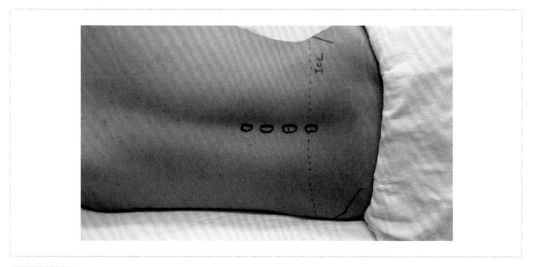

FIGURE 10.9   Lateral decubitus position for lumbar plexus block. Initial surface landmarks include identifying the intercristal line (ICL) and the midline (identified by marking the lumbar spinous processes).

the L5 and L4, and L4 and L3 processes. The PS articular process view appears as a continuous hyperechoic line of "*humps*," with each hump representing the facet joint between the superior and inferior articular process of the successive lumbar vertebrae (Fig. 10.10C).[20] The corresponding intervertebral levels (from S1 to L5 to L4) are noted and marked on the skin at the midpoint of the transducer. The superior and inferior articular processes lie in the coronal plane more posterior than the transverse process and will be seen at a more superficial depth than the corresponding transverse process.

(b) From the L4 and L3 PS articular process view, the transducer is slid laterally until the L4 and L3 transverse processes are identified (typically within

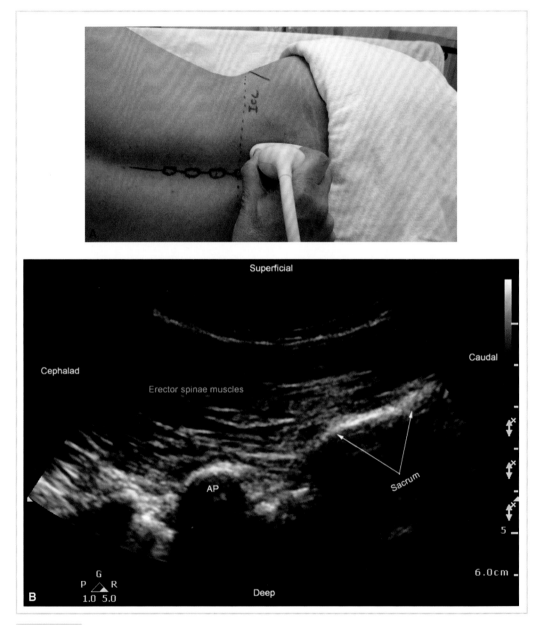

FIGURE 10.10 **A:** The transducer is positioned in a parasagittal orientation over the lumbosacral junction. **B:** Parasagittal long-axis view of the lumbosacral spine. The sacrum is recognizable as a continuous hypoechoic line with posterior acoustic shadowing. **C:** Parasagittal long-axis articular processes view. The articular processes appear as a continuous hypoechoic wavy line of "humps," with each representing the facet joint between a superior and an inferior articular processes. Note that the estimated depth (*horizontal red arrow*) of the articular processes is slightly less than 3.0 cm.

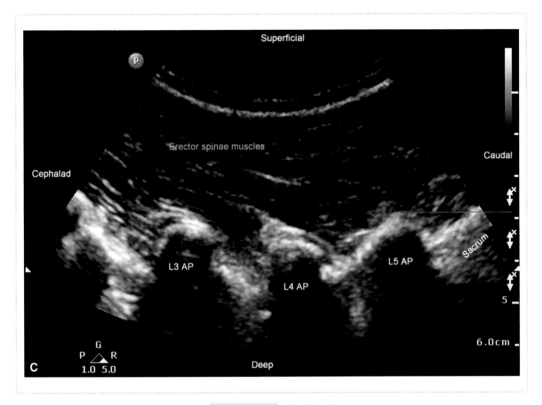

FIGURE 10.10   *(continued)*

2 to 4 cm lateral to the midline) (Fig. 10.11A). The transverse processes appear as short hyperechoic curvilinear structures with "*fingerlike*" posterior acoustic shadowing projecting deep to the transverse processes. The striated PMM, located deep to the transverse processes, is visible in the acoustic (intertransverse) window between the transverse processes[20] (Fig. 10.11B).

(i) The distance (from the midline) of the L4 and L3 transverse processes is noted by marking a vertical line along the long axis of the transducer (Fig. 10.12, red line). The L4 transverse process is placed in the middle (from caudad to cephalad) of the US image, and a line is drawn and extended laterally in the axial plane (Fig. 10.12, yellow line).

(ii) The transducer is then slid slightly cephalad to place L3 processes in the middle of the US image, and a second axial line is extended laterally from the midpoint of the transducer (Fig. 10.12, green line).

(iii) The intersection of the vertical PS (red) and first axial (yellow) lines corresponds to the needle insertion point when the goal of the technique is to initially contact the L4 transverse process.

(iv) In contrast, the black dot along vertical PS (red) line corresponds to the needle insertion point when the needle will be in the interlaminar space (between L4 and L3), and advanced deeper and anterior to the L4 transverse process to reach the lumbar plexus (Fig. 10.12, black dot).

(c) After mapping of the transverse processes, the transducer is then placed transversally on the mid to posterior axillary line, immediately cephalad to

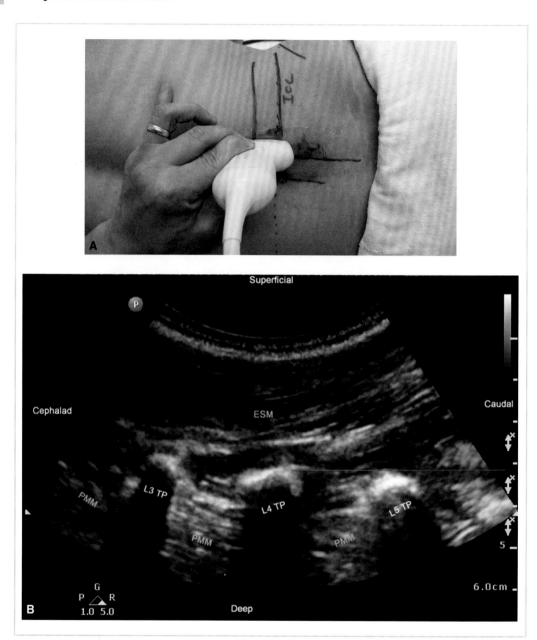

FIGURE 10.11 **A:** The transducer has been moved laterally from the midline over the transverse processes. **B:** Parasagittal long-axis view of the transverse processes (TP). The transverse processes appear as short hyperechoic curvilinear structures with *"fingerlike"* posterior acoustic shadowing projecting deep to the transverse processes. The striated psoas major muscle (PMM), located deep to the transverse processes, is visible in the acoustic (inter-transverse) window between the transverse processes. Note that the estimated depth of the transverse processes is slightly deeper than 3.0 cm (horizontal red line). Erector spinae muscles (ESM).

the iliac crest (Fig. 10.13A). The posterior aspect of the muscles (external and internal oblique and transversus abdominis) of the lateral abdominal wall is visualized (see Chapter 12).

    (i) The transducer is then slid dorsally until the quadratus lumborum muscle (**QLM**) is seen medial to the aponeurosis of the transversus abdominis

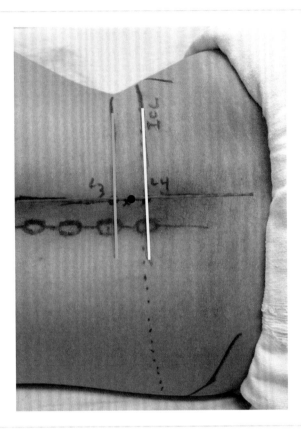

FIGURE 10.12   Surface markings from the per-procedural sonographic mapping of the lumbar plexus block. The red parasagittal line represents the distance from the midline (spinous processes) to the transverse processes. The intersection of the red parasagittal line and the axial yellow line represents the needle insertion point if contact with the L4 transverse process is initially desired. The intersection of the red parasagittal line and the axial green line represents the needle insertion point if contact with the L3 transverse process is desired. The black dot along the red parasagittal line dot represents the inter-transverse window (between the L3 and L4 transverse processes) for the needle insertion point to bypass contacting the L4 transverse process..

muscle. The tendinous insertion of the QLM is located on the lateral tip (apex) of the L4 transverse process.[21,22]

(ii)   With the long axis of the transducer aligned with the previously marked first axial line, the US beam should be insonating the L4 transverse process and associated vertebral body and the surrounding musculature in an axial plane. With the medial aspect of the QLM situated on the apex of the L4 transverse process, the PMM located anterior and the erector spinae muscles (ESM) posterior, respectively, to the transverse processes, a characteristic sonographic pattern (axial *"Shamrock Sign"* view)[21,22] (Figs. 10.13B and 10.14A).

(iii)   The transducer is then tilted slightly cephalad until the transverse process (of L4) disappears. The US beam will insonate across the interlaminar space. The shape of the lateral border of the vertebral body will transition from a relatively flat shape to a more rounded to oval shape. The lateral edge of the vertebral body will appear to protrude into the PMM muscle (Figs. 10.13C and 10.14B).

c. **Ultrasound anatomy**

(1) **Parasagittal articular process view** (Fig. 10.10B, C). The overlapping bony superior and inferior articular processes (forming the facet joints) are visualized as a continuous intensely hyperechoic wavy line of "humps" with posterior acoustic dropout deep to the facet joints. Note that the articular processes lie in a coronal plane more superficial to the corresponding transverse process.

(2) **Parasagittal transverse process view** (Fig. 10.11B). The transverse processes appear as short (noncontiguous) intensely hyperechoic structures with characteristic fingerlike posterior acoustic dropout deep to the transverse processes. The PMM

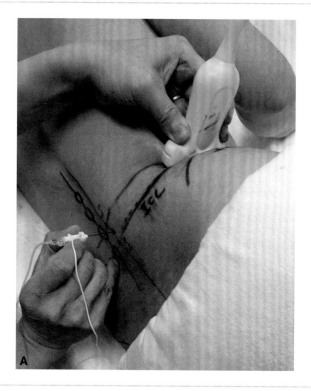

FIGURE 10.13 **A:** Transducer placement (just superior to the iliac crest) and needle insertion point for "Shamrock method" lumbar plexus block. The needle advancement will be from posterior (dorsal) to anterior (ventral). Note the photo is simply a demonstration of the transducer placement and needle placement and was not an actual medical procedure. **B:** Ultrasound view of the "Shamrock method" for lumbar plexus block. The ultrasound beam is insonating the L4 transverse process and vertebral body. The quadratus lumborum muscle (QLM) tendon inserts onto the lateral edge of the L4 transverse process. The erector spinae muscles (ESM) and the psoas major muscle (PMM) are located on the anterior and posterior surfaces, respectively, of the L4 transverse process. The transverse process forms the stem of the Shamrock surrounded by the three muscles (representing the three leaves). The yellow line indicates the direction of needle advancement. **C:** Ultrasound view of the "intertransverse" modified "Shamrock" view. The transducer has been tilted slightly cephalad so that the ultrasound beam is insonating in between the L4 and L3 transverse processes. The L4 vertebral body shape has changed (from the flatter shape in the Shamrock view) to a more oval structure with the lateral edge appearing to "bulge" into the PMM. The yellow line indicates the direction of needle advancement beyond (1 to 2 cm anterior) L4 transverse process.

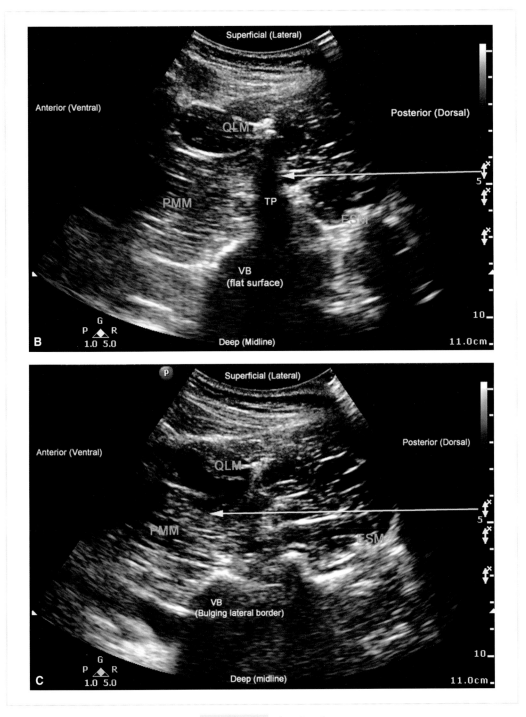

FIGURE 10.13   *(continued)*

is visible deep to the transverse processes in the acoustic (intertransverse) window between the transverse processes. The PMM has the characteristic striated appearance typical of skeletal muscle.

(3) **Axial "Shamrock view"** (Fig. 10.13B). The hyperechoic transverse process projects laterally and forms the stem of the Shamrock. The PMM is located anterior;

the ESM is located posterior; with the medial border of the QLM inserted on to apex of the transverse process forms the outline of the three leaves of a Shamrock.

(4) **Axial intertransverse view** (Fig. 10.13C). The transverse process no longer appears. The lateral edge of the vertebral body has transitioned from a flat shape (in the Shamrock view) to a more rounded to oval shape, and appears to protrude into the substance of the PMM muscle.

d. **Needling technique** (Fig. 10.13A). With the US transducer placed over the iliac crest and the US beam imaging in between L4 and L3 transverse processes (axial intertransverse view), a 21-gauge 100 mm or 20-gauge 150 mm stimulating needle is placed at the previously marked needle insertion point obtained with the PS views.

(1) The peripheral nerve stimulator is set to initially deliver a current output of 1.5 mA (frequency of 2 MHz and pulse duration of 0.1 ms).

(2) The needle is advanced from posterior to anterior in plane to the US beam until it passes 1 to 2 cm anterior to the previously measured depth of the transverse process.

(3) When the needle contacts the lumbar plexus, evoked motor responses of the quadriceps muscle should become visible (quadriceps contraction or patellar ascension). The current output is turned down to between 0.5 and 1.0 mA while maintaining quadriceps contraction.

(4) After the appropriate test injection of either saline or local anesthetic, the quadriceps contraction should disappear. While injecting slowly and incrementally (in 3 to 5 mL aliquots) a total volume of 20 to 35 mL, local anesthetic should be visualized expanding within the PMM.

CLINICAL PEARL Stimulating currents <0.5 mA should not be sought because motor stimulation below this threshold may indicate placement of the needle tip inside a dural sleeve. An injection within the dural sleeve may result in epidural or spinal anesthesia.

CLINICAL PEARL An LPB may be associated with significant discomfort because the needle passes through multiple muscle compartments. Adequate sedation and analgesia are necessary to ensure a still, but cooperative patient.

CLINICAL PEARL Typical onset time is 20 or 30 minutes, depending on the type, concentration, and volume of local anesthetic.

---

e. **Local anesthetic volume.** Typically, a volume of 20 to 35 mL is required to obtain satisfactory local anesthetic distribution (and successful block) around all three branches of the lumbar plexus.[23]

4. **Continuous catheter technique.** If a **continuous catheter technique** is indicated, a larger bore (17- to 18-gauge) Tuohy needle is typically used for initial placement of the needle tip and local anesthetic (20 mL) within the psoas compartment. After local anesthetic distribution (by injection through the needle tip) is ensured, the US transducer is placed aside within the sterile field. A 19- to 20-gauge catheter is inserted through the Tuohy needle and advanced no more than 2 to 3 cm past needle tip. At this point, the US probe is placed over the original site, and an additional 3 to 5 mL of local anesthetic is injected through

the catheter while confirming local anesthetic distribution within the psoas compartment to ensure correct catheter tip position. The needle is then withdrawn over the catheter and fixed in place with a sterile clear adhesive dressing. The proximal end of the catheter is then connected to an infusion pump. The most commonly used local anesthetic utilized is ropivacaine 0.2% with typical infusion volumes from 6 to 10 per hour.

CLINICAL PEARL The needle opening should be directed caudal and laterally to facilitate advancement of the catheter in the direction of the lumbar plexus and minimize the risk of the catheter advancement medially toward the intervertebral foramen. When discontinuing and removing a continuous lumbar plexus catheter, follow the current American Society of Regional Anesthesia recommendations for neuraxial techniques in the anticoagulated patient.[19]

B. **Ultrasound-guided femoral nerve block**

1. **Indications.** The most common indication for FN block is postoperative analgesia after major knee surgery (TKA, anterior-cruciate ligament reconstruction, patellar tendon repair) or open-reduction internal fixation of hip or femoral shaft fractures; anesthesia and analgesia for major surgical procedures below the knee (below the knee amputation [BKA], total ankle replacement) when combined with sciatic nerve block. Operative anesthesia for superficial soft tissue procedures of the anterior thigh (muscle biopsy).

2. **Contraindications.** Usual contraindications to peripheral nerve blocks (i.e., lack of consent, infection at the injection site, allergy to local anesthetics). Preexisting neural compromise is considered a relative contraindication; a careful discussion regarding the potential risks and benefits of performing peripheral nerve blocks in patients with preexisting neural compromise is strongly recommended.[14]

3. **Single-injection technique**
   a. **Patient position.** The patient is supine with the operative leg slightly abducted 10 to 20 degrees and the inguinal region of the operative exposed. Abduction may be difficult and painful in patients with hip or femoral shaft fractures.
   b. **US transducer selection-scanning technique.** A high-frequency linear array transducer (5 to 12 MHz) is typically used for this block. A depth of 3 to 4 cm is adequate to visualize the FN and FA. The US transducer is placed initially at a 90-degree angle to the skin in an axial oblique orientation, parallel to the inguinal crease (Fig. 10.15). The transducer is adjusted (moved slightly cephalad to caudad, medial to lateral, and cephalad to caudad needle angulation) to optimize the appearance of the target structures.
      (1) The most easily recognized structure is the typically **round, pulsatile, non-compressible, and hypoechoic FA**. Medial to the FA is the **larger and easily compressible FV**.
      (2) The **FN is a hyperechoic oval structure located just lateral and slightly deeper to the FA**. The **fascia lata** and **fascia iliaca** are hyperechoic linear structures traveling medial to lateral, superficial, and traveling perpendicular to the short axis (SAX) of the FN and FA (Fig. 10.16A, B). The fascia lata is superficial to the fascia iliaca, and the fascia iliaca is superficial to the FN. As the fascia iliaca courses medially, it thickens to become the iliopectineal ligament and is deep to the FA and FV (Fig. 10.3).
   c. **Ultrasound anatomy** (Fig. 10.16A, B). The FN is most commonly located lateral and adjacent to the FA, but may also be located slightly lateral and deep to the FA. The FN will

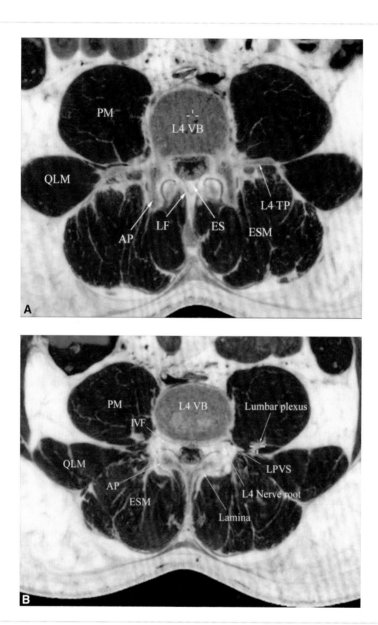

FIGURE 10.14 **A:** Cross-sectional cadaver anatomic section through the L4 vertebral body (L4–VB) and transverse process (L4–TP) corresponding to the "Shamrock method" ultrasound image. **B:** Cross-sectional cadaver anatomic section through the intertransverse process window (between L3 and L4) corresponding to the "intertransverse" modified "Shamrock" view. The intervertebral foramen (IVF), L4 nerve root, and the lumbar plexus (in the posterior part of the PM) are each marked with white arrowheads. ESM, erector spinae muscles; PMM, psoas major muscle; QLM, quadratus lumborum muscle. (From Karmakar MK, et al. Sonoanatomy Relevant for Lumbar Plexus Block in Volunteers Correlated With Cross-sectional Anatomic and Magnetic Resonance Images. *Reg Anesth Pain Med.* 2013;38(5):391–397, Figure 4, p. 393; Figure 5, p. 393.)

appear as a hyperechoic oval to oblong structure, appear triangular, to thin and flat. The hyperechoic FN lays directly on the relatively hypoechoic iliopsoas muscle and deep to the investing fascia iliaca. The fascia iliaca will appear as a thin hyperechoic linear structure running in a horizontal oblique direction from lateral to medial just superficial to the FN.

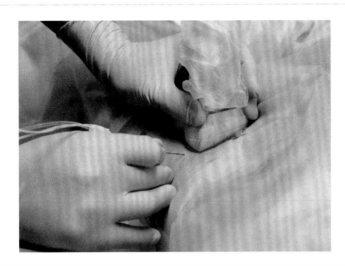

FIGURE 10.15 Patient position, transducer placement, and needle insertion point for ultrasound guided femoral nerve block.

CLINICAL PEARL An anechoic structure coursing laterally off either the profunda femoris or FA is most likely the lateral femoral circumflex artery (LCFA). It will appear to run perpendicular to the SAX appearance of the FN. Color-flow Doppler will identify this as a blood vessel. Simply scan more cephalad to obtain an imaging plane and subsequent needle path that avoids the LFCA.

5

  d. **Needling technique.** A 21-gauge 100 needle is inserted lateral to the transducer and advanced in-plane toward the superiolateral aspect of the FN and just deep to fascia iliaca (Fig. 10.17A). Often, a palpable and visual loss of resistance ("pop") is observed as the needle tip penetrates the fascia iliaca. At this point, after aspiration, a small (1 to 2 mL) aliquot of local anesthetic is injected observing for local anesthetic distribution (seen as an anechoic collection of fluid) around the FN and deep to the fascia iliaca. During the process of incremental aspiration and injection, continuously observe in real time the distribution of the local anesthetic around the FN. Continue the injection until there is satisfactory distribution of local anesthetic around the FN (Fig. 10.17B). Although circumferential distribution of local anesthetic should result in a more complete and rapid onset of block, this has not been rigorously tested in clinical trials. The key is to make sure that the needle tip (and local anesthetic injection) is deep to the fascia iliaca.
  e. **Local anesthetic volume.** A volume of 20 to 25 mL is required to obtain satisfactory local anesthetic distribution around the FN.[24]
 4. **Continuous catheter technique.** If a **continuous catheter technique** is indicated, a larger bore (17- to 18-gauge) Tuohy needle is typically used for initial placement of the needle tip and local anesthetic injection. After local anesthetic distribution (by injection through the needle tip) is ensured, the US transducer is placed aside within the sterile field. A 19- to 20-gauge catheter is inserted through the Tuohy needle and advanced no more than 2 to 3 cm past needle tip. At this point, the US probe is placed over the original site, and an additional 3 to 5 mL of local anesthetic is injected through the catheter while confirming local anesthetic distribution deep to the fascia iliaca to confirm ensure correct catheter tip position. The needle is then withdrawn over the catheter and fixed in place with a sterile

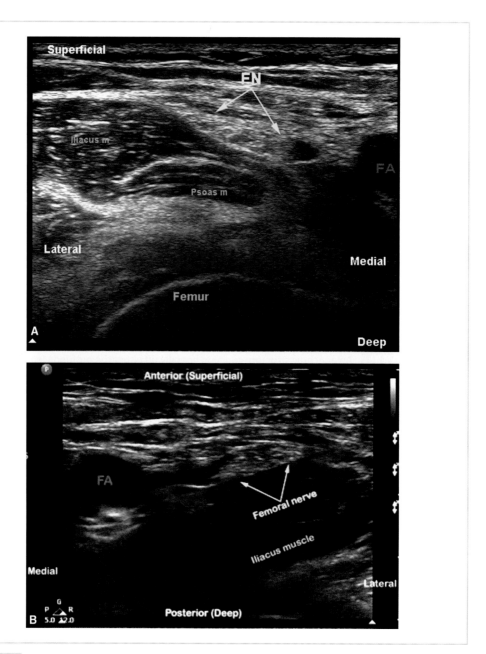

FIGURE 10.16   Ultrasound images of the short-axis view for perivascular femoral nerve block. Note the hyperchoic femoral nerve is located lateral to the hypoechoic femoral artery. The shape of the femoral nerve is typically oval shaped **(A)** with a wider medial to lateral dimension compared to anterior to posterior dimension, but may also be triangular-shaped **(B)**.

clear adhesive dressing. The proximal end of the catheter is then connected to an infusion pump. The most commonly used local anesthetic utilized is ropivacaine 0.2% with typical infusion volumes from 6 to 10 per hour.

5   **CLINICAL PEARL**   The key to successful continuous FN block is placement of the catheter deep to the fascia iliaca. The catheter may be placed either superficial or deep to the FN with no difference in the quality of sensorimotor block, if the catheter tip (and local anesthetic infusion) is placed deep to the fascia iliaca.

CLINICAL PEARL   An efficient technique for placement of continuous femoral catheters begins with "preloading" a 19-guage flexible wire reinforced catheter (will appear hyperechoic because of the metal wire) into the 17-gauge block needle. The proximal end of the catheter is then connected to a 20-mL syringe filled with the desired solution (saline or local anesthetic), and the catheter is flushed and primed (Fig. 10.18A). The catheter tip is then positioned just proximal to the beveled tip of the block needle (Fig. 10.18B). The advantage of preassembling the catheter-needle is that is that once the needle tip enters the femoral perineural compartment (deep to the fascia iliaca, or any other perineural location, or fascial compartment), the catheter may then be advanced beyond the needle without having to place the catheter in the needle.

C. **Ultrasound-guided subsartorial femoral triangle block**

6   **CLINICAL PEARL**   Blockade of the SN, N-VMM, and the posterior branch of the medial femoral cutaneous nerve within the subsartorial apex of the FT is the most common anatomic location for the placement of what has been previously referred to as the adductor canal block (ACB). The original description of US transducer placement was the "midthigh" (halfway between the ASIS and base of the patella). Detailed anatomic dissections of the topography of the course of the SN in the FT and AC support that midthigh transducer placement is within the subsartorial apex of the FT and proximal to the beginning of the AC (defined as the intersection of the medial border of the sartorius muscle and medial border AL).[4,25–27]. Although used interchangeably, most of the published studies on the efficacy of the *"ACB"* for TKA were subsartorial femoral triangle blocks (SSFTB)

6   **CLINICAL PEARL**   Some anesthesiologists may advocate placing *"true adductor canal blocks"* more distal in the thigh, to *"anesthetize just the saphenous nerve and avoid weakness of the quadriceps muscles by sparing the N-VMM."* However, because the N-VMM gives rise to distal sensory branches that innervate the knee capsule, the more proximal SSFTB approach is the anatomically preferred block for optimal anesthesia after TKA.[4]

1. **Indications.** The primary indication (most commonly, utilizing a continuous perineural technique) is postoperative analgesia after TKA and other major surgical procedures of the knee. SSFTB has supplanted continuous femoral nerve block (**CFNB**) for postoperative analgesia after TKA.[28] In the setting of contemporary multimodal analgesia (scheduled perioperative acetaminophen, gabapentin, nonsteroidal anti-inflammatory agents, gabapentinoids, and periarticular local anesthetic infiltration analgesia [**LIA**]), single-injection or continuous subsartorial femoral triangle blocks (**CSSFTB**) provide noninferior analgesia compared to CFNB, but without the associated quadriceps motor block associated with CFNB.[29,30]

2. **Contraindications.** Usual contraindications to peripheral nerve blocks (i.e., lack of consent, infection at the injection site, allergy to local anesthetics). Preexisting neural compromise is considered a relative contraindication; a careful discussion regarding the potential risks and benefits of performing peripheral nerve blocks in patients with preexisting neural compromise is strongly recommended.[18]

3. **Single-injection technique**

   a. **Patient position.** The patient is supine with the operative lower leg slightly abducted and externally rotated. The mid-anteromedial thigh is the most common location for transducer placement.

CLINICAL PEARL Abduction and external location can be facilitated by placement of a 4- to 6-inch bump (rolled towel) on the posteromedial aspect of the midthigh. This position places the anteromedial surface of the midthigh (and transducer placement) in horizontal plane.

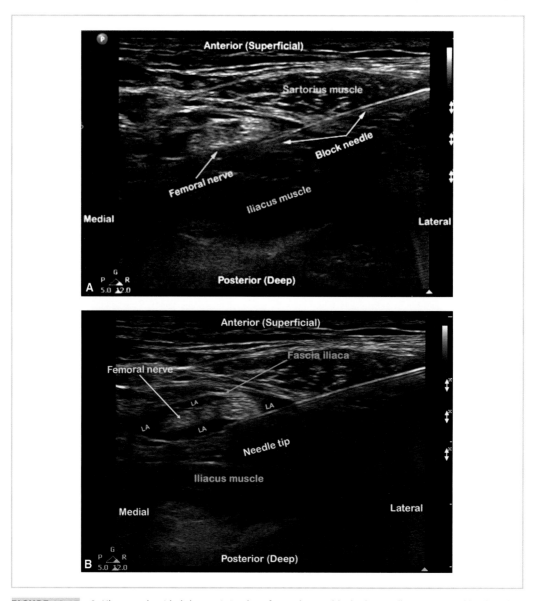

FIGURE 10.17 **A:** Ultrasound-guided short-axis in-plane femoral nerve block. The needle (represented by the *white arrow*) is advanced from a lateral to medial direction and is placed initially just lateral to the femoral nerve and deep to the fascia iliaca. **B:** There is circumferential distribution of local anesthetic (LA) around the femoral nerve. The femoral nerve is located deep to the fascia iliaca (*green arrow*) and superficial to the iliacus muscle.

b. **Ultrasound transducer selection-scanning technique.** A high-frequency linear array transducer (5 to 12 MHz) is typically used for this block. A depth of 3 to 5 cm is adequate for most patients. The US transducer is placed initially at a 90-degree angle, and in an axial orientation over the anteromedial surface of the midthigh. The transducer is adjusted (moved slightly cephalad to caudad, medial to lateral, and cephalad to caudad needle angulation) to obtain and optimize an SAX US image of the target structures.

c. **Ultrasound anatomy** (Fig. 10.19A–C). The major landmark for SSFTB is the **FA**, which is a round, pulsatile, hypoechoic structure located deep to the sartorius muscle. The SN is a small hyperechoic structure adjacent and immediately lateral to the SFA. The compressible **FV** is commonly located directly posterior or posterolateral (and immediately posterior and adjacent to the deep surface of the SN. Within the SSFT, the neurovascular bundle is sandwiched between the adductor muscles (longus and magnus) posteromedially, the VMM anterolaterally, and the sartorius muscle anteromedially. The N-VMM is lateral to the SN and deep to the sartorius muscle (Fig. 10.6).

CLINICAL PEARL The technique begins with "preloading" a 19-guage flexible wire-reinforced catheter (will appear hyperechoic because of the metal wire) into the 17-gauge block needle. The proximal end of the catheter is then connected to a 20-mL syringe filled with the desired solution (saline or local anesthetic), and the catheter is flushed and primed (Fig. 10.19A). The catheter tip is then positioned just proximal to the beveled tip of the block needle (Fig. 10.19B). The advantage of preassembling the catheter-needle is that is that once the needle tip enters the SSFT (or any other perineural location or fascial compartment), the catheter may then be advanced beyond the needle without having to place the catheter in the needle.

d. **Needling technique.** A continuous catheter technique is described because this is the most commonly applied technique for ACB.

After the optimal SAX-view of the SSFT and surrounding muscles are obtained, the preassembled catheter through needle tip is placed 2 to 4 cm lateral to the transducer and advanced in plane toward the SSFT. The most common target for initial needle placement is at the inferior and lateral edge of the SN. When the needle traverses the lateral border of the SSFT, a visible or palpable "loss of resistance" or "pop" is appreciated as the needle tip advances beyond and medial to the VMM. A small test dose of injectate (either local anesthetic or sterile saline is injected) is delivered through catheter tip which should produce an anechoic pool inferior and around the SN. If injectate accumulates within the VMM, the needle tip will have to advanced slightly further to gain access to the SSFT. After the desired volume of solution is injected and the AC has been expanded (to facilitate catheter advancement), the catheter is advanced 3 to 5 cm beyond the needle tip. The needle tip is withdrawn over the catheter, and an additional 2 to 3 mL of injectate is given while observing that the catheter remains within the SSFT.

CLINICAL PEARL If the catheter tip is not easily directly visualized, injection of solution through the catheter, and observing for accumulation of an anechoic pool near the either the SN or FA provides indirect confirmation that the catheter tip is within the SSFT.

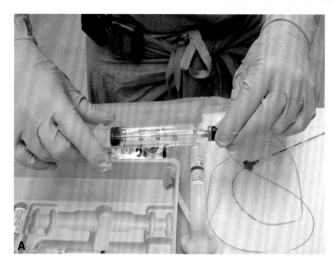

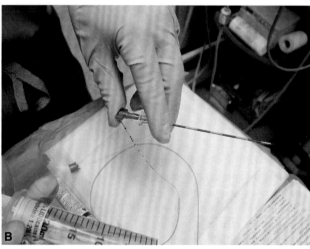

FIGURE 10.18   **A:** The flexible wire-reinforced perineural catheter has already been "preloaded" into the needle. The proximal end of the catheter is connected to the injection syringe. **B:** The catheter is primed until fluid is seen coming from the catheter tip. The catheter tip is positioned just proximal to the beveled end of the block needle.

      e. Local anesthetic volume. For a single-injection technique, 20 mL will fill the SSFT without proximal spread into the FT.[31]

    4. **Continuous catheter technique.** The **continuous catheter technique** has been described in the previous section. Continuous SSFTB is the most commonly used peripheral regional analgesic technique, and many patients are discharged home within 1 to 2 days after TKA. **There are several clinical pearls for management of continuous SSFTBs:**

      a. The timing of when (preoperative vs. postoperative) to place a continuous perineural catheter for SSFTB should be made in conjunction with the surgical team. Practical considerations for preoperative placement include ***theoretical concerns*** of catheter dislodgement during the operation, compression of the catheter next to neurovascular structures by the thigh tourniquet, and the presence of a catheter near the sterile surgical field.

      b. SSFTB block does not provide complete analgesia after TKA, and it is not uncommon for the patients to have mild to moderate discomfort in the postoperative period. The pain may be caused by failure of the SSFTB or it may be caused by pain mediated by either the sciatic and/or ON contribution to the knee. It is difficult to assess for sensory block around the knee because of the surgical dressings and bandages. However, a sensory block along the medial lower leg and over the medial malleolus provides evidence that the SN is blocked within the SSTF.

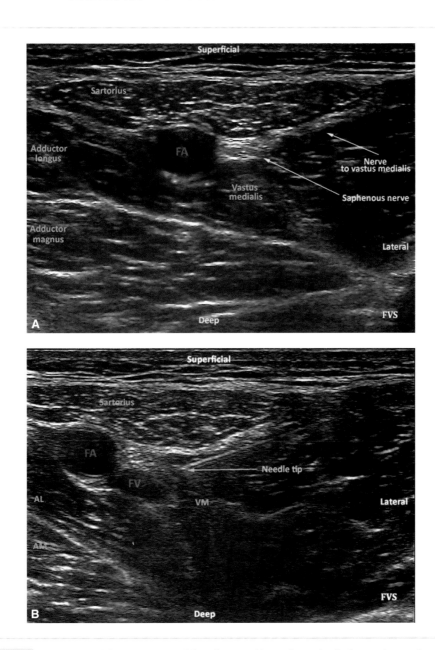

FIGURE 10.19   A: Ultrasound short-axis image of the subsartorial femoral triangle. The hyperechoic saphenous nerve (SN) is located immediately lateral to the SFA. The nerve to the vastus medialis (N-VMM) is located lateral to the SN deep to the sartorius muscle and on the superficial surface of the vastus medialis muscle. **B:** The needle tip is advanced from lateral to medial and is placed beneath and just lateral to the SN. Local anesthetic (LA) is seen on the lateral border of the SN and deep to the N-VMM. The superficial femoral vein (FV) is seen just deep to the SN. **C:** There is circumferential distribution of local anesthetic (LA) around the SN and the N-VMM within the subsartorial femoral triangle.

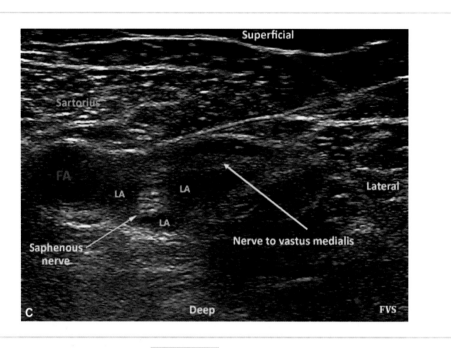

FIGURE 10.19 *(continued)*

    c. SSFTB will typically not result in clinically relevant significant quadriceps motor block and should not contribute to the expected quadriceps motor block associated with TKA. In addition, SSFTB has been demonstrated to provide a clinically relevant increase in quadriceps strength for patients with severe pain after TKA, likely by inhibiting the pain-mediated quadriceps dysfunction.[32]

    d. In the patients with a continuous SSFTB, the delayed onset (12 to 36 hours after beginning the infusion) of increased quadriceps weakness is most likely caused by proximal diffusion of local anesthetic into the FT and resulting blockade of the motor branches to all the quadriceps muscles.[33] The infusion should be temporarily discontinued. If the quadriceps motor block resolves (indicating resolution of a FN block), the infusion may be restarted at a lower rate (and decrease the risk of proximal diffusion), or the SSFT catheter may be removed and replaced more distally. Continued quadriceps weakness 24 to 48 hours after discontinuation of the SSFTB may also represent a rare complication of local anesthetic-induced myotoxicity (of the quadriceps). The weakness may last for 1 to 3 weeks, but will typically resolve completely.[34]

    e. Foot weakness (presenting as lack of plantarflexion or dorsiflexion at the ankle) is not because of SSFTB. Foot weakness (most commonly, a foot-drop) may be caused by persistent blockade of the common peroneal nerve from the periarticular local anesthetic infiltration, or may be due to surgical-induced trauma. Blockade caused by local anesthetic infiltration should resolve within 24 to 48 hours. Persistent foot-drop should prompt further evaluation.

D. Ultrasound-guided obturator nerve block

    1. Indications. Obturator nerve block (**ONB**) is indicated to prevent unwanted adduction of the thigh during transurethral bladder surgery when pharmacologic neuromuscular blockade is not available or contraindicated. Activation of the obturator reflex may result in sudden forceful adduction of the ipsilateral thigh, which may increase the risk of bladder wall perforation or vessel laceration by the resectoscope. Additionally, US-guided ONB may provide additional analgesia (beyond that provided by a subsartorial FT block) after major knee surgery.[35] In the nonoperative setting, ONB is commonly used to treat abductor spasm associated with chronic neurologic disorders.

2. **Contraindications.** Usual contraindications to peripheral nerve blocks (i.e., lack of consent, infection at the injection site, allergy to local anesthetics). Preexisting neural compromise is considered a relative contraindication; a careful discussion regarding the potential risks and benefits of performing peripheral nerve blocks in patients with preexisting neural compromise is strongly recommended.[14]

3. **Single-injection technique**

CLINICAL PEARL   Owing to the significant anatomic variability of the ON, especially regarding the articular branches to the hip joint, USG is the recommended technique of choice.[8] The addition of concurrent PNS has not been shown to improve block success, but does increase block procedure time. To maximize block success and minimize the number of needle passes, targeting the common ON in the interfascial plane between the PM and the OE is the recommended US-guided technique.[9,35,36]

---

   a. **Patient position.** The patient is supine with the operative leg to be blocked slightly abducted and externally rotated.
   b. **US transducer selection-scanning technique.** A high-frequency linear array transducer (5 to 12 MHz) is typically used for this block. A depth of 3 to 5 cm is adequate for most patients. The US transducer is placed initially at a 90-degree angle to the skin in an axial oblique orientation, parallel to the inguinal crease to obtain a view of the FA.
      (1) The transducer is then slid medially along the inguinal crease until the PM is visualized medial to the FV. The transducer is slid further medially until US view demonstrates the characteristic *"Y-shaped"* interfascial plane between the **PM**, **AL**, and **AB** (Fig. 10.20). The PM is located lateral to both the AL and AB. The AD and PD of the ON may be visualized in between the AL and AB and between the AB and **AM**, respectively in this more distal imaging plane.
      (2) The transducer is tilted 40 to 50 degrees cephalad until the intensely hyperechoic (with posterior acoustic dropout) curved structure of the superior pubic ramus is identified deep and lateral to the PM. In this more proximal imaging plane, there is thick hyperechoic fascia deep to the PM and superficial to the OE. The ON is in this interfascial plane (Fig. 10.21).
   c. **Ultrasound anatomy.** The distal SAX imaging plane will show the PM on the lateral aspect of the base of the "Y-shaped" fascial structure. The **AD** and **PD** of the ON appear as small, flattened hyperechoic structures located in between the AM. The AD is between the AL and AB, while the PD is between the AB and AM (Fig. 10.20).

   The SAX proximal interfascial will show the hyperechoic SPR located lateral and deep to the PM. The SPR will appear curvilinear and project an anechoic posterior dropout beneath. The PM is superficial to the OE. The fascia between the PM and OE will appear as a thicker hyperechoic structure extending from lateral to medial from the SPR to the lateral edge of the AB (Fig. 10.21).[36]
   d. **Needling technique.** A 21-guage 100 needle is inserted lateral to the transducer and advanced in-plane from lateral to medial over the SPR and in between the PM and OE. It is not necessary to view the ON because it is often obscured by the thick fascial

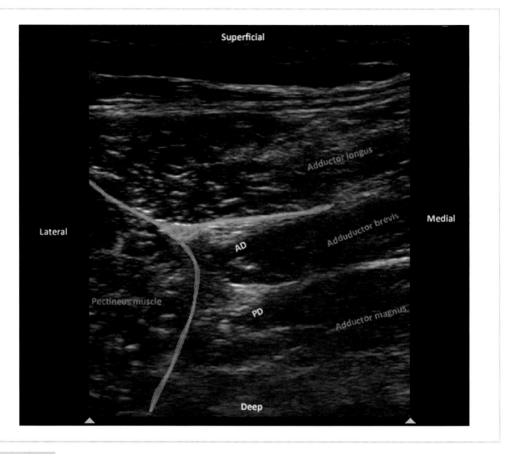

FIGURE 10.20 Short-axis ultrasound image of the distal obturator nerve. A characteristic "Y-shaped" fascial plane (*green line*) is located between the pectineus muscle (located lateral) and the adductor muscles (located medial). The flattened hyperechoic anterior division (AD) and posterior division (PD) of the ON are located between the AL and AB and between the AB and AM, respectively. AB, adductor brevis muscle; AL, adductor longus muscle; AM, adductor magnus; ON, obturator nerve.

between the muscles. A loss of resistance may be appreciated as the needle tip enters the interfascial plane.

    e. **Local anesthetic volume.** 15 mL of local anesthetic will fill the interfascial space and spread proximally to the ON exiting the obturator foramen and distally to the AD and PD of the ON.

  4. Continuous catheter technique. Continuous ON block is rarely indicated in the perioperative setting and will not be described.

E. Ultrasound-guided lateral femoral cutaneous nerve block

  1. Indications. LFCN block is rarely indicated in the acute perioperative setting. Its most common indication is for diagnosis and treatment of the painful chronic mononeuropathy of the LFCN, termed meralgia paresthetica.

  2. Contraindications. Usual contraindications to peripheral nerve blocks (i.e., lack of consent, infection at the injection site, allergy to local anesthetics).

  3. Single-injection technique. The low block success rates of landmark-based (as low as 40%), and/or PNS (85% success rate) techniques are because of the anatomic variability of

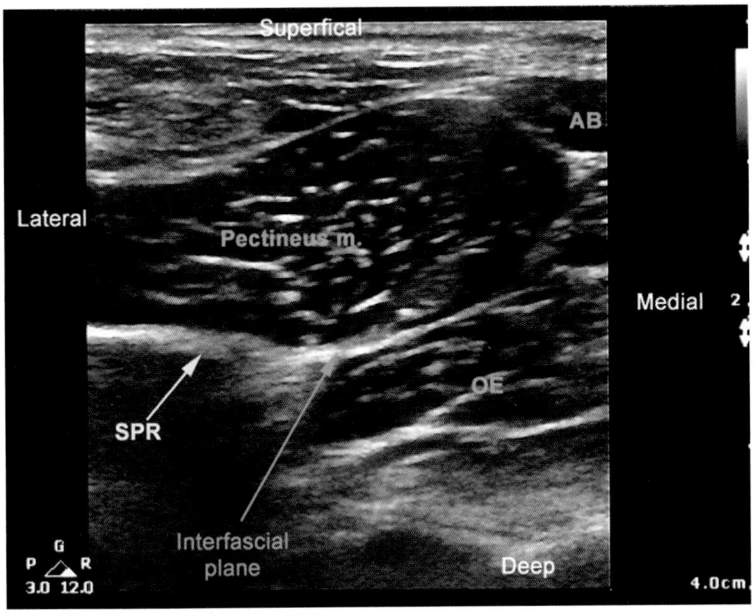

FIGURE 10.21   Short-axis ultrasound image of the proximal interfascial technique for obturator nerve block. The pectineus muscle is located superficial and the obturator externus is located deep to the hyperechoic target fascial plane.

the location and trajectory of the LFCN. USG, however, facilitates direct visualization of either the LCFN or the fascial plane through which the nerve passes.

a. **Patient position.** The patient is in the supine position. The ASIS and the inguinal ligament are marked on the skin to serve as reference points for initial US transducer placement.

b. **Ultrasound transducer selection-scanning technique.** A high-frequency (6 to 13 MHz) linear array transducer is placed in an axial orientation over the ASIS. The ASIS is visualized as a hyperechoic structure with posterior acoustic shadowing. The transducer is then moved distally, and the sartorius muscle is visualized as an inverted triangular structure. The sartorius muscle is directly superficial to the iliac bone, which will be visualized as intensely structure with posterior acoustic dropout (Fig. 10.22). The LFCN will appear as one or more hyperechoic or hypoechoic structures in the SAX view. If the nerve cannot be identified, identify the hyperechoic fascia iliac between the sartorius muscle and the tensor fascia lata.[12,13]

c. **Ultrasound anatomy.** The LFCN will appear as one or more either hyperechoic or hypoechoic structure in SAX view. It is commonly surrounded by a hypoechoic fat pad. If the LCFN cannot be visualized, identify the hyperechoic fascia iliaca located directly superficial to the sartorius and iliacus muscles as a target site for needle placement.

d. **Needling technique.** Owing to the shallow depth of the LCFN, either an SAX in-plane or SAX out-of-plane technique may be used. The needle tip is placed near the LFCN or in between the sartorius muscle and fascia iliaca.

e. **Local anesthetic volume.** 5 to 10 mL of local anesthetic will block the LFCN.

4. **Continuous catheter technique.** Continuous LFCN block is rarely indicated in the perioperative setting and will not be described.

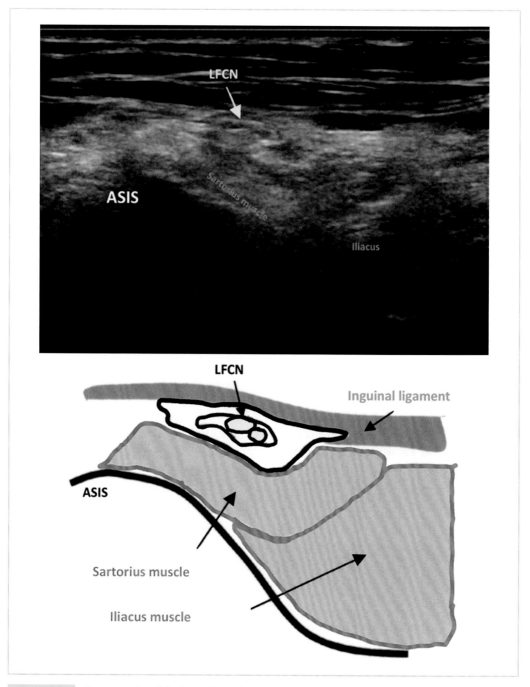

FIGURE 10.22 Short-axis view of the lateral femoral cutaneous nerve (LFCN) just caudal to the anterior superior iliac spine (ASIS). The LFCN is located directly superficial to the sartorius muscle and just deep to the fascia iliaca.

REFERENCES

1. Awad IT, Duggen EM. Posterior lumbar plexus block: anatomy, approaches, and technique. *Reg Anesth Pain Med*. 2005;30:143–149.
2. Farny J, Drolet P, Girard M. Anatomy of the posterior approach to the lumbar plexus block. *Can J Anaesth*. 1994;41:480–485.

3. Birnbaum K, Prescher A, Hebler S, et al. The sensory innervation of the hip joint: an anatomical study. *Surg Radiol Anat.* 1997;19:371–375.
4. Bendtsen TF, Moriggl B, Chan VW, et al. The optimal analgesic block for total knee arthroplasty. *Reg Anesth Pain Med.* 2016;451:711–719.
5. Gustafson KJ, Pinault GCJ, Neville J, et al. Fascicular anatomy of human femoral nerve: implications for neural prosthesis using nerve coffee electrodes. *J Rehabil Res Dev.* 2009;46:973–984.
6. Burckett-St. Laurant D, Peng P, Arango LC, et al. The nerves of the adductor canal and the innervation of the knee: an anatomic study. *Reg Anesth Pain Med.* 2016;41:231–327.
7. Andersen HL, Andersen SL, Tranum-Jensen J. The spread of injectate during saphenous nerve block in the adductor canal block: a cadaver study. *Acta Anaesthesiol Scand.* 2015;59:238–245.
8. Mentzel M, Fleischmann W, Bauer G, et al. Ankle joint denervation. Part 1: anatomy-the sensory innervation of the ankle joint. *Foot Ankle Surg.* 1999;5:15–20.
9. Anagnostopoulou S, Kostopanagiotou G, Paraskeuopoulos T, et al. Anatomic variations of the obturator nerve in the inguinal region: implications in conventional and ultrasound regional anesthesia techniques. *Reg Anesth Pain Med.* 2009;34:33–39.
10. Nielsen TD, Moriggl B, Søballe K, et al. A cadaveric study of ultrasound-guided subpectineal injectate spread around the obturator nerve and its hip articular branches. *Reg Anesth Pain Med.* 2017;42:357–361.
11. Bouaziz H, Vial F, Jochum D, et al. An evaluation of the cutaneous distribution after obturator nerve block. *Anesth Analg.* 2002;94:445–449.
12. Katritsis E, Anagnostopoulou S, Papadopoulos N. Anatomical observations on the accessory obturator nerve (based on 1000 specimens). *Anat Anz.* 1980;148:440–445.
13. Carai A, Fenu G, Sechi E, et al. Anatomical variability of the lateral femoral cutaneous nerve: findings from a surgical series. *Clin Anat.* 2009;22:365–370.
14. Hui GKM, Peng PWH. Meralgia paresthetica: what an anesthesiologist needs to know. *Reg Anesth Pain Med.* 2011;36:156–161.
15. Bodner G, Bernathova M, Galiano K, et al. Ultrasound of the lateral femoral cutaneous nerve: normal findings in a cadaver and in volunteers. *Reg Anesth Pain Med.* 2009;34;265–268.
16. Ilfeld BM. Continuous peripheral nerve blocks: an update of the published evidence and comparison with novel, alternative analgesic modalities. *Anesth Analg.* 2017;124:308–335.
17. Salinas FV. Evidence basis for ultrasound guidance for lower extremity peripheral nerve block: update 2016. *Reg Anesth Pain Med.* 2016;41:261–274.
18. Neal JMN, Barrington MJ, Brull R, et al. The second ASRA Practice Advisory on Neurologic Complications Associated with Regional Anesthesia and Pain Medicine-Executive Summary. *Reg Anesth Pain Med.* 2015;40:401–430.
19. Horlocker TT, Wedel DJ, Rowlingson JC, et al. Executive summary: regional anesthesia in the patient receiving antithrombotic or thrombolytic therapy. American Society of Regional Anesthesia and Pain Medicine Evidence-Based Guidelines (Third Edition). *Reg Anesth Pain Med.* 2010;35:102–105.
20. Chin KJ, Karmakar MK, Peng P. Ultrasonography of the adult thoracic and lumbar spine for central neuraxial blockade. *Anesthesiology.* 2011;114:1459–1485.
21. Karmakar MK, Kwok WH, Soh E, et al. Sonoanatomy relevant for lumbar plexus block in volunteers correlated with cross-sectional anatomical and magnetic resonance images. *Reg Anesth Pain Med.* 2013;38:391–397.
22. Sauter AR, Ullensvang K, Bendtsen TF, et al. Shamrock method: a new and promising technique for ultrasound-guided lumbar plexus block. *Br J Anaesth.* 2013;111 (eLetters Supplement) doi: 10.1093/bja/el_9814.
23. Sauter AR, Ullensvang K, Niemi G, et al. The Shamrock lumbar plexus block: a dose finding study. *Eur J Anaesthesiol.* 2015;32:764–770.
24. Casati A, Baciarello M, Di Cianni S, et al. Effects of ultrasound guidance on the minimum effective anaesthetic volume required to block the femoral nerve. *Br J Anaesth.* 2007;98:823–827.
25. Bendtsen TF, Moriggl B, Chan VW, et al. Redefining the adductor canal block. *Reg Anesth Pain Med.* 2014;39:442–443.
26. Bendtsen TF, Moriggl B, Chan VW, et al. Basic topography of the saphenous nerve in the femoral triangle and the adductor canal block. *Reg Anesth Pain Med.* 2015;40:391–392.
27. Wong WY, Bjorn S, Strid JMC, et al. Defining the location of the adductor canal using ultrasound. *Reg Anesth Pain Med.* 2017;42:241–245.
28. Masaracchia MM, Herrick MD, Barrington MJ, et al. Adductor canal block: changing practice patterns and associated quality profile. *Acta Anaesthesiol Scand.* 2017;61:224–231.

29. Jaeger P, Zaric D, Fomsgaard JS, et al. Adductor canal block versus femoral nerve block for analgesia after total knee arthroplasty: a randomized, double-blind study. *Reg Anesth Pain Med.* 2013;38:526–532.
30. Jaeger P, Nielsen ZJ, Henningsen MH, et al. Adductor canal block versus femoral nerve block and quadriceps strength: a randomized, double-blind, placebo-controlled, c°rossover study in healthy volunteers. *Anesthesiology.* 2013;118:409–415.
31. Jaeger P, Jenstrup MT, Lund J, et al. Optimal volume of local anaesthetic for adductor canal block: using the continual reassessment method to estimate ED95. *Br J Anesth.* 2015;115:920–926.
32. Grevstad U, Mathiesen O, Valentir LS, et al. Effect of adductor canal block versus femoral nerve block on quadriceps strength, mobilization, and pain after total knee arthroplasty: a randomized, blinded study. *Reg Anesth Pain Med.* 2015;40:3–10.
33. Veal C, Auyong DB, Hanson NA, et al. Delayed quadriceps weakness after continuous adductor canal block for total knee arthroplasty. *Acta Anaesthesiol Scand.* 2014;58:362–364.
34. Neal JM, Salinas FV, Choi DS. Local anesthetic-induced myotoxicity after continuous adductor canal block. *Reg Anesth Pain Med.* 2016;41:723–727.
35. Runge C, Borglum J, Jensen JM, et al. The analgesic effect of obturator nerve block added to a femoral triangle block after total knee arthroplasty: a randomized controlled trial. *Reg Anesth Pain Med.* 2016;41:445–451.
36. Taha A. Ultrasound-guided obturator nerve block: a proximal interfascial approach. *Anesth Analg.* 2012;114:236–239.

11

Lower Extremity-Sciatic Nerve Block

Francis V. Salinas

I. **Anatomy**

II. **Drugs**

III. **Approaches and techniques**
  A. **Ultrasound-guided subgluteal approach**
  B. **Ultrasound-guided midfemoral approach**

C. **Ultrasound-guided popliteal approach**

D. **Ultrasound-guided anterior approach**

E. **Ankle block**

KEY POINTS

1. Detailed knowledge of the anatomy of the sciatic nerve, and the osseous and articular innervation of the joints of the lower extremity will allow the operator to select the optimal approach based on the surgical procedure.

2. Ultrasonography has become the predominant technique for sciatic nerve localization.

3. The main approaches to the sciatic nerve block include subgluteal, midfemoral, popliteal, and anterior.

4. Based on the preference/experience of the operator and the coexisting conditions of the patient, the patient may be placed in either the lateral, prone, or supine positions.

5. The deeper approaches to sciatic nerve block (subgluteal and anterior) should be performed with a low-frequency (2 to 5 MHz) curved array ultrasound transducer.

6. Local anesthetic injection deep to the paraneural sheath at the bifurcation of the sciatic nerve consistently provides a more rapid block onset compared to injection external to the paraneural sheath.

7. Ankle block anesthetizes the four terminal peripheral nerve branches of the sciatic nerve, as well as the terminal branch of the femoral nerve (saphenous), and may be successfully performed without ultrasound guidance.

I. **Anatomy.** The sacral plexus is located on the surface of the posterior pelvic wall, anterior to the piriformis muscle. It is formed from the ventral rami of the sacral spinal nerves (S1–S4). It also receives contributions from the lumbar spinal nerves (L4 and L5) via the lumbosacral trunk (Fig. 10.1). The ventral rami enter the pelvis through the anterior sacral foramina and converge to form the sacral plexus. The sacral plexus has a flattened triangular shape with its base oriented lateral to the sacral foramina and its vertex toward the greater sciatic foramen (Figs. 10.1 and 11.1). It lies anterior to the piriformis muscle and posterior to the presacral fascia, which separates it from the intrapelvic viscera. The sacral plexus provides sensory and motor innervation to portions of the lower extremity, including the hip, knee, and ankle joints. The most important branch for lower extremity surgery is the sciatic nerve.

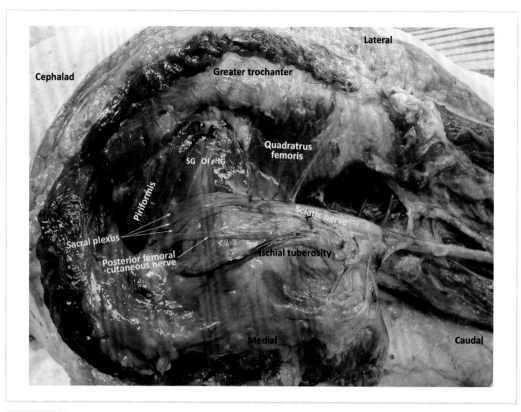

FIGURE 11.1　Cadaver dissection of the sacral plexus and proximal sciatic nerve. SG, superior gemellus; OI, obturator internus; IG, inferior gemellus.

> **CLINICAL PEARL**　Sacral plexus branches that provide articular innervation to the posterior hip joint include the superior gluteal nerve, quadratus femoris nerve, and inferior gemellus nerve. Sacral plexus block combined with lumbar plexus block provides complete sensory block for major hip surgery (hip replacement or hip fracture repair) (1).

A. The lumbosacral trunk (L4 and L5) and the anterior divisions of the S1–S3 ventral rami give rise to the tibial nerve (**TN**), whereas the posterior divisions of S1–S3 ventral rami give rise to the common peroneal nerve (**CPN**). These two distinct nerves travel together to form the sciatic nerve (**SN**). They are independent nerves that do not mix nerve fibers, but they share a common trajectory and common extraneural connective tissue sheath until they physically diverge from each other within the popliteal fossa.

B. As the sciatic nerve exits the pelvis through the infrapiriform foramen at the inferior border of the piriformis, the larger TN is medial and slightly anterior to the CPN. From the point where the sacral plexus first enters the pelvis until the sciatic nerve leaves the gluteal compartment just distal to the ischial tuberosity (IT) of the ischium and greater trochanter (GT) of the femur, it is covered by the mass of the gluteus maximus (Figs. 11.1 and 11.2). Within the gluteal region, the sciatic nerve is located just lateral to the posterior femoral cutaneous nerve and the inferior gluteal artery. Between the IT (medially) and the GT (laterally), the sciatic nerve is in a well-defined intermuscular compartment (*subgluteal compartment*) superficial to the quadratus femoris and deep to gluteus maximus.

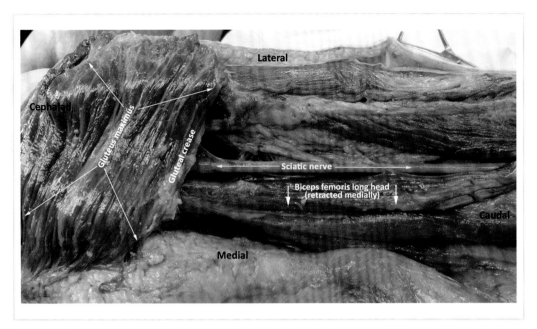

FIGURE 11.2   Cadaver dissection of the trajectory of the sciatic nerve from the proximal thigh to the popliteal fossa. Note the gluteus maximus overlying the proximal sciatic nerve. Note the biceps femoris has been retracted medially.

C. The sciatic nerve descends caudally within the posterior thigh, by passing between the lateral border of the IT and the medial border of the proximal femur (Figs. 11.1 and 11.2). As the sciatic nerve courses into the posterior compartment of the proximal thigh, it lies posterior to the lesser trochanter of the femur. Within the proximal posterior compartment of the thigh, just distal to the inferior border of the gluteus maximus, the sciatic nerve lies on the posterior surface of the adductor magnus muscle immediately lateral to the tendon of the biceps femoris muscle (Figs. 11.2 and 11.3). At this location, the sciatic nerve is relatively superficial and covered only by skin and subcutaneous tissue.

D. Within the midthigh (approximately halfway between the lateral aspect of the GT and the popliteal crease), the sciatic nerve is located posterior and medial to the shaft of the femur in a myofascial plane: dorsal (superficial) to the adductor magnus and ventral (deep) to the belly of the long head of the biceps femoris.

E. As the sciatic nerve continues further distally within the middle third of the posterior compartment of the thigh toward the popliteal fossa, it lies in an intermuscular plane between the adductor magnus and the long head of the biceps femoris muscles (Fig. 11.4).

F. Within the apex of the popliteal fossa, the sciatic nerve is bordered laterally by the long head of the biceps femoris muscle tendon and medially by the semimembranosus–semitendinosus (**SM-ST**) tendons (Figs. 11.3 and 11.4). The divergence of the sciatic nerve into the physically separate TN and CPN components (Figs. 11.3 and 11.4) occurs within the proximal aspect of the popliteal fossa (6 to 9 cm above the popliteal crease, but with a range of 0 to 14 cm), but it may also occur at any point between the sacral plexus and the popliteal crease. Within the popliteal fossa, the sciatic nerve lies posterolateral to the popliteal artery and vein.

II. Drugs

A. The choice of local anesthetic for sciatic nerve block is dependent on the requirements for **onset of anesthesia** and **duration** of analgesia for single-injection techniques, as well as the anatomic

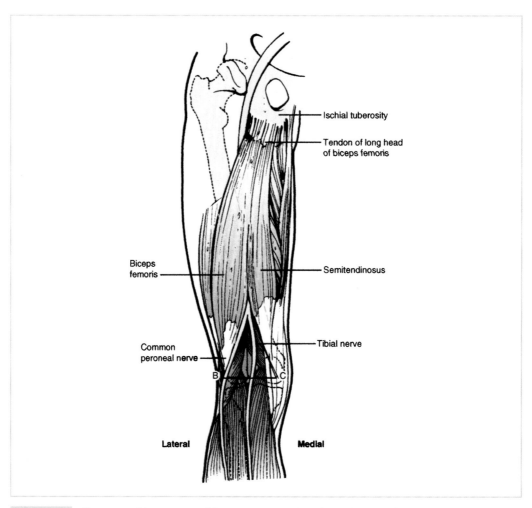

FIGURE 11.3 Illustration of the trajectory of the sciatic nerve and its relationship to the femur and hamstring muscles in the posterior thigh. The medial border of the popliteal fossa is the semi-tendinosis, and the lateral border is the long head of biceps femoris.

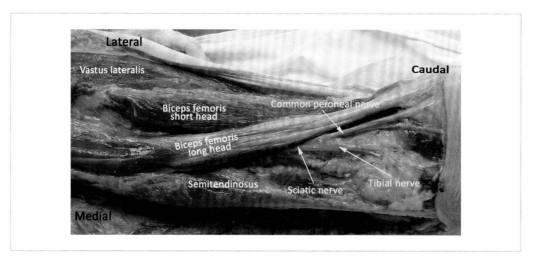

FIGURE 11.4 Cadaver dissection of the distal sciatic nerve in the popliteal fossa. Note the bifurcation of the sciatic nerve into the tibial nerve and common peroneal nerve. Note common peroneal nerve continuing along the lateral border of the popliteal fossa, adjacent to the tendon of the long head of biceps femoris.

location where the block is performed. The sciatic nerve block is different from the individual nerve blocks of the lumbar plexus because the approach (anatomic location) for sciatic nerve block may have an impact on the onset and total local anesthetic mass requirements.

B. Specifically, the proximal approaches to sciatic nerve block have a shorter latency to complete anesthesia and lower total anesthetic requirements compared with the distal popliteal approaches (2). This is likely owing to the difference in the quantitative architecture (ratio of neural tissue and nonneural tissue within and external to the epineurium) between the proximal and distal approaches (3,4).

C. With the advent of **continuous perineural catheter techniques,** the anesthesiologist can extend the anesthetic duration (Tables 11.1 and 11.2) of surgical anesthesia by simply redosing through the indwelling perineural catheter. More commonly, a postoperative infusion of a dilute local anesthetic (e.g., ropivacaine 0.2% or bupivacaine 0.125%) may be used to provide the optimal balance of postoperative analgesia with minimal motor block to facilitate postoperative rehabilitation and recovery. Alternatively, if a neuraxial technique is chosen as the primary anesthetic, a loading dose (10 to 15 mL) of the analgesic infusion of ropivacaine 0.2% may be started intraoperatively. The typical postoperative regimen consists of running the analgesic infusion at 4 to 10 mL/h with or without a patient-controlled bolus of 2 to 5 mL every 20 to 60 minutes based on institutional protocols.

III. **Approaches and techniques**

CLINICAL PEARL The term *approach* refers to the anatomic location where the sciatic nerve is targeted (e.g., subgluteal vs. popliteal). The term *technique* refers to the modality for nerve localization (e.g., ultrasound guidance [USG], peripheral nerve stimulation [PNS], or a combination of both) utilized for a given approach.

2 USG has become the predominant technique for peripheral nerve localization. USG has not only been shown to increase the onset of complete sensory block but also decreases block performance time, block onset time, and local anesthetic requirements compared to PNS (5). There is no evidence to support the routine use of concurrent PNS to supplement a primary USG (*dual-guidance*) technique, especially when the target nerve is well visualized. However, a dual-guidance technique may be useful in two specific circumstances: (1) when target nerve visualization is difficult in specific circumstances, such as increased body habitus, deep nerve location (subgluteal or anterior approach), or anatomic variation and (2) evoked motor responses at current output ≤0.2 mA is highly suggestive of intraneural needle placement, and should prompt slight withdrawal or repositioning of the needle tip prior to local anesthetic injection; however, stimulatory thresholds >0.2 mA do not offer a fail-safe guarantee that the needle tip is extraneural. The sciatic nerve is the longest nerve in the body and **3** may be blocked using the approaches such as subgluteal, anterior, midfemoral, or popliteal levels.

TABLE 11.1 Local anesthetic choices for sacral plexus and proximal sciatic nerve blocks

Local anesthetic (%)	Duration of anesthesia (h)	Duration of analgesia (h)
Lidocaine 1.5–2	3–4	4–6
Mepivacaine 1.5–2	4–5	5–8
Ropivacaine 0.5–0.75	6–12	6–24
Bupivacaine 0.5	8–16	10–24

TABLE 11.2 Local anesthetic choices for distal popliteal sciatic nerve block

Local anesthetic (%)	Duration of anesthesia (h)	Duration of analgesia (h)
Lidocaine 1.5–2	4–5	4–8
Mepivacaine 1.5–2	4–6	6–8
Ropivacaine 0.5–0.75	6–12	12–24
Bupivacaine 0.5	6–12	12–36

4 **CLINICAL PEARL** Although the sciatic nerve is typically *visualized approached* by placing the US transducer on the posterior surface of the thigh, the sciatic nerve may also be *visualized approached* by placing the transducer on the anterior surface of the proximal thigh. The choice of approach will be dictated by the requirements for surgical anesthesia and postoperative analgesia, as well as the ability of the patient to assume the desired position. Although posterior approaches are the most commonly performed techniques, patient factors (morbid obesity, painful fractures, and the presence of casts-fixation devices) may preclude patients from assuming either the lateral decubitus or prone position (6).

A. **Ultrasound-guided subgluteal approach**

1. **Indications.** In combination with a lumbar plexus block (or a combination of femoral, lateral femoral cutaneous, and obturator nerve blocks), complete anesthesia or analgesia for the entire lower extremity from the proximal thigh (distal to the hip joint) to the foot. In combination with a femoral nerve block (or saphenous nerve block above the knee), complete anesthesia or analgesia for the entire lower extremity from below the knee to the foot.

2. **Contraindications.** Usual contraindications to peripheral nerve blocks (i.e., lack of consent, infection at the injection site, allergy to local anesthetics). Preexisting neural compromise is considered a relative contraindication; a careful discussion regarding the potential risks and benefits of performing peripheral nerve blocks in patients with preexisting neural compromise is strongly recommended (6).

3. Single-injection technique
   a. **Patient position.** The patient is typically placed in the lateral decubitus position with a slight forward tilt, hips flexed with the operative side to be blocked uppermost. The dependent limb should be straight, and the operative limb should be slightly flexed at both the hip and the knee. Alternatively, the patient may be placed in the prone position.

4 **CLINICAL PEARL** The choice of patient position will depend on the patient's body habitus, coexisting medical conditions, as well as a preference of the operator.

   b. **Ultrasound transducer selection-scanning technique.** A low-frequency curved array transducer (2 to 5 MHz) is typically used for this block. The US transducer is initially placed at a 90-degree angle to the skin, with the long axis (LAX) of the probe directly over and parallel to a line connecting the IT and GT to obtain a short-axis (SAX) US image of the sciatic nerve (Fig. 11.5A and B).

5 **CLINICAL PEARL** The low-frequency curved array transducer allows greater tissue penetration of the US waves for the deeper location of the sciatic nerve in the subgluteal compartment, as well as providing a wider field of view required to visualize the both the GT and IT.

    c. Ultrasound anatomy (Fig. 11.6). The sciatic nerve appears as a hyperechoic, oval to lip-shaped polyfascicular structure (7,8). Slight adjustments in the transducer position will enhance the anisotropy of the sciatic nerve and optimize its sonographic appearance. The subgluteal compartment is bordered laterally by the GT and medially by the IT, with the sciatic nerve typically located within 3.0 cm lateral to the IT. Both IT and GT appear as intensely hyperechoic curved structures with posterior acoustic dropout. The sciatic nerve is sandwiched deep to the epimysium of the gluteus maximus muscle and superficial to the epimysium of the quadratus femoris muscle. The epimysium of the two muscles forms the subgluteal compartment and appears to suspend the sciatic nerve in between the GT and IT.

    d. Needling technique. Based on the depth of the sciatic nerve, a 100 mm 21-gauge or 150 mm 20-gauge needle is inserted lateral to the lateral aspect of the US transducer (Fig. 11.5). The needle tip is advanced in-plane (SAX-IP) from lateral to medial (Fig. 11.5B), targeting the hyperechoic fascial plane on the lateral boarder of the sciatic nerve (Fig. 11.6). As the needle tip approaches the sciatic nerve, a visible pop or tactile loss of resistance may be appreciated because the needle tip penetrates the fascial plane of the subgluteal compartment. Local anesthetic is injected, and its distribution deep to the gluteus maximus within the subgluteal space, around the sciatic nerve, is observed in real time (Fig. 11.7).

CLINICAL PEARL Because the sciatic nerve may be quite deep in the subgluteal location, the SAX-IP technique may offer no benefit (in terms of needle tip visualization); in this setting, the short-axis out-of-plane (SAX-OOP) technique allows a shorter distance from the skin to the nerve. If the needle tip is still difficult to visualize, injection of small aliquots of either local anesthetic or saline (appearing as anechoic relative to the surrounding tissue) or air (appearing hyperechoic relative to the surrounding tissue) may facilitate the estimation of the depth of the needle tip.

    e. Local anesthetic volume. Typically, a volume of 20 to 30 mL is required to obtain satisfactory local anesthetic distribution around the sciatic nerve within the subgluteal compartment.

  4. Continuous catheter technique. If a **continuous catheter technique** is indicated, a larger bore (17- to 18-gauge) Tuohy needle is typically used for initial placement of the needle tip and local anesthetic within the subgluteal compartment. After local anesthetic distribution (by injection through the needle tip) is ensured, the US probe is placed aside within the sterile field. A 19- to 20-gauge catheter is inserted through the Tuohy needle and advanced no more than 2 to 3 cm past needle tip. At this point, the US probe is placed over the original site, and an additional 3 to 5 mL of local anesthetic is injected through the catheter while confirming local anesthetic distribution around the sciatic nerve to confirm correct catheter tip position. The needle is then withdrawn over the catheter and fixed in place with a sterile clear adhesive dressing. The proximal end of the catheter is then connected to an infusion pump.

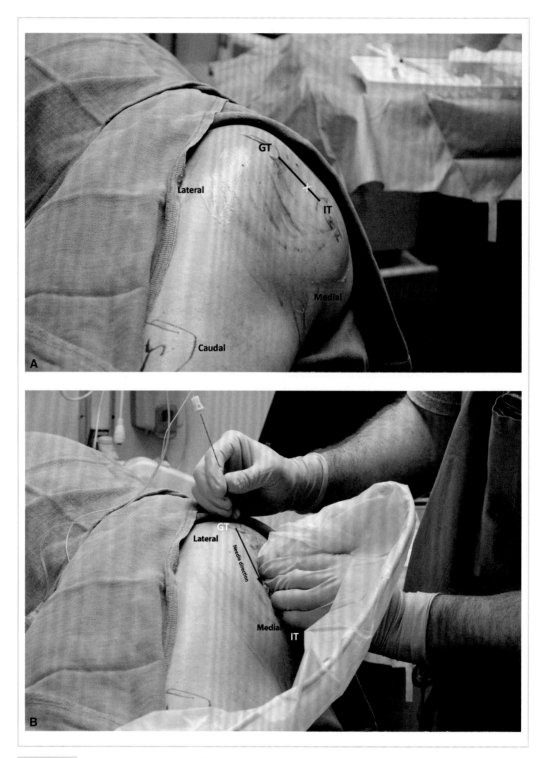

FIGURE 11.5   **A:** Lateral position for the subgluteal approach. The projection for the location of the sciatic nerve between the medial border of the GT and lateral border of the IT is marked by the yellow X. **B:** Ultrasound transducer position, needle placement, and needle direction for SAX-IP technique for subgluteal approach. GT, greater trochanter; IT, ischial tuberosity; SAX-IP, short-axis in-plane.

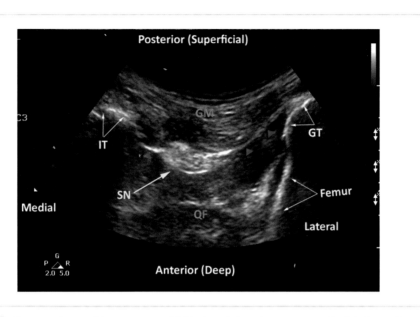

FIGURE 11.6 Short-axis image of the sciatic nerve (SN) in the subgluteal compartment. The SN is located between the IT and GT, and in the intermuscular plane between the GM and QF. Blue arrows highlight the epimysium of the GM and QF. GM, gluteus maximus; GT, greater trochanter; IT, ischial tuberosity; QF, quadratus femoris.

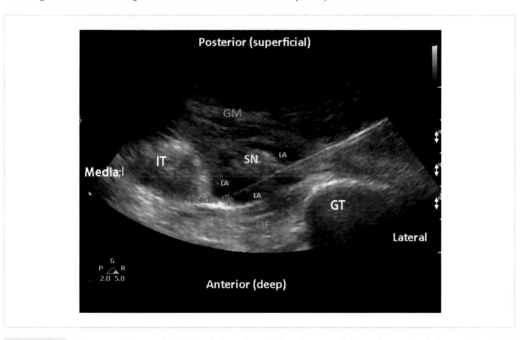

FIGURE 11.7 Ultrasound image of SAX-IP technique for subgluteal approach. Note the needle tip located lateral and just deep to the sciatic nerve (SN). Note the hypoechoic circumferential collection of local anesthetic (LA) around the SN. GM, gluteus maximus; GT, greater trochanter; IT, ischial tuberosity; QF, quadratus femoris; SAX-IP, short-axis in-plane.

   B. Ultrasound-guided midfemoral approach

       1. Indications. In combination with a lumbar plexus block (or combined femoral–obturator nerve blocks), complete anesthesia or analgesia for the entire lower extremity from the knee to the foot. In combination with a femoral nerve block (or saphenous nerve block above the knee), complete anesthesia or analgesia for the entire lower extremity from below the knee to the foot.

CLINICAL PEARL   The midfemoral approach has the advantage of typically being a more superficial block compared to the subgluteal or anterior approach, and may be used when a popliteal approach cannot be performed (because of prior surgery in the popliteal fossa or the presence of a cast covering the latter).

2. **Contraindications.** Usual contraindications to peripheral nerve blocks (i.e., lack of consent, infection at the injection site, allergy to local anesthetics). Preexisting neural compromise is considered a relative contraindication; a careful discussion regarding the potential risks and benefits of performing peripheral nerve blocks in patients with preexisting neural compromise is strongly recommended.

3. **Single-injection technique**
   a. **Patient position.** The patient is placed in the lateral decubitus position with a slight forward tilt, hips flexed with the operative side to be blocked uppermost. The dependent limb should be straight, and the operative limb should be slightly flexed at both the hip and the knee. Alternatively, the patient may be placed in the prone position.
   b. **Ultrasound transducer-scanning technique.** A high-frequency linear array (6 to 15 MHz) transducer is placed perpendicular to LAX of the posterior surface of the midthigh (Fig. 11.8) to obtain an SAX US image of the sciatic nerve.
   c. **Ultrasound anatomy.** The sciatic nerve appears as a hyperechoic polyfascicular structure that is wide and oval flat in shape (7). The sciatic nerve is located superficial (posterior) and medial to the intensely hyperechoic curvilinear line representing the posterior border of the femoral shaft, and sandwiched between the deep surface of the biceps (long head) femoris and the superficial surface of the adductor magnus muscles. The lateral intermuscular septum is visualized as a hyperechoic line traveling from a posterolateral to an anteromedial direction toward the sciatic nerve (9) (Fig. 11.9).
   d. **Needling technique.** Based on the depth of the sciatic nerve, a 100 mm 21-gauge or 150 mm 20-gauge needle is inserted lateral to the lateral aspect of the US transducer (Fig. 11.8B). The needle tip is advanced in-plane from lateral to medial through the vastus lateralis or along the lateral intermuscular septum to initially target the lateral aspect of the sciatic nerve (Fig. 11.10). Local anesthetic is injected, and its distribution deep to the biceps femoris and superficial to the adductor magnus around the sciatic nerve is observed in real time (Fig. 11.11).
   e. **Local anesthetic volume.** Typically, a volume of 20 to 30 mL is required to obtain satisfactory local anesthetic distribution around the sciatic nerve with the midfemoral approach.

4. **Continuous catheter technique.** If a **continuous catheter technique** is indicated, a larger bore (17- to 18-gauge) Tuohy needle is typically used for initial placement of the needle tip and local anesthetic injection. After local anesthetic distribution (by injection through the needle tip) is ensured, the US probe is placed aside within the sterile field. A 19- to 20-gauge catheter is inserted through the Tuohy needle and advanced no more than 2 to 3 cm past needle tip. At this point, the US probe is placed over the original site, and an additional 3 to 5 mL of local anesthetic is injected through the catheter while confirming local anesthetic distribution around the sciatic nerve to confirm correct catheter tip position. The needle is then withdrawn over the catheter and fixed in place with a sterile clear adhesive dressing. The proximal end of the catheter is then connected to an infusion pump.

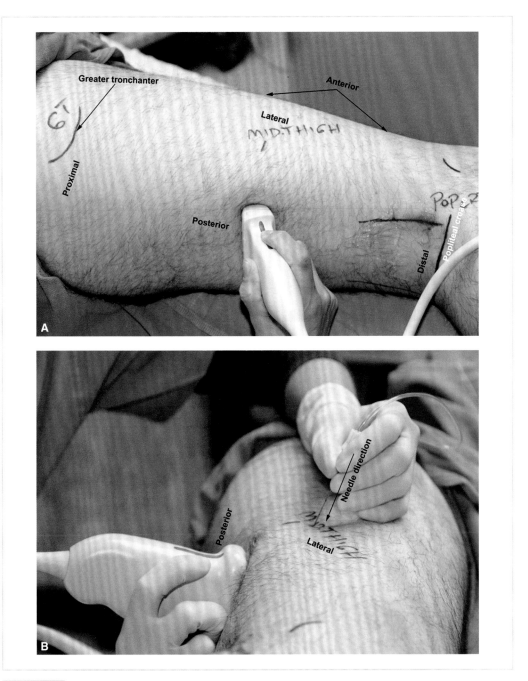

FIGURE 11.8 **A:** Lateral patient position and ultrasound transducer placement for midfemoral approach. **B:** Needle placement along lateral thigh relative to ultrasound transducer position for midfemoral approach. Note the needle trajectory will be perpendicular to the direction of the ultrasound beam.

CLINICAL PEARL If a midfemoral sciatic perineural catheter is indicated, consideration should be given to the possible placement of a midthigh tourniquet. The continuous catheter should then be placed postoperatively. Alternatively, the continuous catheter may be placed preoperatively, and the thigh tourniquet should be adjusted to prevent placement over the catheter insertion site.

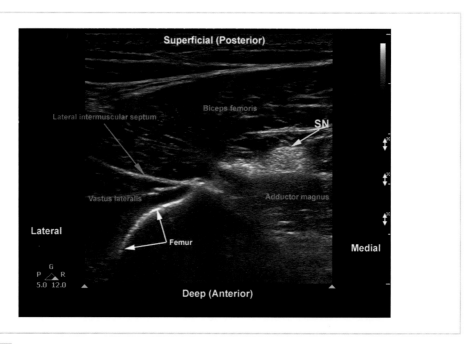

FIGURE 11.9 SAX image of sciatic nerve (SN) at the midfemoral approach. The nerve is in the intermuscular plane between the biceps femoris and adductor magnus. The SN is medial and posterior (superficial) to the posterior border of the femur. SAX, short-axis.

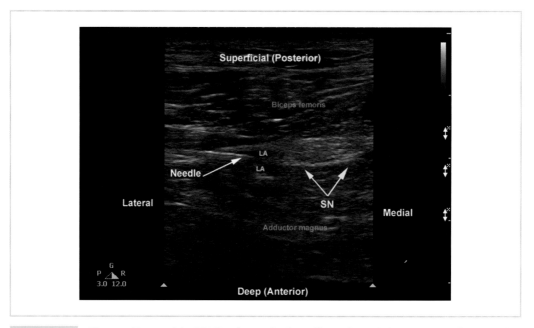

FIGURE 11.10 Ultrasound image of the SAX-IP technique for the midfemoral approach. Note the needle approaches the lateral aspect of the sciatic nerve (SN). LA, local anesthetic; SAX-IP, short-axis in-plane.

C. **Ultrasound-guided popliteal approach**

1. **Indications.** In combination with either a femoral nerve block or a saphenous nerve block (above the knee), complete anesthesia or analgesia for the entire lower extremity from below the knee to the foot, especially when a calf tourniquet is utilized. May be used as the

sole anesthetic–analgesic for foot surgery if the saphenous nerve distribution is not located within the surgical incision and an ankle tourniquet is utilized.

2. **Contraindications.** Usual contraindications to peripheral nerve blocks (i.e., lack of consent, infection at the injection site, allergy to local anesthetics). Preexisting neural compromise is considered a relative contraindication; a careful discussion regarding the potential risks and benefits of performing peripheral nerve blocks in patients with preexisting neural compromise is strongly recommended.

3. **Single-injection technique**
    a. **Patient position.** The patient is typically placed in the lateral decubitus position with a slight forward tilt, hips flexed with the operative side to be blocked uppermost (Fig. 11.12A). The dependent limb should be straight, and the operative limb should be slightly flexed at both the hip and the knee. The patient may also be placed in the prone position (Fig. 11.12B) or in the supine position (with the lower leg elevated on either a surgical mayo stand or pillows to elevate the popliteal fossa of the surface of patient bed-gurney or operating room table) based on the preference of the anesthesiologist and/or the coexisting conditions of the patient.

CLINICAL PEARL   Despite the three different positions for the popliteal fossa approach, they share the same desired US transducer position placement on the posterior distal thigh over the popliteal fossa. The supine position is the most technically challenging because this requires constant "upward pressure" on the US transducer to maintain contact with the skin surface, which can be difficult and fatiguing for the scanning hand-arm of the anesthesiologist.

    b. **Ultrasound transducer-scanning technique.** A high-frequency (6 to 15 MHz) broadband linear array transducer is initially placed perpendicular (Fig. 11.12A and B) to the LAX of the distal thigh (parallel to the popliteal crease). This will allow a SAX view of the popliteal sciatic nerve components and the popliteal vessels. Once the popliteal vessels are identified, the US transducer probe is slowly advanced proximally until the TN is identified. The TN will be located superficially (posteriorly) and slightly lateral to the popliteal artery and vein. As the US probe is advanced further proximally, the CPN will converge from its lateral location within the popliteal fossa toward the TN to form the common SN (Figs. 11.3 and 11.4). The US transducer position should be adjusted to obtain a view of the bifurcation of the sciatic nerve into the TN and CPN.

CLINICAL PEARL   The advantage of this systematic traceback technique, as originally described by Ban Tsui, is threefold (10):
1. The anechoic popliteal vessels may be much more readily visualized than the sciatic nerve and serve as useful landmarks to locate the TN and CPN.
2. The hyperechoic appearance of the sciatic nerve in the apex of the popliteal fossa may be similar in sonographic appearance to the surrounding muscles and tendons. By starting from the distal aspect of the popliteal fossa, the TN may first be identified and then the CPN may be identified, because they converge to form the sciatic nerve.
3. The point at which the TN and CPN converge to form the sciatic nerve should be noted. It has been demonstrated that US-guided deposition of local anesthetic deep to the paraneural sheath at the sciatic nerve bifurcation provides a significantly faster onset of sensory and motor block compared to local anesthetic deposition external to the paraneural sheath (10,11).

6

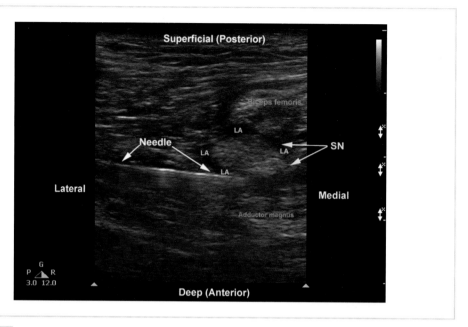

FIGURE 11.11 SAX image of circumferential local anesthetic (LA) distribution around the midfemoral sciatic nerve (SN). SAX, short-axis.

c. **Ultrasound anatomy.** The sciatic nerve appears as a round hyperechoic polyfascicular (honeycomb appearance) structure in the proximal (apex) popliteal fossa (7,10). The sciatic nerve is located superficially (at a depth of 2 to 4 cm) and slightly lateral to the deeper located popliteal artery and vein. The biceps femoris muscle is lateral and the SM-ST muscles are medial, respectively, to the popliteal vessels and sciatic nerve. As the transducer is moved more distally, the TN and CPN will physically diverge from each other and assume an even shallower depth within the distal popliteal fossa. The larger TN courses distally in the midline of the popliteal fossa, whereas the smaller CPN will course distally adjacent and immediately medial to the SM-ST muscles (Fig. 11.13A and B).

CLINICAL PEARL The sciatic nerve exhibits a significant degree of anisotropy because it becomes more superficial as it courses distally within the popliteal fossa. Thus, by angling the beam of the transducer more caudally (toward the foot), this will align the US beam (angle of incidence) closer to a 90-degree angle to the sciatic nerve and optimize the amount of reflection toward the transducer, thus optimizing the sonographic appearance (Fig. 11.14A and B).

d. **Needling technique.** With the SAX-IP technique, the US transducer is placed on the posterior surface of the popliteal fossa, and a 100 mm 21-gauge or 150 mm-20-gauge needle is inserted along the lateral or posterolateral aspect of the distal thigh (Fig. 11.12A and B).

CLINICAL PEARL Prior to inserting and advancing the needle, note the depth of the sciatic nerve on the US screen and insert the needle at the appropriate depth so that the needle will approach the sciatic nerve to as close as a 90-degee angle as possible to the direction of the US beam. This optimizes the US beam angle of incidence to the needle and enhances the amount of specular reflection back to the US probe.

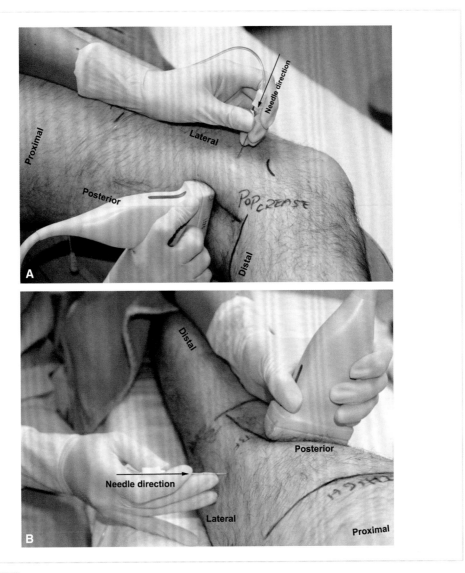

FIGURE 11.12 **A:** Lateral patient position, ultrasound transducer placement, and needle placement–needle direction for SAX-IP technique for popliteal approach. **B:** Prone patient position, ultrasound transducer placement, and needle placement–needle direction for SAX-IP technique for popliteal approach. SAX-IP, short-axis in-plane.

The needle will traverse through the medial border of the biceps femoris muscle as it enters the popliteal fossa and approaches the lateral aspect (CPN) of the SN (Fig. 11.12A). The target location is the either at 12:00 o'clock or 6:00 o'clock position at the cleavage plane between the TN and CPN (Fig. 11.15B). Incremental injection of local anesthetic deep to the paraneural sheath will result in circumferential local anesthetic distribution around both TN and CPN (Fig. 11.15C) (12).

With the SAX-OOP technique, the US transducer is placed in the same initial location as with the SAX-IP technique; the US transducer is placed on the posterior surface of the popliteal fossa. A 100 mm 21-gauge needle is inserted 2 to 3 cm distal to the midpoint of the transducer and is advanced at a 45 to 60 degrees angle targeting where the cleavage plane between the TN and CPN at the 12:00 0'clock position. Incremental injection of local anesthetic deep to the paraneural sheath will result in circumferential local anesthetic distribution around both the TN and CPN.

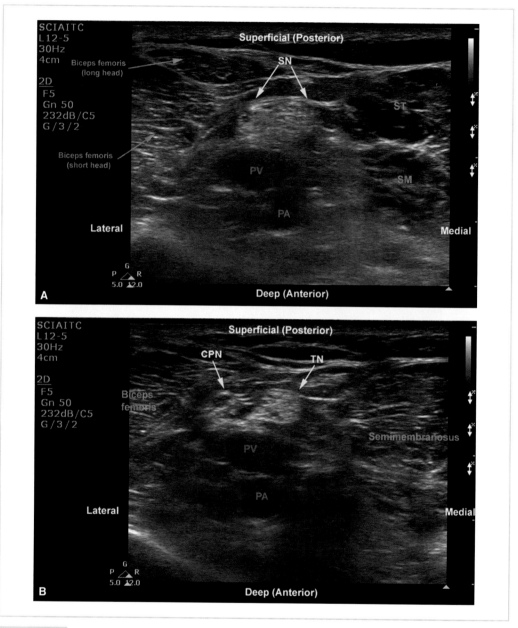

FIGURE 11.13   **A:** SAX image of the sciatic nerve (SN) in the popliteal fossa. The SN is located superficial to the popliteal vein (PV) and popliteal artery (PA). The biceps femoris and the semitendinosis–semimembranosus (ST-SM) form the medial and lateral borders, respectively, of the popliteal fossa. **B:** SAX image of the bifurcation of the sciatic into the tibial nerve (TN) and common peroneal nerve (CPN). Note the cleavage plane between the TN and CPN. SAX, short-axis.

CLINICAL PEARL   The paraneural sheath is often not readily visible prior to local anesthetic injection. Penetration of the paraneural sheath at the cleavage plane between the TN and CPN, followed by subsequent injection should result in separation of the TN and CPN by the local anesthetic, and enhanced visibility of the thin hyperechoic circumferential paraneural sheath enveloping the anechoic local anesthetic surrounding the TN and CPN (12,13). Scanning proximally should demonstrate distention of the paraneural sheath and circumferential local anesthetic distribution around the sciatic nerve.

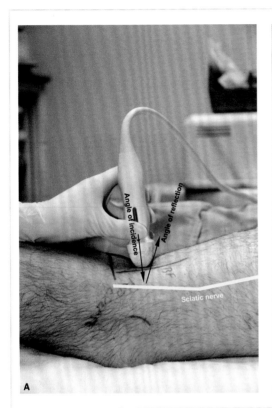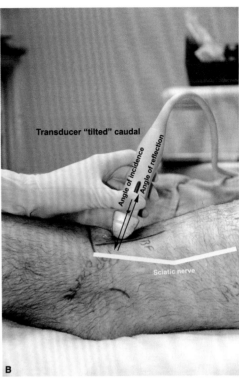

FIGURE 11.14 **A:** Ultrasound transducer placement over the popliteal fossa illustrating the angle of incidence perpendicular to the axial plane of the distal thigh, but not to the course of the distal sciatic nerve. **B:** Ultrasound transducer placement "tilted caudal" over the popliteal fossa illustrating the angle of incidence perpendicular to the course of the distal sciatic nerve.

e. **Local anesthetic volume.** Typically, a volume of 20 to 30 mL is required to obtain satisfactory local anesthetic distribution around the sciatic nerve within popliteal fossa. More recently, subparaneural-targeted injection has been shown to decrease the volume requirements to 15 to 20 mL.

4. **Continuous catheter technique.** If a **continuous catheter technique** is indicated, a larger bore (17- to 18-gauge) Tuohy needle is typically used for initial placement of the needle tip and local anesthetic injection. After local anesthetic distribution (by injection through the needle tip) is ensured, the US probe is placed aside within the sterile field. A 19- to 20-gauge catheter is inserted through the Tuohy needle and advanced no more than 2 to 3 cm past needle tip. At this point, the US probe is placed over the original site, and an additional 3 to 5 mL of local anesthetic is injected through the catheter while confirming local anesthetic distribution within the subparaneural compartment. The needle is then withdrawn over the catheter and fixed in place with a sterile clear adhesive dressing. The proximal end of the catheter is then connected to an infusion pump.

D. **Ultrasound-guided anterior approach**

1. **Indications.** In combination with a lumbar plexus block (or combined femoral–obturator nerve blocks), complete anesthesia or analgesia for the entire lower extremity from the knee to the foot. In combination with a femoral nerve block (or saphenous nerve block above the knee), complete anesthesia or analgesia for the entire lower extremity from below the knee to the foot.

CLINICAL PEARL   The anterior approach to the sciatic nerve block is an advanced technique based on the depth of the sciatic nerve. The advantages of the anterior approach are its simplicity of patient positioning (when the patient cannot assume either a lateral or prone position), the ergonomics of performing a sciatic nerve block in combination with either a femoral or an adductor canal block without having to reposition the patient and prepare an additional sterile field.

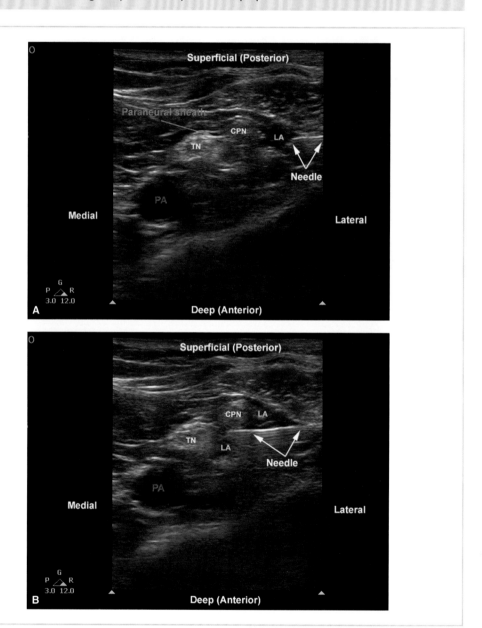

FIGURE 11.15   **A:** SAX-IP technique for the popliteal approach. The needle is advanced from lateral to medial toward the lateral aspect of the CPN. **B:** SAX-IP technique for the popliteal approach. The needle tip is in the cleavage plane between the CPN and TN. **C:** SAX image of circumferential LA distribution after ultrasound-guided subparaneural injection. Note LA is located deep and external to the paraneural sheath. **D:** SAX image of circumferential LA distribution around TN and CPN after ultrasound-guided subparaneural sheath injection. Note LA is located deep and external to the paraneural sheath. The paraneural sheath is quite visible as a hyperechoic structure containing hypoechoic local anesthetic. CPN, common peroneal nerve; LA, local anesthetic; PA, popliteal artery; SAX-IP, short-axis in-plane; TN, tibial nerve.

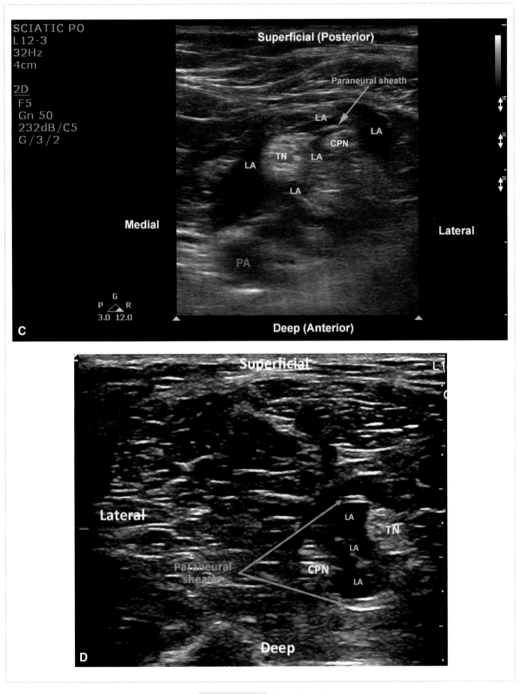

FIGURE 11.15 (continued)

2. **Contraindications.** Usual contraindications to peripheral nerve blocks (i.e., lack of consent, infection at the injection site, allergy to local anesthetics). Preexisting neural compromise is considered a relative contraindication; a careful discussion regarding the potential risks and benefits of performing peripheral nerve blocks in patients with preexisting neural compromise is strongly recommended.

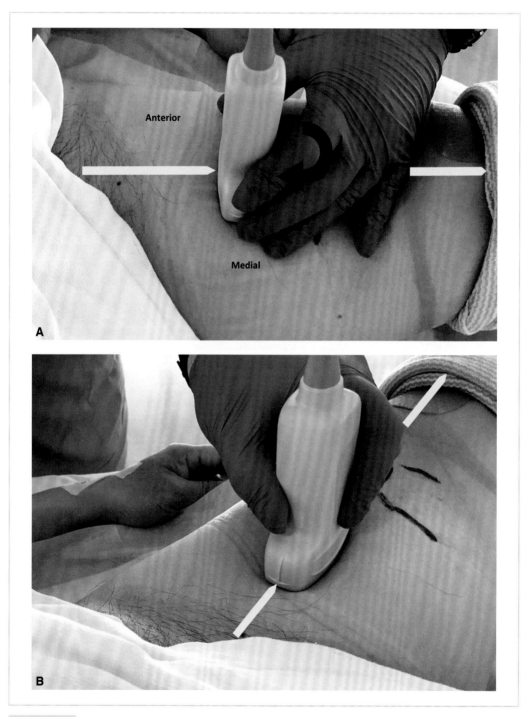

FIGURE 11.16 **A:** Placement of ultrasound transducer placement for SAX imaging of the anterior approach. From this position, the transducer is rotated 90 degrees to obtain the LAX image **(B)**. The yellow arrows indicate the course of the sciatic nerve. **B:** Placement of ultrasound transducer placement for LAX imaging of the anterior approach. The yellow arrows indicate the course of the sciatic nerve. LAX, long-axis; SAX, short-axis.

3. **Single-injection technique**
   a. **Patient position.** The patient is supine with the operative lower extremity slightly abducted and externally rotated at the hip 30 to 45 degrees.
   b. **Ultrasound transducer-scanning technique.** A low-frequency curved array transducer (2 to 5 MHz) is required for this block. The lower frequency allows for a greater depth of penetration, and the curved probe provides a wider field of view required to visualize the femur and the sciatic nerve. The US transducer is placed 8 to 10 cm distal to the inguinal crease on the anterior aspect of the thigh. The US transducer is initially oriented at a 90-degree angle to the skin, with the LAX of the probe perpendicular to the LAX of the thigh (Fig. 11.16A) to initially obtain a SAX view of the sciatic nerve. If visualization of the sciatic nerve is difficult, the transducer is centered either at what appears to be the sciatic nerve medial to intensely hyperechoic proximal to mid shaft of the femur, and then rotated 90 degrees to obtain a LAX view of the sciatic nerve (Fig. 11.16B) (14,15).
   c. **Ultrasound anatomy.** The sciatic nerve often appears as a hyperechoic, oval to elliptical polyfascicular structure posterior (deep), and medial to the hyperechoic femoral shaft. The sciatic nerve is located posterior (deep) to the adductor magnus muscle and anterior (superficial) to the biceps femoris muscle (Fig. 11.17A) (7). The femoral vessels are located within the compartment of the quadriceps muscles superficial and lateral to the sciatic nerve. In the LAX sonographic view, the sciatic nerve appears as a hyperechoic long cable-like structure that runs longitudinally from cephalad to caudad, located in between the adductor magnus and biceps femoris muscles (Fig. 11.17B).
   d. **Needling technique.** If the SAX view of the nerve is acceptable, a 150 mm 20-gauge needle is inserted on the medial aspect of the thigh based on measuring the depth from the surface of the transducer to the sciatic nerve. The needle is inserted at a corresponding depth and advanced in plane from medial to lateral at an angle that should be perpendicular to the trajectory of the US beam. If the LAX view of the sciatic nerve provides a superior view, the needle is inserted 1 to 3 cm cephalad to the cephalad end of the transducer. The needle is then advanced in plane from cephalad to caudad toward the superficial surface of the sciatic nerve. Once the needle is just superficial to the sciatic nerve, local anesthetic is injected and should be observed to spread along the superficial surface of the sciatic nerve.

> **CLINICAL PEARL** With a LAX in-plane technique for the anterior approach, the trajectory of the needle would lead to penetration of the sciatic nerve (in contrast to injecting around the "corners of the nerve" with the more commonly obtained SAX-IP technique). Thus, after initially injecting 10 to 12 mL (deep to the adductor magnus) on the superior surface of the sciatic nerve, the LAX imaging plane just lateral to the sciatic nerve is obtained. Subsequently, the needle trajectory may then be readjusted, and the needle tip advanced from just superficial to (to the pass along lateral aspect of the sciatic nerve) while injecting small aliquots of local anesthetic. The imaging plane may then be readjusted so as to pass along medial border of the sciatic nerve.

   e. **Local anesthetic volume.** Typically, a volume of 20 to 30 mL is required to obtain satisfactory local anesthetic distribution around the sciatic nerve within popliteal fossa.
4. **Continuous catheter technique.** If a **continuous catheter technique** is indicated, a larger bore (17- to 18-gauge) Tuohy needle is typically used for initial placement of the needle tip and local anesthetic injection. After local anesthetic distribution (by injection through the needle tip) is ensured, the US probe is placed aside within the sterile field. A 19- to 20-gauge catheter is inserted through the Tuohy needle and advanced no more than

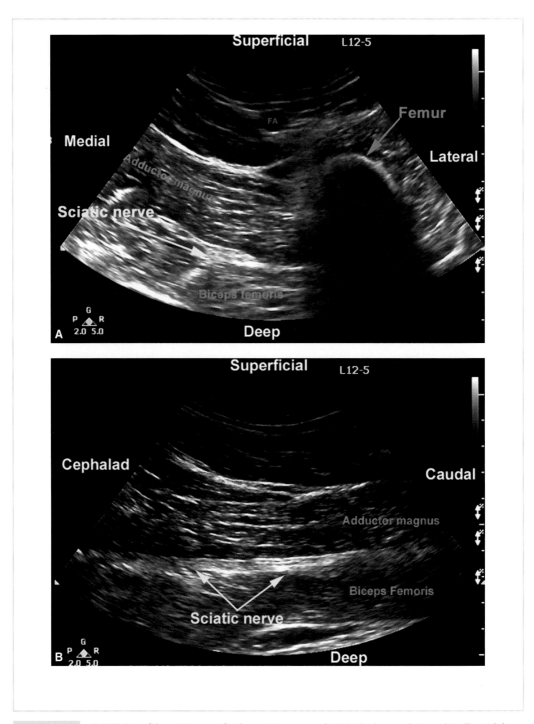

FIGURE 11.17 **A:** SAX view of the sciatic nerve for the anterior approach. Note the hyperechoic oval to ellipsoid shape of the sciatic nerve. The sciatic nerve is in the intermuscular plane between the adductor magnus and biceps femoris, and is medial to the femoral shaft. Note the posterior acoustic dropout created by the femoral shaft FA (femoral artery). **B:** LAX view of the sciatic nerve for the anterior approach. Note the hypoechoic tubular cable-like shape of the sciatic nerve extending from cephalad to caudal in the intermuscular plane between the adductor magnus and biceps femoris. LAX, long-axis; SAX, short-axis.

2 to 3 cm past needle tip. At this point, the US probe is placed over the original site, and an additional 3 to 5 mL of local anesthetic is injected through the catheter while confirming local anesthetic distribution within the subparaneural compartment around the sciatic nerve to confirm correct catheter tip position. The needle is then withdrawn over the catheter and fixed in place with a sterile clear adhesive dressing. The proximal end of the catheter is then connected to an infusion pump.

E. **Ankle block.** The ankle block technique involves blockade of five separate peripheral nerves at the ankle, which include four terminal peripheral nerve branches of the sciatic nerve (posterior tibial, deep peroneal, superficial peroneal, and sural) and the terminal peripheral nerve branch of the femoral nerve (saphenous). Ankle block can be performed without seeking specific nerve localization by paresthesia, motor response, or ultrasonography. A "ring of local anesthetic" is deposited (around the ankle) that blocks all five branches that provide sensory-motor innervation to the foot (Fig. 11.18).

1. **Indications.** Complete anesthesia or analgesia for operative procedures from the mid to distal foot. Will not provide sensory block for an ankle tourniquet.

2. **Contraindications.** Usual contraindications to peripheral nerve blocks (i.e., lack of consent, infection at the injection site, allergy to local anesthetics). Preexisting neural compromise is considered a relative contraindication; a careful discussion regarding the potential risks

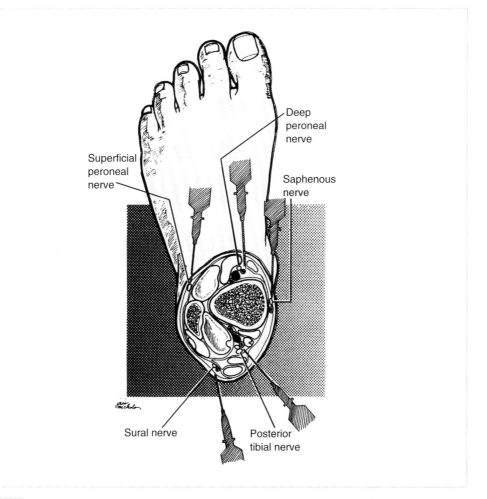

FIGURE 11.18   Axial illustration of the nerve location (and needle injection points) for ankle block.

and benefits of performing peripheral nerve blocks in patients with preexisting neural compromise is strongly recommended.

3. **Technique**

 a. **Posterior tibial nerve.** This can be performed with the patient in the prone or supine positions. If the patient is supine, the knee is flexed to bring the sole of the foot flat on the bed surface. A 1.5 inch 23-to 25 gauge needle is introduced at the level of the medial malleolus just posterior to the pulsation of the posterior tibial artery and anterior to the flexor hallucis longus tendon, and is directed 45 degrees anteriorly to seek a paresthesia of the sole of the foot. If a paresthesia is elicited, the needle is slightly withdrawn and 5 ml of local anesthetic is injected incrementally.

 Alternatively, if no paresthesia is elicited, the needle is advanced until the posterior medial surface of the distal tibia is contacted. 10 ml of local anesthetic is incrementally injected in a fan-shaped area between the medial malleolus and the calcaneal (Achilles) tendon.

CLINICAL PEARL The flexor hallucis longus tendon can be located by asking the patient to plantarflex the toe.

 b. **Sural nerve.** With the patient, still either prone or supine with the knee flexed, 5 mL more is injected superficially behind the lateral malleolus to fill the groove between the malleolus and the calcaneus.

 c. **Saphenous nerve.** Next, 5 mL is injected around the saphenous vein at the level of the medial malleolus between the skin and the bone itself.

 d. **Deep peroneal nerve.** Moving to the front of the ankle, a needle is inserted into the deeper planes below the fascia just lateral to the dorsalis pedis artery at the level of the skin creases, and 5 mL more is injected. If the artery is not palpable, the medial border of the tendon of the extensor hallicus longus (EHL) can be used as a landmark.

CLINICAL PEARL The EHL tendon can be located by asking the patient to dorsiflex the toe.

 e. **Superficial peroneal branches.** A subcutaneous ridge of anesthetic solution is laid down from the anterior tibia at the anterior border of the medial malleolus (overlying the previous injection of the deep peroneal nerve and continuing laterally to meet the previous injection for the sural nerve) to the anterior border of the lateral malleolus. A total of 5 to 10 mL may be required to extend the subcutaneous ring from the medial to lateral malleolus.

REFERENCES

1. Birnbaum K, Prescher A, Hebler S, et al. The sensory innervation of the hip joint: an anatomical study. *Surg Radiol Anat* 1997;19:371–375.
2. Cappelleri G, Aldegheri G, Ruggieri F, et al. Minimum effective anesthetic concentration (MEAC) for sciatic nerve block: subgluteal and popliteal approaches. *Can J Anaesth* 2007;54:283–289.
3. Moayeri N, Groen GJ. Differences in the qualitative architecture of the sciatic nerve may explain differences in potential vulnerability to nerve injury, onset time, and minimum effective anesthetic concentration. *Anesthesiology* 2009;111:1128–1134.

4. Moayeri N, van Geffen GJ, Bruhn J, et al. Correlation among ultrasound, cross-sectional anatomy, and histology of the sciatic nerve: a review. *Reg Anesth Pain Med* 2010;35:442–449.

5. Salinas FV. Evidence basis for ultrasound guidance for lower extremity peripheral nerve block: update 2016. *Reg Anesth Pain Med* 2016;41:261–274.

6. Neal JM, Barrington MJ, Brull R, et al. The second ASRA practice advisory on neurologic complications associated with regional anesthesia and pain medicine: Executive Summary 2015. *Reg Anesth Pain Med* 2015;40:401–430.

7. Chan VW, Nova H, Abbas S, et al. Ultrasound examination and localization of the sciatic nerve: a volunteer study. *Anesthesiology* 2006;104:309.

8. Karmakar MK, Kwok WH, Ho AM, et al. Ultrasound-guided sciatic nerve block: description of a new approach at the subgluteal space. *Br J Anaesth* 2007;98:390–395.

9. Barrington MJ, Lai SK, Briggs CA, et al. Ultrasound-guided midthigh sciatic nerve block-a clinical and anatomical study. *Reg Anesth Pain Med* 2008;33:369–376.

10. Tsui BC, Finucane BT. The importance of ultrasound landmarks: a traceback approach using the popliteal vessels for identification of the sciatic nerve. *Reg Anesth Pain Med* 2006;31:481–482.

11. Vloka JD, Hadzic A, April E, et al. The division of the sciatic nerve in the popliteal fossa: anatomical implications for popliteal nerve block. *Anesth Analg* 2001;92:215–217.

12. Andersen HL, Andersen SL, Tranum-Jensen J. Injection inside the paraneural sheath of the sciatic nerve: direct comparison among ultrasound imaging, macroscopic anatomy, and histologic analysis. *Reg Anesth Pain Med* 2012;37:410–414.

13. Karmakar MK, Shariat AN, Pangthipampai P, et al. High definition ultrasound imaging defines the paraneural sheath and the fascial compartments surrounding the sciatic nerve at the popliteal fossa. *Reg Anesth Pain Med* 2013;38:447–451.

14. Dolan J. Ultrasound-guided anterior sciatic nerve block in the proximal thigh: an in-plane approach improving the needle view and respecting fascial planes. *Br J Anesth* 2013;110:319–320.

15. Tsui BC. Ultrasound-guided anterior sciatic nerve block using a longitudinal approach: expanding the view. *Reg Anesth Pain Med* 2008;33:275–276.

12

Truncal Blocks

Ki J. Chin and Monica Liu

KEY POINTS

1. When used within the framework of a multimodal regimen, truncal blocks provide effective analgesia for a wide variety of surgical procedures involving the chest and abdomen.

2. Truncal blocks are generally safe to perform and result in fewer side effects than neuraxial blocks.

3. Except for thoracic paravertebral blocks (TPVB), truncal blocks provide somatic but not visceral analgesia.

4. Each specific truncal block anesthetizes only part of the chest or abdomen. Thus, the choice of technique must be carefully tailored to the surgical procedure.

5. Bilateral truncal blocks are required in surgical procedures involving the midline.

6. Most truncal blocks target fascial planes (where nerves travel) instead of the actual nerves. This confers safety and simplicity at the expense of some interindividual variability in intensity and extent of sensory blockade.

7. Transversus abdominis plane (TAP), rectus sheath, quadratus lumborum (QL), and ilioinguinal/iliohypogastric nerve blocks provide analgesia for the anterolateral abdominal wall.

8. Thoracic paravertebral, pectoral (PECS 1 and 2), and serratus plane blocks provide analgesia for the anterolateral chest wall and thoracic cage.

I. Anatomy. Detailed knowledge of the muscular and fascial layers of the chest and abdominal wall, and the path taken by nerves within these layers, is essential to perform ultrasound-guided truncal blocks successfully.

II. Anatomy of the anterolateral abdominal wall (Fig. 12.1)

    A. The layers of the abdominal wall consist of skin, subcutaneous tissue, muscles and their associated fascia, and parietal peritoneum.

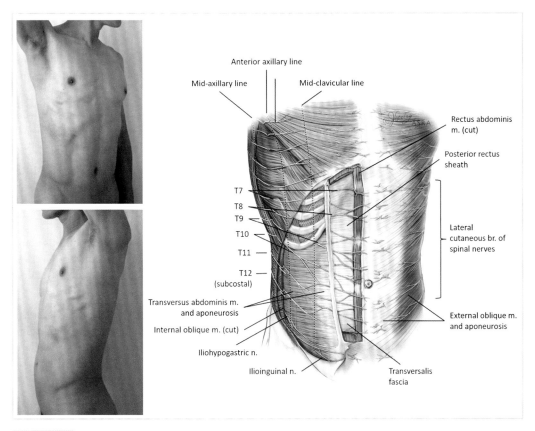

FIGURE 12.1 Surface anatomy, muscular layers, and nerves of the anterolateral abdominal wall. The external and internal oblique muscles and aponeuroses have been cut away on the right to show the transversus abdominis plane (TAP). The lateral cutaneous branches arise from their respective spinal nerves at or posterior to the mid-axillary line and supply the skin of the lateral abdominal wall up to the midclavicular line. The T7–T9 nerves enter the TAP at or medial to the midclavicular line. Communicating branches between the spinal nerves give rise to neural plexuses within the TAP and the rectus sheath. The rectus sheath is absent midway between the umbilicus and pubis. (Image Copyright 2017 American Society of Regional Anesthesia and Pain Medicine. Used with permission. All rights reserved.)

B. The three flat muscles have their origins on the ribs and on the dense thoracolumbar fascia of the back. They wrap around laterally to encase the abdominal contents (Fig. 12.1).

   1. **External oblique.** The largest and most superficial flat muscle with fibers that run inferomedially.

   2. **Internal oblique.** Runs deep to the external oblique with fibers that travel superomedially.

   3. **Transversus abdominis.** The deepest of the three flat muscles with fibers that run transversely.

C. In the anterior part of the abdominal wall, these three muscles taper off into aponeuroses that blend together to form the rectus sheath, which encases the vertically oriented rectus abdominis muscle. The **rectus abdominis** is a paired muscle separated by the linea alba along the midline of the abdomen. The linea alba results from the aponeurotic fusion of all three flat muscles.

D. The anterior layer of the rectus sheath is formed from the aponeuroses of the external oblique and the internal oblique muscles. The posterior layer is formed from the aponeuroses of the internal oblique and transversus abdominis muscles. The posterior rectus sheath ends midway between the umbilicus and pubic symphysis, at the arcuate line, where only the transversalis fascia separates the rectus abdominis muscle from the peritoneal cavity (Fig. 12.1).

E. **The rectus abdominis has tendinous attachments to the anterior rectus sheath that gives rise to the appearance of a "six pack"; the posterior rectus sheath compartment is not segmented.**

F. **The transversalis fascia runs deep to the transversus abdominis muscle, separating it from the parietal peritoneum, and is continuous with the fascia iliaca inferiorly, the endothoracic fascia superiorly, and the anterior layer of the thoracolumbar fascia posteriorly.**

G. **The anterior abdominal wall is innervated by the T6–T12 intercostal nerves and the L1 nerve (Fig.** 12.1). At the angle of each rib, the intercostal nerves give off lateral cutaneous branches, which subsequently emerge in the mid-axillary line to supply the lateral chest and abdominal wall.

H. **The main nerve trunks continue anteriorly and run in the transversus abdominis plane (TAP), a neurovascular fascial plane between the internal oblique and transversus abdominis muscles.** Within the TAP, the nerves form a plexus (1); this constitutes the target point for TAP blocks.

I. **Upon reaching the edge of the rectus sheath (the linea semilunaris), the nerves pierce the latter and lie within the posterior rectus sheath where further branching and communication occur; this constitutes the target point for rectus sheath blocks.** The nerves terminate in anterior cutaneous branches that ascend through the medial half of the rectus abdominis muscle to innervate the skin and subcutaneous tissue. One should note that the area adjacent to the abdominal midline is supplied by overlapping innervation from both sides.

J. **It is also important to remember that the T6–T9 nerves supplying the upper abdomen only emerge from the costal margin and enter the TAP medial to the anterior axillary line.** The T6 nerve emerges just lateral to the linea alba, whereas the T7–T9 nerves emerge at increasingly lateral locations (Fig. 12.1). The **subcostal TAP block** targets the T6–T9 nerves by injecting local anesthetic within the TAP **medial** to the anterior axillary line.

K. **In contrast, the T10–T12 nerves enter the TAP more laterally, between the mid-axillary and anterior axillary lines.** The **lateral TAP block** primarily targets these nerves by injecting local anesthetic in a more lateral location within the TAP at the level of the mid-axillary line.

L. **The ilioinguinal and iliohypogastric nerves, which originate from the lumbar plexus, enter the TAP in the region of the anterior third of the iliac crest and exit the TAP through the internal oblique muscle at a variable location medial to the anterior superior iliac spine (ASIS) (Fig.** 12.2).

M. **Both the TAP and rectus sheath are highly vascularized.** The main arteries within the TAP are descending branches of the lower thoracic intercostal arteries and ascending branches of the deep circumflex arteries. The rectus sheath contains the superior and deep epigastric arteries.

CLINICAL PEARL   The rich vascular supply of the TAP and rectus sheath increases the risk of local anesthetic systemic absorption and toxicity (especially in the context of high doses of local anesthetic). Thus, appropriate precautions must be taken while injecting local anesthetic in these planes. In particular, it is recommended that epinephrine, 5 µg/mL, can be added to the local anesthetic, and that patients be closely monitored for at least 30 minutes after the block's performance.

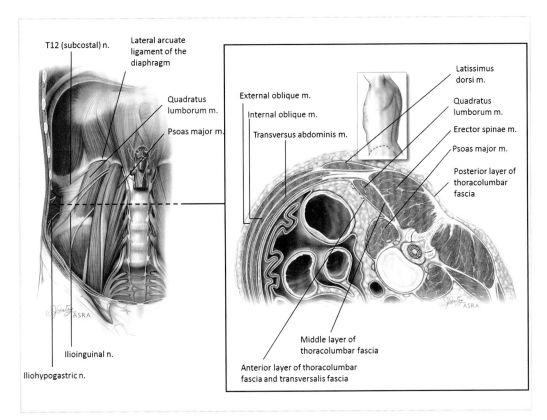

FIGURE 12.2 The anatomy of the posterolateral abdominal wall. The external oblique muscle tapers off into a free edge that abuts the latissimus dorsi muscle. The internal oblique and transversus abdominis muscles taper off into aponeuroses that blend into the thoracolumbar fascia. The thoracolumbar fascia divides into three layers (anterior, middle, and posterior) to encase the quadratus lumborum (QL) and erector spinae muscles. The ilioinguinal and iliohypogastric nerves are L1 branches of the lumbar plexus that emerge from the lateral border of psoas major muscle to run over the anterior surface of QL and transversus abdominis muscles. They ascend into the transversus abdominis plane along the anterior half of the iliac crest. Medial to the anterior superior iliac spine, the nerves continue to ascend and pierce the internal oblique muscle and external oblique aponeurosis. (Image Copyright 2017 American Society of Regional Anesthesia and Pain Medicine. Used with permission. All rights reserved.)

III. Anatomy of the posterior abdominal wall

A. The posterolateral abdominal wall is formed by the external oblique, internal oblique, and transversus abdominis muscles; their aponeuroses; as well as the psoas major and quadratus lumborum (QL) muscles (Fig. 12.2).

B. The QL muscle attaches inferiorly to the iliac crest and runs posterior to the lateral arcuate ligament of the diaphragm to attach to the 12th rib. It is covered on its ventral surface by the anterior layer of the thoracolumbar fascia and transversalis fascia and on its dorsal surface by the middle layer of the thoracolumbar fascia.

C. The thoracolumbar fascia is a tough membranous sheet that envelopes these muscles and consists of anterior, middle, and posterior layers (Fig. 12.2). The anterior layer blends with the **transversalis fascia** and separates the QL and psoas major muscles. The middle layer blends laterally with the aponeuroses of transversus abdominis and internal oblique muscles and separates the QL and erector spinae muscles. The posterior layer is formed from the aponeuroses of the latissimus dorsi and serratus posterior muscles. These layers and the intermuscular planes provide a potential path for local anesthetic (injected around the QL muscle) to spread superiorly toward the thoracic paravertebral space and the spinal nerves.

> **CLINICAL PEARL** The posterior tapering off of the internal oblique and transversus abdominis muscle into their aponeuroses is an important ultrasonographic landmark for the QL block.

IV. Anatomy of the paravertebral space

A. **Spinal nerves exit the spinal canal through the intervertebral foramina, which lie approximately midway between the transverse processes of adjacent vertebrae.**

B. **The transverse processes constitute the critical bony landmarks for paravertebral blocks.** They cannot be palpated but must be located in relation to the spinous processes. Their relationship to the latter varies along the length of the spine (Fig. 12.3).

   1. For thoracic vertebrae, the steep angle and bulbous tip of the spinous process mean that its cephalad edge lies at the level of the transverse process of the *inferior* vertebra.

   2. For lumbar vertebrae, the cephalad edge of the spinous process is at the level of the transverse process of the *same* vertebra.

   3. The 11th and 12th thoracic vertebrae represent a transition point between thoracic and lumbar vertebrae. The spinous processes of the T11–T12 vertebrae are elongated like those belonging to lumbar vertebrae, but their cephalad edge does not quite extend to the lower edge of their own transverse processes.

C. **The thoracic paravertebral space is a wedge-shaped anatomical compartment bound medially by the vertebral bodies, intervertebral discs and foramen; anterolaterally by the endothoracic fascia, parietal pleura (T2–T10/11), and diaphragm (T10/11–T12); and posteriorly by the transverse processes and superior costotransverse ligaments.**

   1. The paravertebral space contains fat, extrapleural fascia, segmental nerve roots dividing into ventral and dorsal rami, the sympathetic chain, rami communicantes, and radicular vessels (Fig. 12.4).

   2. It communicates with the contiguous paravertebral spaces (superiorly and inferiorly), the epidural space (medially), and the intercostal space (laterally).

   3. The **superior costotransverse ligament** joins the inferior aspect of the transverse process (above) with the superior aspect of the neck of the rib (below).

   4. The **endothoracic fascia** (deep fascia of the thorax) divides the paravertebral space into anterior and posterior compartments. The sympathetic chain can be found in the anterior compartment (i.e., the "extrapleural" paravertebral space), whereas the intercostal nerves and vessels lie in the posterior compartment (i.e., the "subendothoracic" paravertebral space).

> **CLINICAL PEARL** The pleura curves anteriorly as it approaches the neuraxial midline, and consequently, the thoracic paravertebral space widens. This not only reduces the risk of pleural puncture but also decreases pleural visibility on ultrasound.

V. Anatomy of the anterolateral thoracic wall

A. **The major muscles of the anterolateral chest wall are the pectoralis major, pectoralis minor, and serratus anterior muscles (Fig.** 12.5).

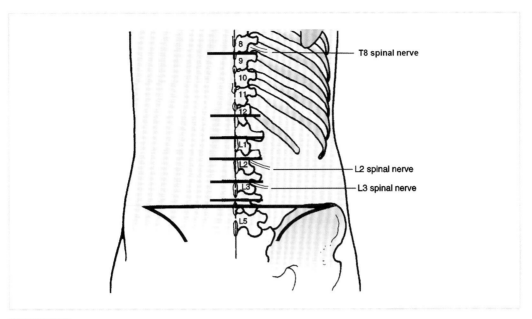

FIGURE 12.3 Bony anatomy relevant to the paravertebral block. The steep thoracic spinous processes mean that a transverse line drawn from the cephalad edge of the spinous process of one vertebra (e.g., T8) will intersect the transverse process of the vertebra below (T9). The spinal nerve roots emerge inferior to the transverse processes of the vertebrae for which they are named.

1. The **pectoralis major** is a thick triangular-shaped muscle that originates from the medial half of the clavicle and the lateral sternum and inserts into the lateral lip of the bicipital groove of the humerus. It is innervated by the medial and lateral pectoral nerves.

2. The **pectoralis minor** is a smaller triangular-shaped muscle that lies deep to the pectoralis major. It originates from the 3rd to 5th ribs near the costal cartilages and inserts on the medial border and superior surface of the coracoid process of the scapula. It is innervated by the medial pectoral nerve.

3. The **serratus anterior** is a large digitated muscle covering the anterolateral wall of the thorax. It lies superficial to the ribs and intercostal muscles. It originates from the upper borders of the first eight ribs laterally and inserts on the ventral surface of the medial border of the scapula. Its motor innervation is provided by the long thoracic nerve, which arises from C5–C7 roots of the brachial plexus.

B. **The lateral pectoral nerve (C5–C7) and medial pectoral nerve (C8–T1) arise from the lateral and medial cord of the brachial plexus, respectively.** The lateral pectoral nerve enters the intermuscular plane between the pectoral muscles in close proximity to the pectoral branch of the thoracoacromial artery. The medial pectoral nerve lies deep to the pectoralis minor muscle and pierces the latter to innervate the inferior aspect of the pectoralis major.

C. **The chest wall is also innervated by the lateral and anterior branches of the upper thoracic intercostal nerves (Fig.** 12.4). The thoracic intercostal nerves arise from the ventral rami of spinal nerves and travel anteriorly between the intercostal muscles. They give off a lateral cutaneous branch at the angle of the rib, which emerges over the serratus anterior muscle to supply the lateral aspect of the chest wall and the axilla (Fig. 12.5). The main nerve trunks continue anteriorly and pierce the internal intercostal and pectoralis major muscles in the parasternal area before terminating in anterior cutaneous branches.

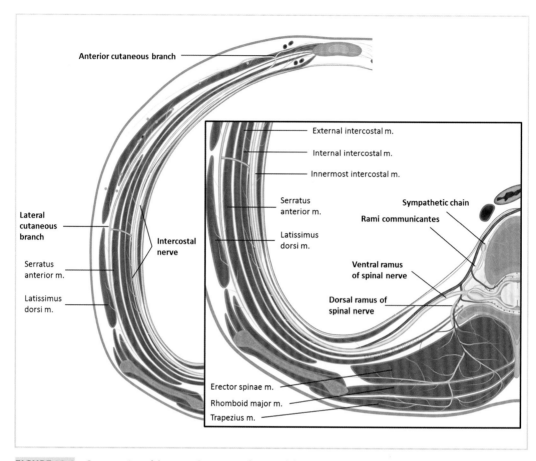

FIGURE 12.4 Cross-section of thorax and anatomy of a typical thoracic spinal nerve. As the spinal nerve emerges from the intervertebral foramen, it divides into a ventral and dorsal ramus. The branches of the dorsal ramus supply the muscles and skin of the back. The ventral ramus continues anteriorly as the intercostal nerve, giving off a lateral cutaneous branch (close to the angle of the rib), which emerges in the mid-axillary line to innervate the lateral thoracoabdominal wall. The terminal anterior cutaneous branch emerges close to the midline to innervate the anterior thoracoabdominal wall. (Image adapted and used with permission from Maria Fernanda Rojas Gomez.)

  D. **The skin overlying the clavicle and the periclavicular chest wall is innervated by the supraclavicular nerves, which originate from the superficial cervical plexus.**

  VI. Drugs. Local anesthetic volume constitutes the primary consideration in truncal blocks because analgesic efficacy inherently depends on local anesthetic spread within the fascial plane. Typical injectates range between 15 and 30 mL in adults. The choice of local anesthetic solution and concentration should respect maximum recommended doses, with calculations based on lean rather than actual bodyweight. Long-acting local anesthetics, such as ropivacaine and bupivacaine, are most commonly used for truncal blocks.

CLINICAL PEARL With truncal blocks, there exists a large surface area for potential vascular absorption of local anesthetic into the systemic circulation. The addition of epinephrine, e.g., 5 μg/mL, is recommended to reduce the local anesthetic peak plasma concentration, and the patient should be observed for potential signs and symptoms of local anesthetic systemic toxicity for a minimum of 30 to 45 minutes after truncal blocks.

3 **CLINICAL PEARL**   With the exception of thoracic paravertebral blocks (TPVB), truncal blocks provide somatic analgesia only. Visceral pain should be managed with alternative modes of analgesia including opioids, acetaminophen, and nonsteroidal anti-inflammatory drugs.

VII. Techniques

    A. **Ultrasound-guided TAP block**

4

        1. **Indications**
            a. **Subcostal TAP block.** Analgesia for upper abdominal (T6–T9) wall surgery.
            b. **Lateral TAP block.** Analgesia for lower abdominal (T10–T12) wall surgery.

        2. **Contraindications**
            a. Usual contraindications to peripheral nerve blocks (i.e., lack of consent, local infection at the injection site, and allergy to local anesthetic agent)

        3. **Single-injection technique**
            a. **Subcostal TAP block.** The patient is positioned supine. Place a linear ultrasound transducer parallel to the costal margin lateral to the rectus sheath (Fig. 12.6). Identify the transversus abdominis muscle, which lies deep to rectus abdominis muscle (medially) and deep to internal oblique muscle (laterally). Infiltrate the subcutaneous tissues with local anesthetic. Using an in-plane technique, direct an 80- or 100-mm short-beveled needle in a posterolateral direction away from the midline, injecting local anesthetic in the fascial plane between the rectus abdominis/internal oblique and transversus abdominis muscles. A local anesthetic volume of 15 to 20 mL is typically used.
            b. **Lateral TAP block**. The patient is positioned supine or with a slight lateral tilt for a more posterior approach. Place a linear ultrasound transducer in a transverse orientation in the mid-axillary line between the iliac crest and costal margin to identify the external oblique, internal oblique, and transversus abdominis muscles (Fig. 12.6). Infiltrate the subcutaneous tissues with local anesthetic. Using an in-plane technique, direct an 80- or 100-mm short-beveled needle in an anterior-to-posterior direction through the external oblique and internal oblique muscles to reach the TAP. Inject local anesthetic to hydrodissect and expand the fascial plane between the internal oblique and transversus abdominis muscles. A local anesthetic volume of 15 to 20 mL is typically used.

CLINICAL PEARL   The location at which the T6–T9 nerves emerge into the TAP signifies that a lateral TAP block will not anesthetize the upper abdomen. In fact, the area supplied by the T6 and T7 nerves is probably best anesthetized using a rectus sheath block (because the T6–T7 nerves emerge very close to the midline).

5 **CLINICAL PEARL**   Performing bilateral injections in both subcostal TAP and lateral TAP locations is necessary to block the entire anterior abdominal wall (2). Midline incisions necessitate bilateral blocks because of the overlapping innervation by nerves originating from both sides.

        4. **Continuous technique.** The needle approach and sonographic target for continuous subcostal or lateral TAP block are similar to the ones described for the single-injection techniques. If perineural catheters are placed preoperatively, a more lateral needle insertion site will minimize interference with the surgical field. Standard steps for perineural catheter

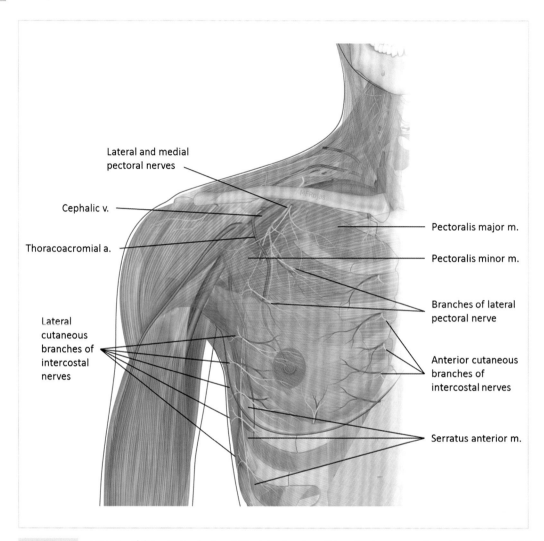

FIGURE 12.5   Anatomy of the anterior chest wall. The lateral and medial pectoral nerves are branches of the brachial plexus that pierce and innervate the pectoral muscles and the superolateral quadrant of the anterior chest wall. The cephalic vein and thoracoacromial artery lie in close proximity to the pectoral nerves in the plane between the pectoralis major and minor muscles. The axilla and the anterolateral aspect of the chest wall are innervated by the lateral cutaneous branches of the intercostal nerves (T1–T5), which arise close to the angle of the rib and ascend through the intercostal and serratus anterior muscles, emerging into a subcutaneous location in the mid-axillary line. The anteromedial aspect of the chest wall is innervated by the terminal anterior cutaneous branches of the T1–T5 intercostal nerves. (Image adapted and used with permission from Maria Fernanda Rojas Gomez.)

insertion should be employed (*vide supra*). A local anesthetic infusion rate of 5 to 8 mL/h is typically used. In depth discussion of perineural catheters can be found in Chapter 2.

CLINICAL PEARL   If the external oblique, internal oblique, and transversus abdominis muscles cannot be clearly identified on ultrasound, start the scan close to the midline to identify the linea alba and the rectus abdominis, and then slide the transducer laterally to visualize the linea semilunaris and the transition into the three muscle layers.

CLINICAL PEARL Expansion of the TAP space with injection of local anesthetic will aid catheter insertion and placement.

B. Ultrasound-guided rectus sheath block

1. **Indications.** Analgesia for surgery involving midline abdominal wall incisions through the rectus abdominis muscle (e.g., umbilical or epigastric hernia repair). Bilateral blocks are always required.

2. **Contraindications.** Usual contraindications to peripheral nerve blocks (*vide supra*).

3. **Single-injection technique.** The patient is positioned supine. Place the linear transducer in a transverse orientation above the umbilicus to identify the linea alba and the rectus muscles

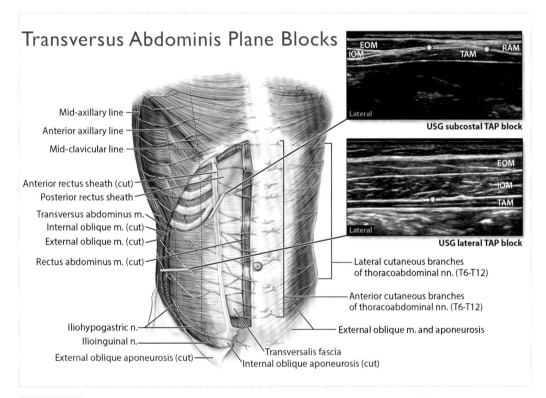

FIGURE 12.6 Anatomy of the anterolateral abdominal wall and the ultrasound-guided (USG) subcostal and lateral transversus abdominis plane (TAP) blocks. The **USG subcostal TAP block** targets the T6–T9 nerves where they emerge into the TAP caudad to the costal margin. The transducer is placed parallel and adjacent to the costal margin (blue line). Closer to the midline, the TAP is the plane between rectus abdominis muscle (RAM) and transversus abdominis muscles (TAM). In this location, the external oblique (EOM) and internal oblique (IOM) muscles exist as aponeuroses, which contribute to the formation of the anterior rectus sheath. The EOM and IOM become visible as the transducer is moved more laterally along the costal margin. Injection may be performed at multiple points along the costal margin (circles). Alternately, using an in-plane technique, a needle can be continuously advanced between the RAM/IOM and the TAM (with concomitant local anesthetic injection). Note that the lateral cutaneous branches of the thoracoabdominal nerves are not covered by the block. The **USG lateral TAP block** targets the T10–T12–L1 nerves. The transducer is placed in a transverse orientation in the mid-axillary line between the costal margin and iliac crest. Local anesthetic injection is performed in the TAP between the IOM and TAM (circle), with the needle usually inserted in an anterior-to-posterior direction. The TAM has a characteristic darker hypoechoic appearance and is significantly thinner than the IOM. (Image Copyright 2017 American Society of Regional Anesthesia and Pain Medicine. Used with permission. All rights reserved.)

on either side. Slide the transducer laterally to identify the linea semilunaris, marking the lateral aspect of the rectus sheath and rectus abdominis muscle (Fig. 12.7). Infiltrate the subcutaneous tissues with local anesthetic. Using an in-plane technique, direct an 80-or 100-mm short-beveled needle in a lateral-to-medial direction to enter the lateral aspect of the posterior rectus sheath compartment (Fig. 12.8). Deposit the local anesthetic between the rectus muscle and posterior rectus sheath. A local anesthetic volume of 15 to 20 mL is commonly used per side. For larger incisions, it is reasonable to perform injections above and below the umbilicus (a total of four injections) to ensure adequate spread. However, care must be taken to remain superior to the arcuate line and not to exceed maximum recommended local anesthetic doses.

CLINICAL PEARL   Because the anterior abdominal wall moves with diaphragmatic excursion, TAP and rectus sheath blocks may be technically challenging if the patient breathes rapidly and deeply. Therefore it is often easier to perform these blocks under general anesthesia. The risk of nerve injury is regarded as low.

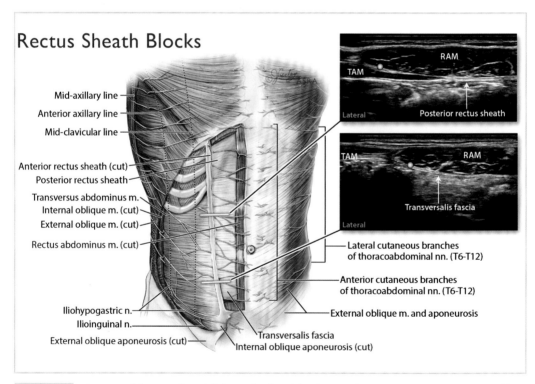

Rectus Sheath Blocks

RAM
TAM
Lateral
Posterior rectus sheath

TAM
RAM
Transversalis fascia
Lateral

Mid-axillary line
Anterior axillary line
Mid-clavicular line

Anterior rectus sheath (cut)
Posterior rectus sheath
Transversus abdominus m.
Internal oblique m. (cut)
External oblique m. (cut)
Rectus abdominus m. (cut)

Lateral cutaneous branches of thoracoabdominal nn. (T6-T12)

Anterior cutaneous branches of thoracoabdominal nn. (T6-T12)

External oblique m. and aponeurosis

Iliohypogastric n.
Ilioinguinal n.
External oblique aponeurosis (cut)
Transversalis fascia
Internal oblique aponeurosis (cut)

FIGURE 12.7   Anatomy of the anterolateral abdominal wall and the ultrasound-guided rectus sheath block. This block targets the terminal muscular branches and anterior cutaneous branches of the thoracoabdominal nerves. The transducer is placed in a transverse orientation superior to the umbilicus to visualize the lateral aspect of the rectus abdominis muscle (RAM) and rectus sheath. Close to the costal margin, the transversus abdominis muscle (TAM) is often visible dorsal to the RAM. If the transducer is placed caudad to the midpoint between the umbilicus and pubic symphysis, the posterior rectus sheath is absent and the dorsal surface of RAM is bound by its epimysium and transversalis fascia. Local anesthetic injection is performed in the posterior rectus sheath compartment between the lateral aspect of the RAM and its deep investing layer of fascia (circles) to target the nerves before they ascend through the RAM into their subcutaneous location. (Image Copyright 2017 American Society of Regional Anesthesia and Pain Medicine. Used with permission. All rights reserved.)

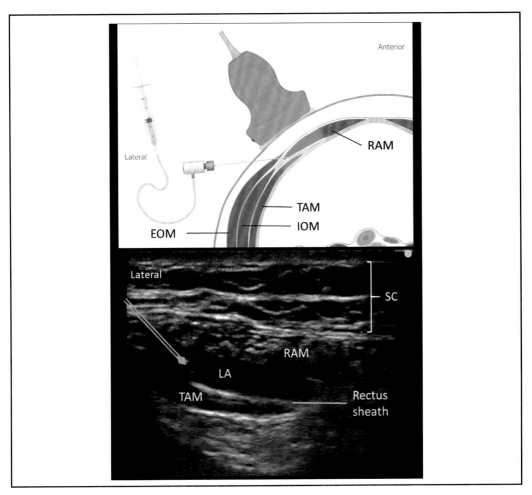

FIGURE 12.8 Ultrasound-guided rectus sheath block. The transducer is placed in a transverse orientation just above the umbilicus to visualize the lateral edge of the RAM. Using an in-plane technique, the needle is advanced aiming for LA spread between the RAM and the hyperechoic line of the posterior rectus sheath. EOM, external oblique muscle; IOM, internal oblique muscle; LA, local anesthetic; RAM, rectus abdominis muscle; SC, subcutaneous tissue; TAM, transversus abdominis muscle. (Image reproduced with permission from Maria Fernanda Rojas Gomez and KJ Chin Medicine Professional Corporation.)

    4. Continuous technique. The sonographic target for continuous rectus sheath block is identical to the one described for the single-injection technique—the fascial plane between the lateral aspect of the rectus abdominis muscle and the posterior rectus sheath. The needle may be inserted in a lateral-to-medial direction as described above, or it may be inserted in a superior-to-inferior direction to thread the catheter along the length of the rectus sheath rather than across the latter. Standard steps for perineural catheter insertion should be employed (*vide supra*). A local anesthetic infusion rate of 5 to 8 mL/h is typically used. In depth discussion of perineural catheters can be found in Chapter 2.

C. Ilioinguinal–iliohypogastric nerve block

    1. Indications. Analgesia for surgery involving incisions in the inguinal and suprapubic area (T12–L1 dermatomes) of the anterior abdominal wall (e.g., inguinal hernia repair, caesarean delivery)

2. **Contraindications.** Usual contraindications to peripheral nerve blocks (*vide supra*).

3. **Ultrasound-guided single-injection technique.** The patient is positioned supine. Place the linear transducer slightly superior and posterior to the ASIS, parallel to an imaginary line connecting the ASIS and the umbilicus. The three muscular layers of the anterolateral abdominal wall are visualized adjacent to the acoustic shadow of the iliac crest. The ilioinguinal and iliohypogastric nerves are often visible as hyperechoic structures adjacent to the iliac crest in the TAP (Fig. 12.9). The ascending branch of the deep circumflex iliac artery and subcostal (T12) nerve can also be visualized in this plane but in a more medial location. Infiltrate the subcutaneous tissues with local anesthetic. Using an in-plane technique, direct a 50- or 80-mm short-beveled needle in a medial-to-lateral direction. Inject local anesthetic in the fascial plane between the internal oblique and transversus abdominis muscles. A local anesthetic volume of 10 to 12 mL is typically used in the adult patient.

CLINICAL PEARL   If the ilioinguinal/iliohypogastric nerves cannot be visualized, local anesthetic injection to distend the TAP close to the iliac crest will result in a successful block.

CLINICAL PEARL   Although TAP, rectus sheath, and ilioinguinal/iliohypogastric nerve blocks all provide analgesia for the anterior abdominal wall, for more "targeted" local anesthetic spread, we recommend the use of rectus sheath blocks for midline abdominal surgery, particularly for vertical incisions above the umbilicus, and ilioinguinal/iliohypogastric nerve blocks for incisions in the T12/L1 territory.

D. **Ultrasound-guided QL block** (3,4–6). There exist two different approaches to the ultrasound-guided QL block: the posterior QL block (or "QL2" block) and the transmuscular (or anterior) QL block. These relatively new truncal blocks constitute alternatives to the ultrasound-guided TAP block and may offer more extensive analgesia (7,8). Research into their mechanism of action is ongoing, but it appears that paraspinal and paravertebral spread of local anesthetic (rather than spread within the TAP) may account for the clinical efficacy of the posterior and transmuscular QL block, respectively (9).

1. **Indications.** Analgesia for surgery of the lower abdomen and periumbilical area.

2. **Contraindications.** Usual contraindications to peripheral nerve blocks (*vide supra*).

3. **Ultrasound-guided posterior QL block (single-injection technique).** The patient is positioned supine, or lateral with the side to be blocked uppermost. A curvilinear transducer is recommended, but a linear transducer may also be used in slim patients. Place the transducer in a transverse orientation in the mid-axillary line between the iliac crest and the costal margin and identify the three flat muscles of the anterolateral abdominal wall. Trace the muscles posteriorly until the internal oblique and transversus abdominis muscles taper into their aponeuroses and the middle layer of thoracolumbar fascia, visible as a hyperechoic line posterior to the QL muscle (Fig. 12.10). Infiltrate the subcutaneous tissues with local anesthetic. Using an in-plane technique, direct an 80- or 100-mm short-beveled needle in an anterior-to-posterior direction, passing through the external oblique muscle until the tip is positioned between the thoracolumbar fascia and QL muscle. Inject local anesthetic to distend this plane, in order to spread over the posterior surface of the QL muscle. A volume of 20 to 25 mL is typically used in the adult patient.

Ilioinguinal-Iliohypogastric Blocks

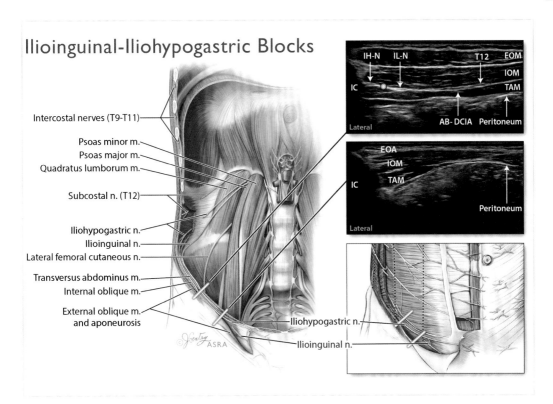

FIGURE 12.9 Anatomy of the ultrasound-guided II-N and IH-N nerve block. The IH-N and II-N emerge from the lateral border of psoas major muscle. They initially pass over the ventral surface of quadratus lumborum, before traveling under the dorsal aspect of TAM and its aponeurosis. Both nerves pierce the TAM to enter the TAP at a variable location posterior to the ASIS. The transducer is positioned parallel and superior/posterior to an imaginary line connecting the umbilicus and the ASIS (upper blue line). The edge of the transducer rests against the IC, which can be seen as an acoustic shadow. In this position, the three muscular layers of the abdominal wall are visible. The II-N and IH-N are located in the TAP between the IOM and TAM and can be found very close to the IC. The ascending branch of the deep circumflex iliac artery (AB-DCIA) travels more medially in the TAP, as does the subcostal nerve (T12). Injection of local anesthetic is performed in the TAP close to the IC (circle), avoiding the nerves if they are visible. The block should not be performed medial and inferior to the ASIS (lower blue line) because the IH-N and II-N are ascending to the surface in this location and not consistently located in any musculofascial plane. AB-DCIA, ascending branch of deep circumflex iliac artery; ASIS, anterior superior iliac spine; EOM, external oblique muscle; IC, iliac crest; IH-N, iliohypogastric nerve; II-N, ilioinguinal nerve; IOM, internal oblique muscle; TAM, transversus abdominis muscle; TAP, transversus abdominis plane. (Image Copyright 2017 American Society of Regional Anesthesia and Pain Medicine. Used with permission. All rights reserved.)

4. **Ultrasound-guided transmuscular QL block (single-injection technique).** The patient is sitting or positioned lateral with the side to be blocked uppermost. Place a curvilinear transducer in a transverse orientation in the posterior axillary line between the iliac crest and the costal margin to identify the tapering of the internal oblique and transversus abdominis muscles into their aponeuroses and the middle layer of thoracolumbar fascia, visible as a hyperechoic line posterior to the QL muscle. Increase the depth of penetration on the ultrasound machine until the acoustic shadows of the lumbar vertebral body and transverse process are visualized (Fig. 12.10). Identify the psoas major muscle lying adjacent to the vertebral body and anterior to the QL muscle. Infiltrate the subcutaneous tissues with local anesthetic. Using an in-plane technique, direct an 80- or 100-mm short-beveled needle in a posterior-to-anterior direction, passing through the QL muscle until the tip is positioned between the QL and psoas major muscles. Inject local anesthetic to distend this plane in

order to spread over the anterior surface of the QL muscle, thus separating it from psoas major muscle. A volume of 20 to 25 mL is typically used in the adult patient.

> **CLINICAL PEARL**   An adequate volume of injection is important because the mechanism of action of the transmuscular QL block involves local anesthetic spread cranially into the thoracic paravertebral space (9).

> **CLINICAL PEARL**   Local anesthetic spread to the branches of the lumbar plexus (which course over the anterior surface of the QL muscle) is possible, and this may result in lower limb weakness. Patients should be carefully assessed and fall precautions, implemented when ambulating for the first time after the block.

5. **Continuous technique.** The needle approach and sonographic target are the same as described for the single-injection technique. Standard steps for perineural catheter insertion should be employed (*vide supra*). A local anesthetic infusion rate of 5 to 8 mL/h is typically used. In depth discussion of perineural catheters can be found in Chapter 2.

E. **Thoracic paravertebral block** (10–12)

1. **Indications.** Anesthesia or analgesia for unilateral breast or chest wall procedures, thoracic trauma, and abdominal surgery. It may also be used for video-assisted thoracoscopic surgery or thoracotomy, especially when thoracic epidural analgesia is contraindicated or undesirable (13). The level at which the block is performed must match the surgical site. A single-injection TPVB of 15 to 20 mL will usually anesthetize up to two dermatomes cephalad and two dermatomes caudad to the level of injection, although this is subject to interindividual variability. Alternatively, multiple injections of 3 to 5 mL at separate levels may be performed to ensure adequate spread to the desired nerve territories.

> **5**
> **CLINICAL PEARL**   Because innervation overlaps across the midline, areas near the latter may not be adequately blocked by unilateral TPVBs. Similarly, there exists considerable overlap between adjacent dermatomes on the same side. Thus, it is almost always necessary to inject a large volume of local anesthetic (single-injection technique) or to perform blocks one dermatomal level above and below the desired level(s) to ensure adequate anesthesia of the targeted dermatome(s) (multiple-injection technique).

2. **Contraindications.** Usual contraindications to peripheral nerve blocks (*vide supra*).

3. **Ultrasound-guided parasagittal in-plane TPVB (single-injection technique).** The patient can be placed in a seated, prone, or lateral decubitus position. Place the linear transducer in a sagittal plane approximately 5 cm from the midline. Identify the acoustic shadow of the ribs, internal intercostal membrane, and pleura. Slide the transducer medially to identify the bony transition from rib to transverse process. The transverse process is always more superficial than the rib and displays a less-rounded profile. The pleura also often becomes less visible deep to the transverse processes compared with the ribs because it curves anteriorly toward the midline. Aim to visualize the superior costotransverse ligament between contiguous transverse processes—a slight lateral tilt of the transducer may facilitate its identification (Fig. 12.11). Infiltrate the skin with local anesthetic at the

Quadratus Lumborum Block

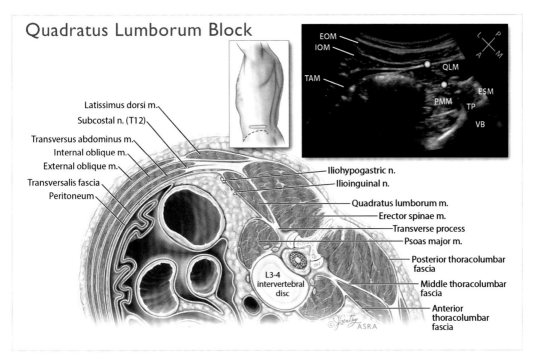

FIGURE 12.10   Anatomy of the posterior abdominal wall and the ultrasound-guided QL block. The EOM ends in a free edge, which abuts the latissimus dorsi muscle. The IOM and TAM end in aponeuroses that blend with the thoracolumbar fascia. The thoracolumbar fascia itself divides into three layers (posterior, middle, and anterior) that envelop the QLM and ESM. The QL block is performed by placing a curvilinear transducer on the posterolateral aspect of the abdominal wall in a transverse oblique orientation, between the iliac crest and the costal margin (blue line). Key landmarks for identifying the QLM are the VB, TP, and PMM. At the L3–L4 level, the large intestine in the peritoneal cavity may be seen deep to the abdominal wall muscles (as depicted in this figure); at the L2–L3 level, the kidney is usually visible in the retroperitoneal space. The circles indicate targets for local anesthetic injection either anterior or posterior to the QLM. EOM, external oblique muscle; ESM, erector spinae muscle; IOM, internal oblique muscle; PMM, psoas major muscle; QL, quadratus lumborum; QLM, quadratus lumborum muscle; TAM, transversus abdominis muscle; TP, transverse process; VB, vertebral body. (Image Copyright 2017 American Society of Regional Anesthesia and Pain Medicine. Used with permission. All rights reserved.)

inferior border of the transducer, and using an in-plane technique, advance an 80-mm short-beveled needle in a cephalad-to-caudad direction. Pass the needle tip through the superior costotransverse ligament. Inject a 15- to 20-mL bolus of local anesthetic solution, aiming for ventral (downward) displacement of the pleura.

CLINICAL PEARL   Steep needle angulation may be required to enter the thoracic paravertebral space without striking the inferior transverse process. An alternative strategy is to rotate the transducer away from a strict parasagittal orientation into a slightly oblique one such that the caudad end of the transducer overlies the rib rather than the transverse process. The lower height of the rib permits a shallower needle trajectory to reach the thoracic paravertebral space (Fig. 12.11).

4.   **Ultrasound-guided transverse in-plane TPVB (single-injection technique).** The patient can be positioned in a seated, prone, or lateral decubitus position. With the linear transducer in a transverse orientation over the midline, identify the acoustic shadows of the spinous process, transverse process, and rib. Position the tip of the transverse process in the middle of the image. Rotate the transducer slightly to an oblique transversal position along the long

axis of the rib and slide the transducer slightly inferiorly, enabling visualization of the pleura, the superior costotransverse ligament, and the "thumb-like" contour of the transverse process (Fig. 12.12). Infiltrate the skin at least 2 cm lateral to the tip of the transverse process. Insert an 80-mm short-beveled needle in a lateral-to-medial direction to penetrate the superior costotransverse ligament. The needle tip should not be advanced once it is obscured by the shadow of the tip of the transverse process. Inject a 15- to 20-mL bolus of local anesthetic solution, striving for ventral (downward) displacement of the pleura.

CLINICAL PEARL Hydrolocation with frequent 0.5 mL aliquots of normal saline or 5% dextrose should be used to track the needle tip as it is advanced toward the thoracic paravertebral space. Because the needle tip pierces the superior costotransverse ligament and enters the thoracic paravertebral space, this injection will produce ventral (downward) displacement of the pleura; the desired local anesthetic dose can be injected at this point.

5. **Continuous technique.** Both ultrasound-guided methods described above may be used for catheter placement. If the transverse in-plane technique is used, the catheter should not be advanced more than 2 cm beyond the needle tip to avoid inadvertent entry into the intervertebral foramen. The sagittal in-plane technique may minimize the risk of this complication; however, the catheter should not be advanced more than 3 cm beyond the needle tip because its direction and path become unpredictable. Standard steps for perineural catheter insertion should be employed (*vide supra*). A local anesthetic infusion rate of 5 to 8 mL/h is typically used. In depth discussion of perineural catheters can be found in Chapter 2.

CLINICAL PEARL Catheter advancement in the paravertebral space can be met with resistance. Injecting a 5- to 10-mL bolus of local anesthetic solution (to dilate the space) can facilitate the process. If the catheter threads very easily, the needle and/or catheter may have penetrated the pleural cavity.

F. **Pectoral (PECS) block** (14)
   1. **Indications**
      a. **PECS 1 block.** Targets the lateral and medial pectoral nerves and provides analgesia for simple mastectomy and anterior chest wall procedures
      b. **PECS 2 block.** Targets the lateral and medial pectoral nerves and the lateral cutaneous branches of intercostal nerves to provide analgesia for anterolateral breast or chest wall surgery extending into the axilla (e.g., sentinel lymph node biopsy, modified radical mastectomy)
   2. **Contraindications.** Usual contraindications to peripheral nerve blocks (*vide supra*)
   3. **Single-injection technique**
      a. **PECS 1.** The patient is positioned supine. Place the linear transducer obliquely over the midclavicular region of the thoracic wall. From superficial to deep, identify the pectoralis major muscle, pectoralis minor muscle, axillary artery, axillary vein, and pleura. Locate the thoracoacromial artery along with the lateral pectoral nerve in the intermuscular plane between the pectoral muscles. Infiltrate the subcutaneous tissues with local anesthetic. Using an in-plane technique, direct a 50-mm short-beveled needle in a superomedial to inferolateral direction until the tip is positioned between the pectoral muscles (Fig. 12.13). Inject the local anesthetic aiming for a spread within this fascial plane. A volume of 10 to 20 mL is typically used.

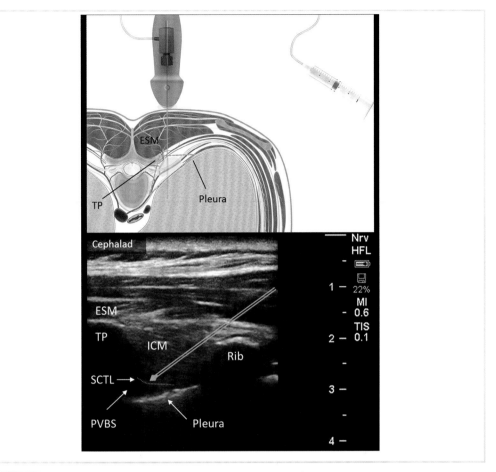

FIGURE 12.11   Ultrasound-guided parasagittal in-plane approach to the thoracic paravertebral block. The transducer is placed in a longitudinal parasagittal orientation at the desired vertebral level, and the tip of the TP is visualized deep to ESM. The pleura is visible as a hyperechoic line, and the SCTL presents as a fainter hyperechoic line (dotted line added for clarity). The PVBS is the dark triangular area between the two structures. Note that the transducer has been rotated into a slight oblique orientation, so that its caudad end is displaced laterally. This brings the lower rib, rather than its corresponding TP, into view; the rib has a lower profile than the TP, which allows a shallower needle trajectory. Using an in-plane technique, the needle is advanced through the ICM to pierce the SCTL and enter the thoracic paravertebral space. The endpoint consists of ventral pleural displacement with local anesthetic injection. ESM, erector spinae muscle; ICM, intercostal muscles; PVBS, paravertebral space; SCTL, superior costotransverse ligament; TP, transverse process. (Image adapted and used with permission from Maria Fernanda Rojas Gomez and Amit Pawa.)

    b. **PECS 2**. The PECS 2 block is a combination of the PECS 1 block and serratus plane block (*vide infra*) performed with the same needle pass. The patient and transducer are set up similarly as for the PECS 1 block and the same anatomy, identified. Perform a PECS 1 block as described above with an 80-mm short-beveled needle and inject 10 mL of local anesthetic in the intermuscular plane between the pectoralis major and minor muscles. Subsequently, continue to slide the transducer laterally and inferiorly until serratus anterior muscle is visualized deep to pectoralis minor at the level of the 3rd rib. Using an in-plane technique, advance the needle through the pectoralis minor muscle to enter the plane superficial to serratus anterior muscle. Inject a 15- to 20-mL bolus of local anesthetic aiming for spread within this fascial plane (Fig. 12.14).

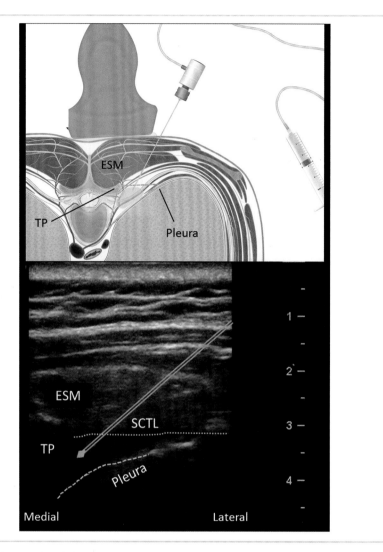

FIGURE 12.12   Ultrasound-guided transverse in-plane approach to the thoracic paravertebral block. The transducer is placed in a transverse orientation at the desired vertebral level, and the tip of the TP is visualized deep to ESM. The pleura presents as a hyperechoic line that curves inferomedially deep to the TP. Using an in-plane technique, the needle is advanced in a lateral-to-medial direction to pierce the SCTL and enter the thoracic paravertebral space. The endpoint consists of pleural displacement downward with local anesthetic injection. ESM, erector spinae muscle; SCTL, superior costotransverse ligament; TP, transverse process. (Image adapted and used with permission from Maria Fernanda Rojas Gomez and Amit Pawa.)

CLINICAL PEARL   Local anesthetic injection superficial to the serratus anterior muscle can cause tracking into the axilla and disruption of the surgical tissue planes around the lymph nodes. To circumvent this possibility, the second injection in the PECS 2 block can be performed in the fascial plane deep to the serratus anterior muscle.

G. **Serratus plane block** (15)

1. **Indications.** Analgesia for surgery or trauma of the anterolateral thoracic wall (e.g., breast surgery, rib fractures).

2. **Contraindications.** Usual contraindications to peripheral nerve blocks (*vide supra*).

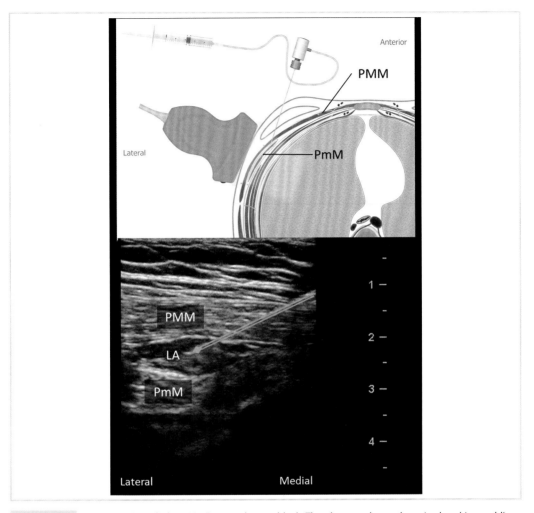

FIGURE 12.13 Ultrasound-guided "PECS 1" pectoral nerve block. The ultrasound transducer is placed in an oblique orientation on the anterolateral chest wall (caudad to the clavicle) to visualize the PMM and PmM. Using an in-plane technique and a lateral-to-medial direction, the needle tip is positioned between PMM and PmM. The endpoint consists of LA spread in the intermuscular plane between these two muscles. This anesthetizes the medial and lateral pectoral nerves. The thoracoacromial artery and cephalic vein are often visible in this plane as well. LA, local anesthetic; PMM, pectoralis major muscle; PmM, pectoralis minor muscle. (Image adapted and used with permission from Maria Fernanda Rojas Gomez and Amit Pawa.)

3. **Single-injection technique.** The patient is placed in the lateral decubitus position with the side to be blocked uppermost. The arm is extended at the shoulder and adducted across the chest to expose the lateral chest wall. Place the linear transducer in a parasagittal plane just inferior to the clavicle and identify the 2nd and 3rd ribs. Slide the transducer laterally and inferiorly to identify the 4th and 5th ribs and align the transducer with the posterior axillary line. In this location, the latissimus dorsi muscle will be overlying the serratus anterior muscle, which in turn overlies the ribs and intercostal muscles (Fig. 12.15). Infiltrate the subcutaneous tissues with local anesthetic. Using an in-plane technique, direct an 80-mm short-beveled needle in a superior-to-inferior direction until the tip is positioned between the latissimus dorsi muscle and the serratus anterior muscle. Inject local anesthetic to distend this plane (superficial to the serratus anterior muscle). Alternatively, in cases where bony analgesia is desired, the needle needs only to be advanced deeper into the plane between the serratus

anterior muscle and the rib/intercostal muscle. This injection **deep** to the serratus anterior muscle will also prevent local anesthetic tracking into the axilla and disruption of surgical planes. A local anesthetic volume of 20 to 30 mL is typically used.

4. **Continuous technique.** The needle approach and sonographic target are similar to those described for the single-injection technique. The catheter tip can be placed either superficial or deep to the serratus anterior muscle depending on the desired effect. Standard steps for perineural catheter insertion should be used (*vide supra*). A local anesthetic infusion rate of 5 to 8 mL/h is typically used. In depth discussion of perineural catheters can be found in Chapter 2.

CLINICAL PEARL   Although TPVBs, PECS, and serratus plane blocks all provide effective analgesia for breast surgery, the latter two techniques are preferred because of their technical simplicity and (potentially) lower risk of complications (16).

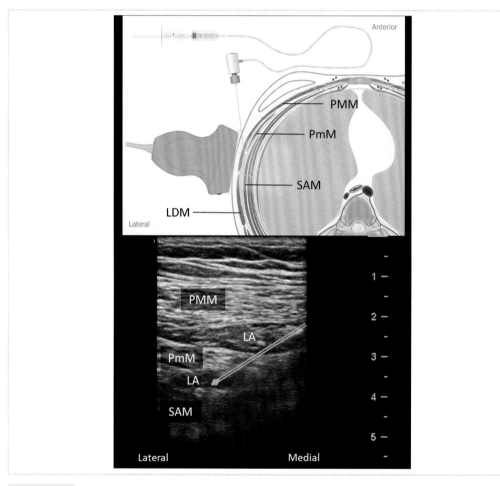

FIGURE 12.14   Ultrasound-guided "PECS 2" pectoral nerve block. The ultrasound transducer is placed in an oblique orientation on the anterolateral chest wall (caudad to the clavicle) to visualize the PMM and PmM. The transducer is moved laterally until the SAM can be found dorsal to the pectoralis minor muscle. Using an in-plane technique and a lateral-to-medial direction, the needle tip is positioned between PmM and SAM. The endpoint consists of LA spread in the intermuscular plane between PmM and SAM. This is usually combined with LA injection between PMM and PmM (i.e., the PECS 1 block; see Figure 12.13). LA, local anesthetic; LDM, latissimus dorsi muscle; PMM, pectoralis major muscle; PmM pectoralis minor muscle; SAM, serratus anterior muscle. (Image adapted and used with permission from Maria Fernanda Rojas Gomez and Amit Pawa).

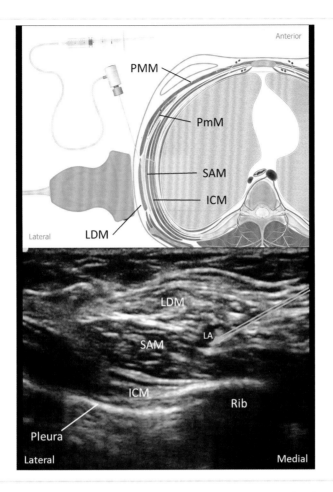

FIGURE 12.15 Ultrasound-guided serratus plane block. The ultrasound transducer is placed in an oblique transverse or longitudinal orientation in the mid-axillary or posterior axillary line to visualize the LDM overlying the SAM. Using an in-plane technique, the needle is positioned between the LDM and SAM. The endpoint consists of local anesthetic spread in the intermuscular plane between the LDM and SAM. ICM, intercostal muscle; LA, local anesthetic; LDM, latissimus dorsi muscle; PMM, pectoralis major muscle; PmM, pectoralis minor muscle; SAM, serratus anterior muscle. (Image adapted and used with permission from Maria Fernanda Rojas Gomez and KJ Chin Medicine Professional Corporation.)

VIII. Complications. Local anesthetic systemic toxicity deserves particular consideration as a complication in the context of truncal blocks. To achieve adequate local anesthetic spread and a successful block, relatively large volumes must be administered in highly vascularized fascial planes. It is important to respect maximum local anesthetic doses, particularly in smaller patients and in the setting of multiple-injection techniques.

A detailed consideration of block complications can be found in Chapter 14. Complications specific to truncal blocks are listed in Table 12.1.

TABLE 12.1 Complications of specific truncal blocks

Block	Complication
Transversus abdominis plane	Visceral trauma
Rectus sheath	Visceral trauma

(continued)

TABLE 12.1   Complications of specific truncal blocks (*continued*)

Block	Complication
Ilioinguinal and iliohypogastric	Visceral trauma Pelvic hematoma Femoral nerve block
Quadratus lumborum	Lumbar plexus block Retroperitoneal hematoma
Paravertebral	Pleural puncture/pneumothorax Epidural spread Dural puncture Intrathecal injection Hypotension
Pectoral	Thoracoacromial artery injection Pleural puncture/pneumothorax Axillary fascia puncture
Serratus plane	Pleural puncture/pneumothorax

ACKNOWLEDGMENTS

The authors wish to acknowledge the contributions of Christopher M. Bernards, MD, who authored chapter "Paravertebral Block" in the previous edition, and Dr. Maria Fernanda Rojas Gomez, who provided assistance with many of the illustrations.

REFERENCES

1. Rozen WM, Tran TMN, Ashton MW, et al. Redefining the course of the thoracolumbar nerves: a new understanding of the innervation of the anterior abdominal wall. *Clin Anat* 2008;21:325–333.
2. Borglum J, Jensen K, Christensen AF, et al. Distribution patterns, dermatomal anesthesia, and ropivacaine serum concentrations after bilateral dual transversus abdominis plane block. *Reg Anesth Pain Med* 2012;37:294–301.
3. Chin KJ, McDonnell JG, Carvalho B, et al. Essentials of our current understanding: abdominal wall blocks. *Reg Anesth Pain Med* 2017;42:133–183.
4. Blanco R, McDOnnell JG. Optimal point of injection: the quadratus lumborum I and II blocks. Anaesthesia 2013;68. http://www.respond2articles.com/ANA/forums/post/1550.aspx. Accessed April 5, 2017.
5. Dam M, Hansen CK, Borglum J, et al. A transverse oblique approach to the transmuscular quadratus lumborum block. *Anesthesia* 2016;71:603–604.
6. Hansen CK, Dam M, Bendtsen TF, et al. Ultrasound-guided quadratus lumborum blocks: definition of the clinical relevant endpoint of injection and the safest approach. *A A Case Rep* 2016;6:39.
7. Blanco R, Ansari T, Riad W, et al. Quadratus lumborum block versus transversus abdominis plane block for postoperative pain after cesarean delivery: a randomized controlled trial. *Reg Anesth Pain Med* 2016;41:757–762.
8. Murouchi T, Iwasaki S, Yamakage M. Quadratus lumborum block: analgesic effects and chronological ropivacaine concentrations after laparoscopic surgery. *Reg Anesth Pain Med* 2016;41:146–150.
9. Dam M, Morrigl B, Hansen CK, et al. The pathway of injectate spread with the transmuscular quadratus lumborum (TQL) block—a cadaver study. *Anesth Analg* 2017. doi: 10.1213/ANE.0000000000001922.
10. Batra RK, Krishnan K, Agarwal A. Paravertebral block. *J Anaesth Clin Pharmacol* 2011;27:5–11.
11. Greengrass RA, Duclas R. Paravertebral blocks. *Int Anesth Clin* 2012;50:56–73.
12. Krediet AC, Moayeri N, van Geffen G, et al. Different approaches to ultrasound-guided thoracic paravertebral block. *Anesthesiology* 2015;123:459–474.
13. Yeung JH, Gates S, Naidu BV, et al. Paravertebral block versus thoracic epidural for patients undergoing thoracotomy. *Cochrane Database Syst Rev* 2016;2:CD009121.

14. Blanco R, Fajardo M, Parras T. Ultrasound description of PECS II (modified PECS I): a novel approach to breast surgery. *Rev Esp Anestesiol Reanim* 2012;59:470–475.

15. Yeung JH, Gates S, Naidu BV, et al. Paravertebral block versus thoracic epidural for patients undergoing thoracotomy. *Cochrane Database Syst Rev* 2016;2:CD009121.

16. Bolin ED, Harvey NR, Wilson SH. Regional anesthesia for breast surgery: techniques and benefits. *Curr Anesthesiol Rep* 2015;5:217–224.

13

Head and Neck Blocks

Roderick J. Finlayson

KEY POINTS

1. Awake intubation can be the safest course of action in the presence of a difficult airway (1).

2. Adequate airway anesthesia will enhance patient cooperation and greatly facilitate awake intubation.

3. Sensory innervation of the airway is divided into three zones supplied by the trigeminal, glossopharyngeal, and vagal nerves.

4. Topical anesthesia is sufficient for most clinical situations. However, nerve blocks can provide additional analgesia when, particularly, stimulating procedures are planned.

5. Total local anesthetic doses should be closely monitored during airway anesthesia in order to avoid toxicity.

6. Cervical plexus blocks are commonly used in conjunction with brachial plexus blocks to provide surgical anesthesia and postoperative analgesia for shoulder and clavicle surgeries.

7. Cervical plexus blocks can also be used to provide anesthesia for carotid endarterectomy. Not only do they allow the patient's neurologic status to be monitored, they also confer greater hemodynamic stability and result in shorter hospital stay than general anesthesia.

8. Superficial and intermediate cervical plexus blocks provide greater safety and efficacy than deep cervical plexus blocks for carotid endarterectomy.

9. Facial nerve blocks can provide anesthesia for minor cosmetic procedures as well as laceration repairs and are particularly suited for pediatric analgesia.

10. Although the three trigeminal branches can be blocked proximally at the pterygopalatine fossa, a distal approach is associated with fewer complications.

I. Airway blocks

    A. Anatomy

        1. Sensory fibers of the nasal mucosa arise from the middle division of the trigeminal nerve (i.e., cranial nerve V) by means of the sphenopalatine ganglion (Fig. 13.1). The latter lies

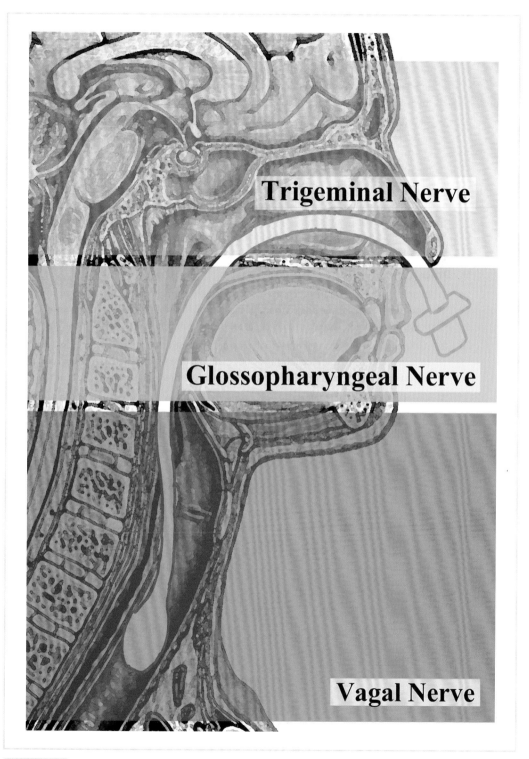

FIGURE 13.1   Sensory innervations of the airway. The trigeminal nerve (i.e., cranial nerve V) supplies the nasal mucosa, superior portion of the pharynx, uvula, and tonsils; the glossopharyngeal nerve (i.e., cranial nerve IX) supplies the oropharynx, supraglottic regions, and posterior portion of the tongue; and the vagus nerve (i.e., cranial nerve X) supplies the larynx and trachea.

under the nasal mucosa posterior to the middle turbinate. Fibers from this ganglion also provide sensory innervation to the superior portion of the pharynx, uvula, and tonsils. These fibers can be anesthetized with transmucosal topical application of local anesthetic.

2. The glossopharyngeal nerve (i.e., cranial nerve IX) provides sensory innervation to the oropharynx, supraglottic region, and posterior portion of the tongue (Fig. 13.1). This nerve can be blocked by topical anesthesia or direct submucosal injection of local anesthetic behind the tonsillar pillar.

3. Sensation in the larynx itself above the vocal cords is provided by the superior laryngeal nerve. The latter departs from the main vagus nerve (i.e., cranial nerve X) in the carotid sheath and courses anteriorly, sending an internal branch that penetrates the thyrohyoid membrane. Behind the latter, the nerve subdivides to provide sensory innervation to the vocal cords, epiglottis, and arytenoids (Fig. 13.1).

4. Below the vocal cords, sensory innervation is provided by branches of the recurrent laryngeal nerve, which originates from the vagus nerve. The recurrent laryngeal nerve also provides motor fibers to all but one of the intrinsic laryngeal muscles. Topical (or transtracheal) anesthesia can efficiently anesthetize the recurrent laryngeal nerve.

B. **Drugs**

1. In order to facilitate transmucosal absorption, higher concentrations of local anesthetics are required for topical anesthesia than for perineural infiltration. As it is readily available and presents a favorable toxicity profile, lidocaine in concentrations of 4% to 10% is commonly used.

2. Although there exists evidence that plasma concentrations are significantly lower with topical application than local infiltration, care must be taken when exceeding a total dose of 300 mg in adult patients. (See section "Complications")

3. Use of topical vasoconstrictors can be beneficial because they reduce bleeding. A vasoconstricting nasal spray (oxymetazoline 0.05%) can be applied before the local anesthetic, or alternatively, 0.25% phenylephrine can be added to the lidocaine solution.

C. **Techniques**

1. **Topical anesthesia**
   a. **Nasal mucosa.** Cotton pledgets soaked in 4% lidocaine on long applicators are inserted bilaterally into both nares and directed posteriorly along the inferior and middle turbinates until they contact the posterior pharyngeal wall and sphenoid bone, respectively (Fig. 13.2). This technique provides anesthesia to the sphenopalatine ganglion, usually within 5 minutes.
   b. **Mouth and pharynx.** A total of 4 mL of 4% lidocaine is placed in an atomizer and the tongue, sprayed with local anesthetic. The patient is then instructed to gargle with the residue. Next, the (anesthetized) tongue is grasped with a dry gauze sponge and gently held with one hand. The patient is then instructed to pant vigorously (like a puppy) whereas the rest of the local anesthetic is sprayed into the posterior pharynx with each inspiration.
   c. **Trachea.** A transtracheal injection can be used to provide tracheal anesthesia (Fig. 13.3). Alternatively, if a fiber-optic bronchoscope is being used to facilitate intubation, a similar volume of 4% lidocaine can be injected through the distal port once the trachea is visualized (2).

2. **Nerve blocks**
   a. **Lingual branches of glossopharyngeal nerve.** The tongue is retracted medially with a tongue depressor to reveal the inferior curve of the anterior tonsillar pillar (Fig. 13.4). A 25-gauge spinal needle is used to inject 2 mL of 1% lidocaine 0.5 cm below the mucosa at a point 0.5 cm lateral to the base of the tongue itself. The longer length of the spinal

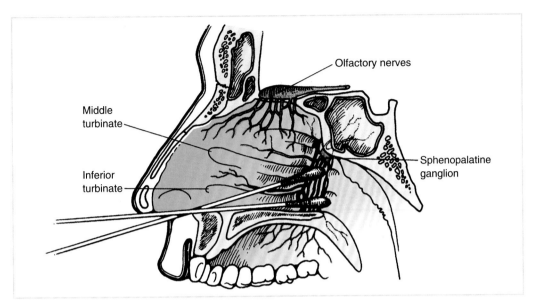

FIGURE 13.2 Nasal airway anesthesia. Cotton pledgets soaked in local anesthetic are inserted along the inferior and middle turbinates to produce anesthesia of the underlying sphenopalatine ganglion by transmembrane diffusion of the solution. Wide pledgets are needed to provide maximal topical anesthesia and vasoconstriction of the nasal mucosa as well.

needle will allow easier control by permitting the syringe to remain outside the mouth. Aspiration is performed before injection to detect intravascular placement. Bilateral infiltrations are required to block both lingual branches of the glossopharyngeal nerve.

   b. **Superior laryngeal nerve.** Patient's head is extended. The thyroid cartilage and hyoid bone are identified. The index finger retracts the skin down over the superior ala of the thyroid cartilage, and the skin is wiped with an alcohol swab. A 23- or 25-gauge needle connected to a 5-mL syringe filled with 1% lidocaine is inserted into the tip of the cartilage. The index finger then releases the skin traction, and the needle is "walked off" the cartilage superiorly and is inserted just through the firm thyrohyoid membrane. The tip now lies in the loose areolar tissue plane beneath the membrane (Fig. 13.5). After (negative) aspiration, 2.5 mL of 1% lidocaine is injected into the plane beneath the membrane. This sequence is repeated on the opposite side. Alternatively, the needle can be inserted into the posterior (greater) cornu of the hyoid bone and "walked off" the bone (caudad) onto the membrane.

CLINICAL PEARL

   • Airway anesthesia can be performed with the patient in the supine position, but it is often more comfortable if done with the patient's head slightly elevated or in the sitting position.
   • Topical anesthesia is usually sufficient for awake intubation. Nerve blocks are associated with greater risk but may be indicated in specific situations where greater suppression of the gag reflex is required (e.g., direct rigid laryngoscopy).
   • If sedation is not contraindicated, an agent such as dexmedetomidine (which has minimal respiratory depression) can be used.
   • Nasal mucosal anesthesia is useful if nasal intubation is planned and the addition of a vasoconstrictor will help reduce mucosal bleeding.

- Anesthesia of the mouth and oropharynx will allow introduction of both the laryngoscope and tube down to the level of the epiglottis
- Anesthesia of the larynx and trachea (by blockade of the branches of the vagus nerve or by transtracheal injection) allows the patient to tolerate insertion of the tube and fiber-optic scope below the cords without coughing, thus reducing the significant cardiovascular response usually associated with tracheal intubation. However, blockade of laryngeal/tracheal sensation may be contraindicated if there is a risk of vomiting and aspiration.

5   D. **Complications**

1. **Local anesthetic toxicity** is a concern when performing airway anesthesia because multiple sites are blocked using both topical and injected lidocaine (3). The recommended dose for topical lidocaine is 3.5 mg/kg or 300 mg. Caution is warranted when administering large doses in higher risk patients, such as the elderly and those with reduced liver function. Resuscitation equipment should be at hand, and the patient has to be monitored closely during the block and for at least 20 minutes after its completion.

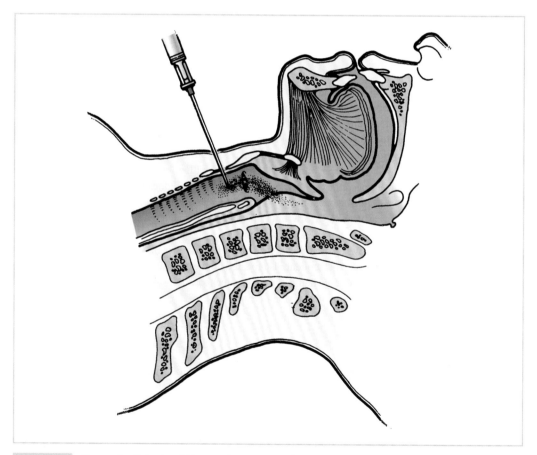

FIGURE 13.3   Transtracheal injection. A 20-gauge intravenous catheter is introduced through the cricothyroid membrane. After tracheal entry is confirmed by air aspiration, the metal introducer is removed, and a syringe is connected to the plastic needle, which is left in place. Four milliliters of local anesthetic is injected as the patient inspires; the inward air flow will carry the solution down the trachea, and the usual cough reflex will spread it up to the undersurface of the vocal cords.

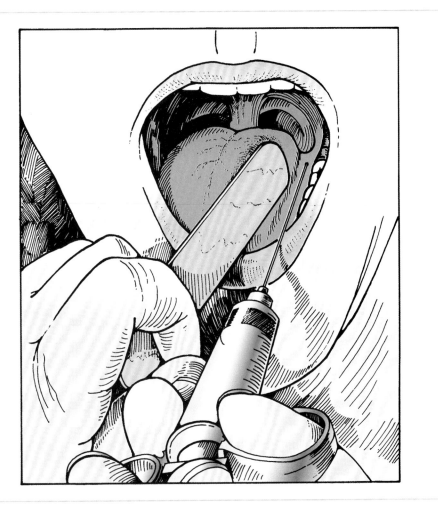

FIGURE 13.4 Glossopharyngeal nerve (lingual branch) block. The tongue is pushed medially with a tongue depressor, and a spinal needle is inserted into the base of the anterior tonsillar pillar, 0.5 cm lateral to the base of the tongue and advanced 0.5 cm deep. After (negative) aspiration, 2 mL of local anesthetic is injected. Both sides need to be anesthetized for adequate blunting of the gag reflex. A three-ring syringe makes aspiration easier, and the use of a spinal needle allows better visualization of the injection site while the hand remains outside the mouth.

2. **Epistaxis** may occur even with the use of a nasal vasoconstrictor. Gentle insertion and generous lubrication of the tube will reduce this possibility, whereas the presence of a deformity or coagulopathy will increase the risk.

3. **Aspiration** of gastric contents may occur if anesthesia of the cords and trachea is carried out in the presence of reflux or active vomiting. These techniques should be used with caution (or not at all) if there is a significant risk of aspiration.

II. Cervical plexus blocks

A. Anatomy

1. The cervical plexus originates from the anterior rami of the C1–C4 spinal nerves and gives rise to both superficial and deep branches.

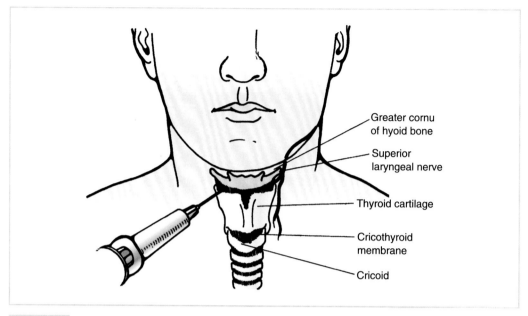

FIGURE 13.5   Superior laryngeal nerve block. The 23- to 25-gauge needle is introduced into the superior border of the lateral wing of the thyroid cartilage. It is then gently advanced off the cartilage to drop through the thyrohyoid membrane. After (negative) aspiration, 2 to 3 mL of local anesthetic is injected into the space below the membrane.

2. Cervical plexus blocks are typically performed at the C4 level, where the nerves course in a groove between the longus capitis and middle scalene muscles, before emerging along the posterior border of the sternocleidomastoid (SCM) muscle (4).

3. Deep branches innervate muscles of the anterior neck as well as the diaphragm (phrenic nerve), whereas superficial branches provide cutaneous sensation to the ear, neck, mandibular angle, shoulder, and clavicle.

4. Branches of the superficial cervical plexus include the great auricular, lesser occipital, transverse cervical, and supraclavicular nerves.

CLINICAL PEARL   Cervical plexus blocks are classified as superficial, intermediate, and deep, based on the final needle tip position relative to the superficial (investing) and deep (prevertebral) cervical fascias. Superficial blocks are confined to the subcutaneous tissues, whereas intermediate blocks target the space between the investing and prevertebral facial layers (i.e., the posterior cervical space). In contrast, deep blocks target the space below the prevertebral fascia.

B. **Drugs**
    All local anesthetics will present a slightly decreased duration of action because of the increased vascularity found in the soft tissues of the neck. Intermediate- or long-acting aminoamide agents are appropriate for surgery. Ropivacaine 0.25% to 0.5% and bupivacaine 0.25% are sufficient to anesthetize the sensory nerves of the cervical plexus. If supplementation is required during surgery, 1% lidocaine can be used.

6   C. **Techniques**
    Patients are placed supine with the head turned toward the nonoperative side.

1. **Landmark-based superficial cervical plexus block**
   a. An "X" is marked at the midpoint of the posterior border of the SCM muscle, where it is often intersected by the external jugular vein.
   b. After aseptic preparation, a skin wheal is made at the "X."
   c. A 5-cm (2-in.) needle is introduced through the skin wheal, and local infiltration is performed along the posterior border of the SCM muscle 4 cm (1.5 in.) above and below the level of the "X" (Fig. 13.6). A total volume of 10 mL is commonly used.

2. **Ultrasound-guided intermediate cervical plexus block**
   a. A high-frequency linear transducer is placed on the anterolateral aspect of the neck at the level of the upper pole of the thyroid cartilage (Fig. 13.7).
   b. The sonographic target is the hyperechoic band representing the fusion of the investing and prevertebral fascias (i.e., the posterior cervical space), which can be found between the SCM muscle laterally and the levator scapula muscle medially (5,6) (Fig. 13.8).
   c. Color duplex Doppler should be used to scan the target area and projected needle path in order to detect the presence of incidental blood vessels.
   d. Using an in-plane technique, a 5-cm (2-in.) block needle is inserted at the posterior border of the SCM muscle and advanced toward the fascial band (Figs. 13.7 and 13.8).
   e. A local anesthetic volume of 5 to 10 mL is then injected with resultant dilation of the posterior cervical space.

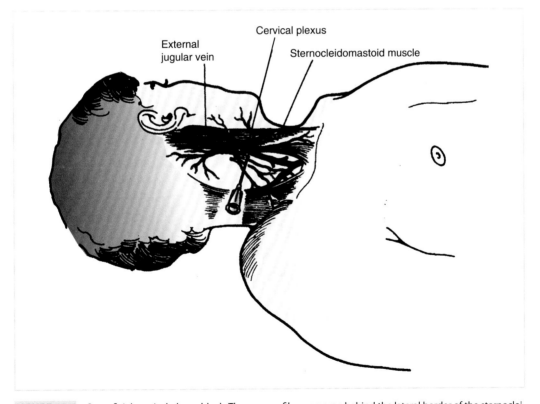

FIGURE 13.6 Superficial cervical plexus block. The sensory fibers emerge behind the lateral border of the sternocleidomastoid muscle. A needle inserted at its midpoint (usually where the external jugular vein crosses the muscle) can be directed superiorly and inferiorly to block all the terminal branches.

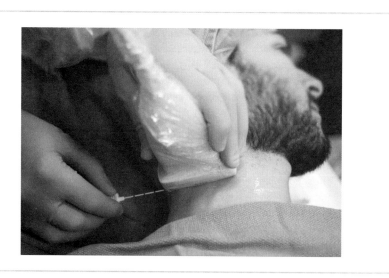

FIGURE 13.7 Ultrasound probe placement for an in-plane approach of the intermediate cervical plexus block. The patient is supine with his head turned toward the nonoperative side.

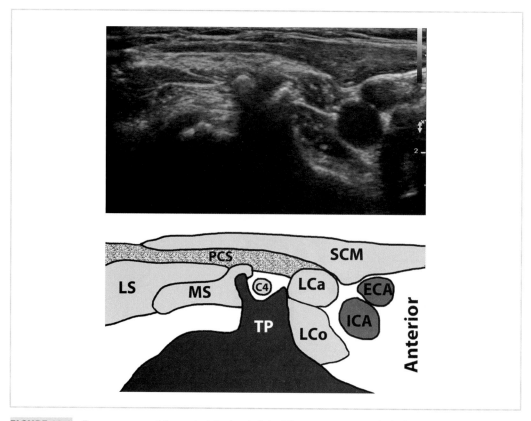

FIGURE 13.8 Transverse scan of the neck at the level of the C4 transverse process (TP). The posterior cervical space (PCS), i.e., the target for the intermediate cervical plexus block, can be seen between the levator scapulae (LS) and sternocleidomastoid (SCM) muscles. The C4 nerve root (C4) emerges between the middle scalene (MS) and longus capitis (LCa) muscles. The anterior scalene muscle is typically small and difficult to identify at this level. The carotid artery bifurcation into internal (ICA) and external carotid arteries (ECA), as well as the longus colli muscle, can be visualized anteriorly.

> **CLINICAL PEARL**
> - Unlike its superficial and intermediate counterparts, deep cervical plexus blocks target both motor and sensory pathways. However, there is no evidence that motor blockade improves surgical conditions. Furthermore, deep blocks are associated with a greater risk of complications (7).
> - For carotid endarterectomy, intraoperative block supplementation with local infiltration is often required, because structures such as the carotid sheath may receive innervation from the vagal and glossopharyngeal nerves.

D. **Complications**

1. Vascular breach remains the most common complication after cervical injection procedures and can result in **hematomas** as well as **local anesthetic toxicity**. Routine pre-procedural Duplex color Doppler scanning and careful in-plane needling technique can minimize these risks. In addition, injections should be done in small increments (1.0 to 1.5 mL), with careful monitoring of the patient's mental status. Real-time visualization of local anesthetic spread can provide further reassurance.

2. **Phrenic nerve blockade** may occur in patients undergoing intermediate cervical plexus blocks. Most patients can tolerate unilateral diaphragmatic paresis; however, those with preexisting contralateral phrenic nerve dysfunction or limited pulmonary function can experience respiratory failure. Bilateral blocks should be avoided for this reason.

3. **The recurrent laryngeal nerve** is also commonly blocked, leading to transient unilateral **vocal cord paresis**. This should not be problematic unless the opposite nerve is blocked or damaged. In such a scenario, airway obstruction can occur.

4. Other complications that have been reported with deep cervical plexus blocks, such as **vertebral artery puncture and spinal anesthesia**, should not occur with properly performed intermediate or superficial cervical plexus blocks because they do not breach the deep (prevertebral) cervical fascia.

III. **Facial blocks**

A. **Anatomy**

1. The face, forehead, and anterior two-thirds of the top of the head are innervated by the three branches of the trigeminal nerve (i.e., cranial nerve V). Terminal branches include the supraorbital, supratrochlear, infraorbital, and mental nerves.

2. **Supraorbital nerve** exits the orbit through the **supraorbital notch**, which is located near the middle of the supraorbital rim directly above the pupil when the patient looks straight ahead (Fig. 13.9). The supraorbital nerve supplies the upper eyelid, forehead, and scalp to the vertex.

3. **Infraorbital nerve** exits the maxilla through the **infraorbital foramen**, which lies just below the infraorbital rim, in line with the pupil when the patient looks straight ahead (Fig. 13.9). The infraorbital nerve provides sensory innervation to the cheek, lower eyelid, nasal ala, and upper lip.

4. **Mental nerve** is the terminal sensory branch of the inferior alveolar nerve. It exits the mandible through the **mental foramen**, which lies in line with the pupil (when the patient looks straight ahead) and approximately midway between the alveolar and inferior mandibular borders (Fig. 13.9). The mental nerve innervates the lower lip and chin.

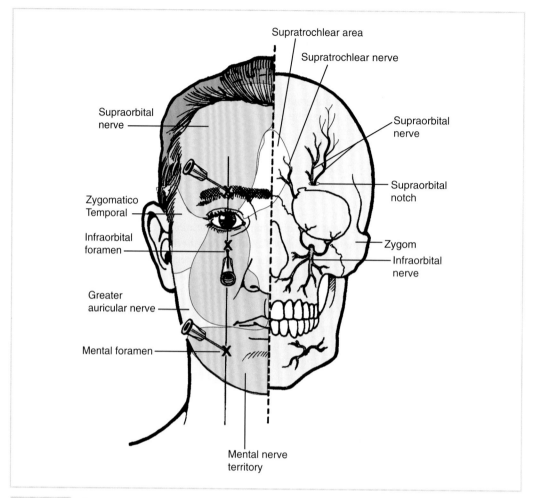

FIGURE 13.9   Cutaneous innervation of the face. Most of the face and forehead are innervated by the terminal branches of the ophthalmic (supraorbital, supratrochlear), maxillary (infraorbital), and mandibular (mental) nerves. The foramina through which the supraorbital, infraorbital, and mental nerves emerge lie along a straight line passing through the pupil when the subject looks straight ahead.

B. Drugs

   1.   All local anesthetics employed for peripheral nerve blocks are appropriate for nerve blocks of the face. However, because only sensory nerves require anesthesia, more dilute concentrations (e.g., lidocaine 1%, bupivacaine 0.25%) can be used.

C. Techniques

   1.   The three trigeminal terminal branches provide cutaneous innervations to the face and can be anesthetized where they exit their respective foramina (Fig. 13.9).

   2.   **Supraorbital nerve block.** With the patient looking straight ahead, the supra-orbital notch can be palpated along the supraorbital rim directly above the pupil. A 22- or 25-gauge needle is inserted at the supraorbital foramen (not into it). Two milliliters of local anesthetic are injected.

   3.   **Infraorbital nerve block.** With the patient looking straight ahead, the infraorbital foramen lies just below the orbital rim. A skin wheal is raised approximately 0.5 cm (0.25 in.) below the infraorbital foramen. A 22- or 25-gauge needle is directed cephalad toward the foramen (because the foramen angles cephalad). Two milliliters of local anesthetic is injected.

4. **Mental nerve block.** With the patient looking straight ahead, the mental foramen can be palpated in line with the pupil at a point midway between the upper and lower borders of the mandible. A 22- or 25-gauge needle is appropriate. The canal of the mental nerve angles medially and inferiorly. It is therefore more easily approached by entering the skin approximately 0.5 cm (0.25 in.) lateral and superior and angling the needle toward the foramen. Two milliliters of local anesthetic is injected.

CLINICAL PEARL   When performing these blocks, it is important not to penetrate the foramen, because this may damage the exiting nerve and may cause a hematoma by breaching the accompanying artery.

D. **Complications**

1. **Nerve injury** is rare but can occur, particularly, if the needle tip penetrates the foramen during injection. **Hematomas and intravascular injections** are also possible because of the high vascularity found in facial soft tissues.

ACKNOWLEDGMENTS

The author wishes to acknowledge the contributions of Michael F. Mulroy, MD, who authored the chapter "Airway, cervical plexus, and Facial Block" in the previous edition.

REFERENCES

1. Apfelbaum JL, Hagberg CA, Caplan RA, et al. Practice guidelines for management of the difficult airway, an updated report by the American Society of Anesthesiologists Task Force on Management of the Difficult Airway. *Anesthesiology* 2013;118:251–270.
2. Simmons ST, Schleich AR. Airway regional anesthesia for awake fiberoptic intubation. *Reg Anesth Pain Med* 2002;27:180–192.
3. Reasoner DK, Warner DS, Todd MM, et al. A comparison of anesthetic techniques for awake intubation in neurosurgical patients. *J Neurosurg Anesth* 1995;7:94–99.
4. Usui Y, Kobayashi T, Kakinuma H, et al. An anatomical basis for blocking of the deep cervical plexus and cervical sympathetic tract using an ultrasound-guided technique. *Anesth Analg* 2010;110:964–968.
5. Leblanc I, Chterev V, Rekik M, et al. Safety and efficiency of ultrasound-guided intermediate cervical plexus block for carotid surgery. *Anaesth Crit Care Pain Med* 2016;35:109–114.
6. Tran DQ, Dugani S, Finlayson RJ. A randomized comparison between ultrasound-guided and landmark-based superficial cervical plexus block. *Reg Anesth Pain Med* 2010;35:539–543.
7. Pandit JJ, Satya-Krishna R, Gration P. Superficial or deep cervical plexus block for carotid endarterectomy: a systematic review of complications. *Br J Anaesth* 2007;99:159–169.

Complications Associated with Regional Anesthesia

Joseph M. Neal

KEY POINTS

1. The provision of regional anesthesia must balance its positive benefits with the risk of associated complications. Most regional anesthetic complications are indeed expected, short-lived side effects associated with local anesthetic effects. Fortunately, life-altering complications are extremely rare.

2. Because of their rarity, it is difficult to determine accurately the true incidence of regional anesthesia–associated complications. Even when the incidence is known, it is often difficult to deconstruct causation as a function of anesthetic, surgical, and/or patient factors.

3. Neurologic injuries are the most feared and devastating regional anesthetic complications. Injuries to the neuraxis demand rapid diagnosis and intervention to preserve function. Transient postoperative peripheral nerve symptoms are common, but long-term injury is rare. Other causes of neurologic injury include direct neural trauma, inflammation, and/or ischemia.

4. Local anesthetic systemic toxicity (LAST) ranges from minor symptoms of central nervous system excitation to life-threatening seizure and/or cardiac arrest. Ultrasound guidance reduces the frequency of LAST throughout its continuum. When a major LAST event occurs, resuscitation is markedly different from that of ischemic cardiac arrest. Lipid emulsion therapy is an effective antidote.

5. Bradycardia and hypotension are expected sequelae of neuraxial anesthesia that pose little problem if managed expeditiously. However, the potential for cardiovascular collapse is always present.

6. Although ultrasound guidance has reduced the incidence and intensity of hemidiaphragmatic paresis, and likely has reduced the incidence of pneumothorax, it has not completely eliminated these complications.

7. Local anesthetics find their way to various unintended destinations. The result can be nuisance side effects such as hoarseness or Horner syndrome. Conversely, devastating complications can occur if neuraxial spread of local anesthetic is unrecognized and not treated promptly.

8. Postdural puncture headache (PDPH) is a risk of neuraxial techniques. Small-gauge, atraumatic tip spinal needles reduce PDPH risk, as does avoidance of spinal anesthesia in patients less than 30 years old. Epidural blood patch is an effective treatment. Perhaps the greatest risk of PDPH is misdiagnosis when the patient's headache is actually from a more sinister neurologic process.

I. Introduction

A. Patient injury associated with regional anesthesia ranges from mere nuisance to life altering. Bruising from axillary brachial plexus block or temporary hoarseness from unintended local anesthetic spread to the recurrent laryngeal nerve may be distressing to the patient, but will resolve fully and quickly. Conversely, clinicians and patients fear permanent nerve injury or death from local anesthetic systemic toxicity (LAST). Life-altering injuries associated with regional anesthesia are extremely rare.

B. Regional anesthesia–related complications are difficult to study because their low frequency makes it difficult to accrue enough patients in randomized controlled trials to achieve sufficient statistical power from which to draw conclusions about incidence, etiology, and risk. Consequently, much of the literature of rare regional anesthesia complications comes from large observational studies or small case reports. Recommendations for avoiding injury are often based on expert opinion derived from analysis of case reports, small case series, or pharmacokinetic inference. Retrospective reviews or voluntary reporting to a central registry suffer from reporting bias (clinicians may choose not to report their serious complications or they may dismiss minor complications as too trivial to merit reporting). Such sources often lack the accuracy, detail, or follow-up necessary to characterize causation, risk, and recovery. Even large prospective studies may fail to ask the right questions or to follow patients long enough to identify late-developing problems. For example, Philips et al.'s (1) classic prospective study of 10,440 patients undergoing lidocaine spinal anesthesia in the 1960s did not detect what came to be recognized in the 1990s as transient neurologic symptoms (TNS) (2).

C. **Accurate determination of incidence is difficult for rare complications**—the number depends on how the data were derived. For example, in Sweden a young woman undergoing labor analgesia has a 1 per 200,000 risk for epidural hematoma. Yet that same woman at age 70 and undergoing spinal anesthesia for total knee arthroplasty is at 1 per 3,800 risk for the same complication because degenerative spine disease has reduced the cross-sectional area of her spinal canal, thereby leaving little room for both blood and spinal cord (3).

D. Difficulties associated with incidence estimation aside, most contemporary studies report **the approximate long-term perioperative nerve injury per regional block as 2–4/10,000 (4); severe LAST as 2.5/10,000 (5); and serious neuraxial infection as 0.2–0.3/10,000 (3).**

E. Studies from the Mayo Clinic (6) and elsewhere (7,8) suggest that the decision to perform a **regional anesthetic *per se* does not place patients at higher risk** for perioperative nerve injury.

II. Neurologic injury

A. **Overview**
Central to understanding perioperative nerve injury is appreciating its multifactorial nature. When a needle and drug are used near a nerve that subsequently sustains injury, temporal proximity makes it tempting to blame the complication on the regional anesthetic. Although **regional anesthesia** can cause neural injury, **it is directly responsible for injury in only 10% to 15% of cases (4)**. The vast majority of perioperative nerve injury is surgery-related,

often from trauma to the nerve, traction, or compression. Patient comorbidity influences risk for perioperative nerve injury, including sex, extremes of body habitus, and medical conditions such as diabetes mellitus, hypertension, and tobacco abuse (8,9).

> **CLINICAL PEARL**   Regional anesthesia is rarely the cause of perioperative nerve injury. Surgical and/or patient factors are more likely than not responsible for the injury. From the patient's perspective, it is the injury that is most important, not who or what is to blame. Collaborative patient care is in everyone's best interest.

B. Hemorrhagic complications

1. Spinal hematoma is a potentially devastating complication that can occur spontaneously, but has also been linked to neuraxial block procedures.

2. Specific guidelines for the management of regional anesthetics in patients who are receiving antithrombotic or thrombolytic therapy are complex, updated periodically, and difficult to retain in one's memory. Therefore, anesthesiologists are referred to the latest version of the American Society of Regional Anesthesia and Pain Medicine's (ASRA) practice advisory on this topic (10) (www.asra.com) and/or ASRA's smart phone app (ASRA Coags; iOS or Android).

3. **Key concepts related to the prevention of hemorrhagic complications include the following**:

   a. Multiple anticoagulants increase risk.

   b. Traumatic or prolonged needle placement increases risk, but a small amount of blood during placement does not mandate case cancellation.

   c. Renal failure increases risk by reducing the clearance of some anticoagulants, particularly the oral anti-Xa inhibitors (rivaroxaban, apixaban, edoxaban) and direct thrombin inhibitors (dabigatran).

   d. Bleeding can occur not just with needle or epidural catheter placement, but also with catheter removal.

   e. Although aspirin and nonsteroidal anti-inflammatory drugs are considered low risk for regional anesthetic techniques, the same may not apply to large-needle, interventional pain medicine procedures such as intrathecal pumps or spinal cord stimulators.

   f. Patients with ankylosing spondylitis or severe spinal stenosis may be at higher risk for neurologic compromise should bleeding occur within the limited cross-sectional area of their spinal canal.

4. All patients with indwelling neuraxial catheters should undergo **scheduled neurologic evaluation** of lower-extremity sensory and motor function at least every 4 hours. Patients at high risk or heightened concern should be evaluated every 1 to 2 hours.

5. **Timely diagnosis of spinal hematoma is paramount** because the chances for meaningful recovery diminish rapidly when surgical decompression is delayed more than 8 hours after initial symptom presentation. The severity of neurologic deficit is predictive of ultimate recovery. Back pain and bowel/bladder symptoms may be present, but are not universal. Of particular concern is sensory or motor deficit outside of the block's expected distribution, for example, lower leg or foot weakness in the presence of a thoracic epidural. Numbness or weakness suspected to arise from local anesthetic action may be addressed by turning the epidural drug infusion down or off, but the patient must be reexamined within an hour. Failure to respond to these measures demands immediate neuroimaging (magnetic resonance imaging [MRI] preferred if immediately available; computerized tomography if not) and referral to a neurosurgeon.

C. **Infectious complications**

1. Epidural abscess or meningitis can complicate **neuraxial anesthetics**. Epidural abscess may be indolent initially and present as low-grade fever or mild back pain. Signs and symptoms may then escalate rapidly to include severe back pain, weakness, and/or bowel or bladder dysfunction. Meningitis presents with fever, headache, nuchal rigidity, and/or photophobia.

2. Bacterial colonization at the injection or catheter site is common with **peripheral nerve blocks**, especially in the axilla or femoral region. True infection is rare—3% or fewer catheters show signs of localized infection, and even fewer develop deep infection that requires drainage or antibiotics.

3. **Key to infection prevention is handwashing**, jewelry removal, and the use of a face mask during the procedure (11). Blocks should not be performed through infected skin. Data strongly support the superiority of chlorhexidine/alcohol mixtures for skin disinfection.

4. Infection **risk is increased** when catheters are used for more than 3 to 5 days, in trauma or critical care unit patients, and when the patient develops systemic infection. Regional techniques should not be undertaken, or should be delayed, in patients with untreated sepsis.

5. As with spinal hematoma, correct diagnosis and rapid intervention are paramount to circumvent paralysis or death, which may occur in up to 30% of patients with meningitis.

D. **Direct neural trauma**

1. Direct injury to the spinal cord or spinal nerves by needles or catheters has been reported as a 5 per million neuraxial anesthetic event (3). The structure that is injured is determined by needle trajectory (Fig. 14.1).

2. **Awareness of anatomic factors may lower the risk of direct spinal cord trauma**. Risk is increased by the practitioner's inaccuracy in determining vertebral levels, especially in large patients or those with poor vertebral landmarks. This risk may be mitigated in challenging patients by using ultrasound to determine vertebral level (see Chapter 6 for details). Midline gaps in the mid-to-high thoracic ligamentum flavum occur in up to 20% of patients, thereby negating the expected resistance to epidural needle advancement. The posterior-to-anterior dimension of the epidural space narrows progressively from 4 to 12 mm in the lumbar spine to fewer than 2 mm in the high thoracic spine (12).

3. The spinal cord has no sensory innervation and that to the meninges is inconsistent. Consequently, **cases have been reported of needle entry into the spinal cord without warning**, even in unsedated patients (12). Injection of substances into the spinal cord usually elicits pain.

4. If direct spinal cord trauma is suspected because of an intense, nonresolving paresthesia or new neurologic deficit, immediate MRI is recommended. If spinal cord injury is confirmed, some experts recommend administering high-dose steroids in consultation with a neurologist or neurosurgeon (4).

5. Needle-related injury of the peripheral nerves is exceptionally rare, in part because nerves tend to move away from approaching needles or catheters. Similar to the spinal cord, paresthesia may or may not herald nerve injury. Injury can occur in the absence of warning signs (9).

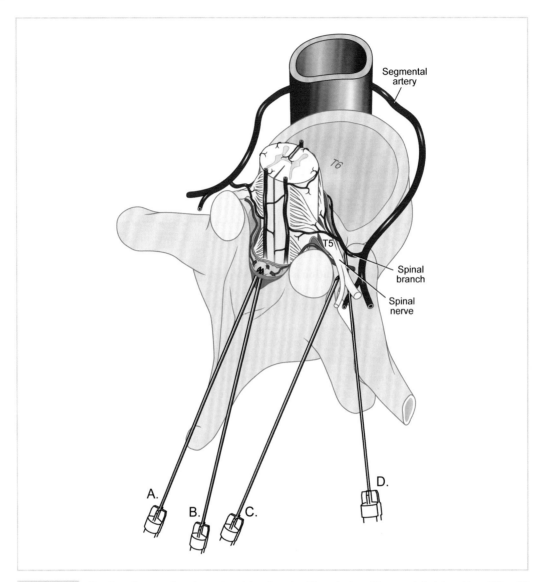

FIGURE 14.1 Needle trajectory often determines injury location. The spinal cord is potentially injured by midline **(A)** and paramedian **(B)** approaches. Spinal nerves are potentially injured by unintended lateral deviation of needles **(C)** or by planned lateral trajectory, such as with the transforaminal approach **(D)**. (From Neal JM, Rathmell JP. *Complications of Regional Anesthesia and Pain Medicine.* 2nd ed. Philadelphia, PA: Lippincott Williams & Wilkins; 2013, used with permission.)

   E. **Neurotoxicity**

   1. All **local anesthetics** are neurotoxic and capable of producing permanent neurologic injury. Neurotoxicity increases with local anesthetic concentration and exposure time, that is, reduced drug clearance. Clinically relevant local anesthetic doses and concentrations rarely produce injury in normal individuals or uncompromised neural tissues. (The chapters on regional block techniques recommended doses and concentrations of local anesthetic for specific blocks.) Preservative-free **opioids** are not neurotoxic.

   2. **Adjuvants such as epinephrine do not cause nerve injury in isolation**, but worsen it by prolonging local anesthetic clearance and thus exposure time. Dexmedetomidine and

clonidine have undergone extensive neurotoxicity studies and are believe to be nontoxic. Dexamethasone is less well studied; some experts advise caution in diabetic patients.

3. **Excipients, preservatives, and disinfectants**. Commonly used and dosed preservatives or excipients are not neurotoxic (13). There is no evidence that disinfectants such as chlorhexidine/alcohol are neurotoxic when used properly, but they should be allowed to dry before needle placement. Care should be taken to avoid disinfectant splashing onto block trays, needles, or drugs.

4. **Extreme care should also be taken to avoid injection of unintended substances during single-injection techniques or into continuous delivery systems**. Precautions include proper labelling of syringes and drugs, reading and re-reading labels before injection, and avoidance of superfluous stopcocks or port access on catheters that subserve a neural structure.

5. **Peripheral nerve injury**
   a. The precise etiology of regional anesthetic-associated peripheral nerve injury is unknown. **Classic theory suggests a dual mechanism** by which a needle or catheter disrupts the perineurium, thereby exposing denuded axons to the neurotoxic effects of local anesthetic (which is nontoxic to intact axons) (Fig. 14.2).
   b. An additional postulated etiology of peripheral nerve injury involves localized or diffuse inflammation (see Postsurgical Inflammatory Neuropathies)
   c. Because needle or catheter injury may expose the axons to neurotoxic agents, **most experts recommend avoiding needle-to-nerve contact during peripheral nerve block placement.** Nevertheless, ultrasound studies of patients in whom initial nerve localization was accomplished using peripheral nerve stimulation (PNS) confirm unintended intraneural needle placement more often than appreciated previously. The fact that these patients rarely suffer injury is likely a function of the high proportion of nonneural connective tissue present within a nerve's cross-sectional microanatomy, resistance of the perineurium to needle penetration, and acknowledgment that direct needle injury may not play as significant a role in nerve injury as once thought.
   d. Although ultrasound guidance (UG) helps avoid unintended subepineurial needle placement, **there is no evidence that ultrasound use *per se* has reduced the incidence of anesthesia-related nerve injury** from that previously reported with PNS alone (14). Some experts advocate localizing peripheral nerves with both UG and PNS. This opinion is based on extrapolated evidence from human supraclavicular and popliteal sciatic block studies that demonstrate a motor response elicited at 0.2 mA or less is consistent with subepineurial needle placement, whereas a response at 0.5 mA or greater is most often indicative of extraneural needle placement (9). Nevertheless, there is no evidence that combining UG with PNS reduces nerve injury, but it does increase procedural time without concomitant increasing block success (Fig. 14.3).
   e. Patient report of paresthesia or pain associated with needle-to-nerve contact or unintended intraneural injection is inconsistent, but when it happens serves as yet another safety monitor. For this reason, **the use of regional anesthesia in anesthetized or deeply sedated adults is discouraged (4)**. However, regional anesthesia is performed routinely in anesthetized children.
   f. **Diagnosis and treatment**
      (1) Postoperative neurologic symptoms after peripheral nerve block are reported in up to 20% of patients the day after surgery, diminish to 3% at 1 month, and to 2–4/10,000 at 9 to 12 months.
      (2) Most sensory symptoms will resolve within days to weeks and can be managed expectantly.

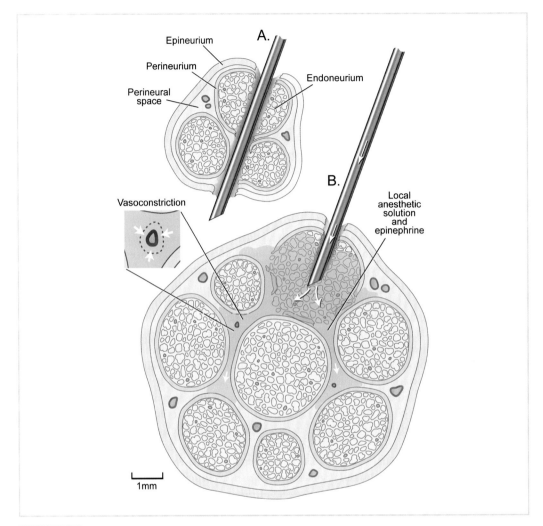

FIGURE 14.2 Peripheral nerves can be injured directly by needles **(A)**. More often, peripheral nerve injury is believed to involve a dual mechanism of needle disruption of the protective perineurium, which then allows previously innocuous local anesthetic to exert neurotoxic effects on denuded axons within the fascicles **(B)**. Epinephrine worsens injury by reducing drug clearance (inset). (From Neal JM, Rathmell JP. *Complications of Regional Anesthesia and Pain Medicine.* 2nd ed. Philadelphia, PA: Lippincott Williams & Wilkins; 2013, used with permission.)

> **(3) More worrisome signs and symptoms include complete nerve deficit at the end of surgery, motor signs, recrudescence of block after initial resolution, and/or severe pain**. Any of these presentations should be treated as an emergency because expanding hematoma, constricting bandages or casts, and so forth can often be rectified with full symptom resolution.
>
> **(4)** When the injury fails to resolve or has worrisome components, early referral to a neurologist is warranted. Although electrophysiologic studies do not change for 2 to 3 weeks after an injury, consideration may be given to early, bilateral studies when the injury is severe.
>
> **(5)** Neuropathic pain should be treated with opioids and/or gabapentinoids, plus referral to a neurologist or chronic pain physician.

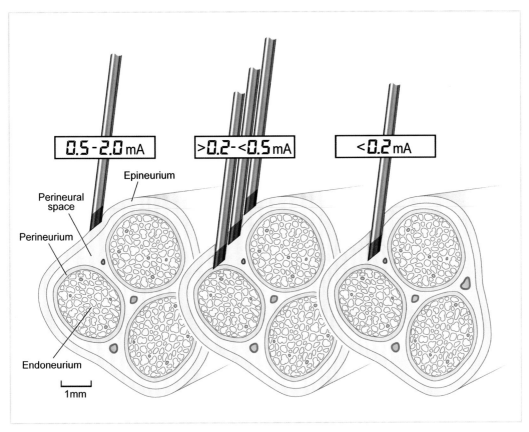

FIGURE 14.3 Peripheral nerve stimulation can be an additional monitor to lessen the risk of peripheral nerve injury. As extrapolated from human studies of supraclavicular and popliteal sciatic block, motor response at 0.5 mA or greater is usually indicative of extraneural needle placement, whereas a motor response less than 0.2 mA usually indicates subepineurial needle location. A motor response between 0.2 and 0.5 mA is not definitive for either location. (From Neal JM, Rathmell JP. *Complications of Regional Anesthesia and Pain Medicine.* 2nd ed. Philadelphia, PA: Lippincott Williams & Wilkins; 2013, used with permission.)

6. **Cauda equina syndrome**
   a. The cauda equina may be particularly susceptible to neurotoxic injury because intrathecal nerve roots have no protective covering and a long transit course, thereby increasing their surface area (Fig. 14.4). Cauda equina syndrome (CES) from presumed local anesthetic neurotoxic injury is rare and poorly understood. One study observed CES in 0.2/10,000 neuraxial anesthetics. In this report, 28% of CES cases were associated with spinal stenosis, whereas the remaining cases were unremarkable in terms of local anesthetic dose, concentration, adjuvant use, and subsequent neuroimaging (3).
   b. CES has been linked to supernormal doses of local anesthetic and/or local anesthetic maldistribution within the lumbosacral intrathecal sac, as manifested by dense sacral but no lumbar–thoracic anesthesia.
   c. CES is also postulated to be the result of inflammation brought on by the anesthetic or surgical procedure, the drugs used, patient characteristics, or yet unknown factors.
   d. Because of CES association with supernormal doses, it is recommended that failed spinal anesthetics not be redosed, or if they are, that the total local anesthetic dose does not exceed the recommended maximum for a single injection.

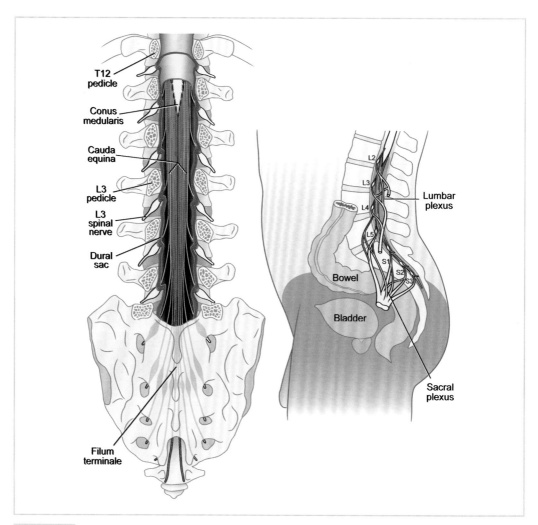

FIGURE 14.4 The cauda equina is believed to be susceptible to neurotoxicity because of its long transit and denuded intrathecal spinal nerve roots. Cauda equina syndrome typically involves bowel and bladder dysfunction with varying degrees of saddle anesthesia and lower-extremity weakness. (From Neal JM, Rathmell JP. *Complications of Regional Anesthesia and Pain Medicine.* 2nd ed. Philadelphia, PA: Lippincott Williams & Wilkins; 2013, used with permission.)

F. Spinal cord ischemia and infarction

1. Ischemic injury or infarction of the spinal cord is a decidedly rare and poorly understood event. Although ischemia and infarction can affect any portion of the spinal cord, the most common variety is anterior spinal artery syndrome (ASAS). Most ASAS presents spontaneously in patients at risk for vascular disease (hypertension, tobacco abuse, advanced age). When ASAS or other forms of spinal ischemia present in the setting of a neuraxial block, the latter is often invoked as the causative event.

2. ASAS presents classically as sudden or rapidly progressive motor and sensory deficit (pain and temperature) with preserved posterior column functions (proprioception, vibration, fine touch). Varied presentations can occur, such as slower, progressive onset rather than sudden lower-extremity muscle flaccidity.

3. **Key points related to spinal cord ischemia** include the following:
   a. Direct needle injury to the anterior spinal artery cannot occur without the needle traversing the spinal cord. However, needles and catheters placed lateral to the vertebrae may injure spinal arteries or radicular arteries that supply the spinal cord (Fig. 14.5).
   b. Because the lower thoracic and lumbosacral spinal cord is supplied by the single arterius radicularis magnus, deficits involving the lower spinal cord and conus medullaris are most common.
   c. Despite being invoked as the agent that causes ischemia, **epinephrine** in clinically used concentrations does not adversely affect spinal cord blood flow (SCBF) (15).

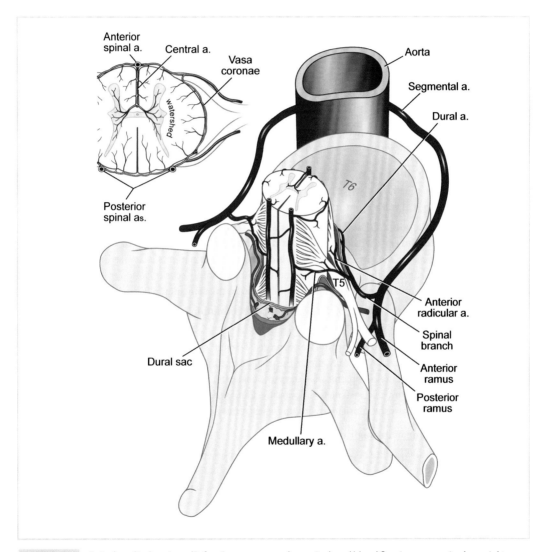

FIGURE 14.5   Spinal cord ischemia and infarction can occur when spinal cord blood flow is compromised, as might occur from needle trauma to the lateral feeding arteries (spinal branch, radicular arteries) or the posterior spinal arteries. Note that the anterior spinal artery cannot be damaged without first traversing the spinal cord. A limited number of medullary arteries supply to spinal cord, especially in the thoracolumbar area. When their flow is compromised, the anterior spinal artery is often affected and places the anterior two thirds of the spinal cord at risk. (From Neal JM, Rathmell JP. *Complications of Regional Anesthesia and Pain Medicine*. 2nd ed. Philadelphia, PA: Lippincott Williams & Wilkins; 2013, used with permission.)

   d. The contribution of **hypotension** to spinal cord ischemia is poorly understood and believed not to be a factor in the majority of patients. However, there may exist a subset of patients in whom a mean arterial pressure (MAP) of 60 to 65 mm Hg is below their lower limit of autoregulation, thereby leading to pressure-passive SCBF. Because the autoregulatory curve for SCBF mirrors that of cerebral blood flow, one may infer from studies of cerebral stroke that **prolonged periods of blood pressure 30% to 40% below baseline MAP might place a very small subset of patients at risk for spinal cord ischemia**. This phenomenon is likely most relevant in patients with reduced oxygen-carrying capacity, as may occur with anemia, sickle cell disease, hyperventilation, a tight spinal canal, and the like (12).

   4. Neuroimaging may be normal in the early hours after suspected spinal cord ischemia. If the diagnosis is suspected (or later confirmed on MRI), the patient may benefit from improving SCBF by lowering spinal cerebrospinal fluid (CSF) pressure via lumbar drain placement. Many experts do not recommend steroid therapy in the setting of ischemic neurologic injury. Neurologic consultation is encouraged.

> **CLINICAL PEARL**   Even though hypotension is unlikely to be a factor in spinal cord ischemia in the vast majority of patients, there are few reasons to permit a patient's MAP to fall 20% to 30% below baseline during provision of a neuraxial anesthetic. When such diminution of MAP occurs, it should not be allowed to remain at those levels, especially for times exceeding 20 minutes.

   G. **Postsurgical inflammatory neuropathies**

   1. Postsurgical inflammatory neuropathies **(PSIN) (16) typically present hours to days after surgery with a neurologic distribution inconsistent with that expected from block- or surgery-related nerve damage**. These patients may present with mono- or poly-neuropathies, plexopathies, or with mixed motor–sensory lesion patterns. The sensory and motor deficits may or may not fall within the same neural territory.

   2. Early recognition of PSIN is crucial because **immunomodulation therapies** might improve the disease's overall course.

   3. **Neuralgic amyotrophy (Parsonage–Turner syndrome)** is a unique inflammatory neuropathy that typically affects the upper extremity. Neuralgic amyotrophy often begins as excruciating neuropathic pain days to weeks after surgery. As the pain subsides, the patient develops muscle weakness and wasting. Pain, sensory, and motor involvement often do not follow patterns consistent with upper-extremity innervation.

   H. **Preexisting neurologic disease**

   1. The advisability of performing regional anesthesia on a patient with preexisting neurologic disease has been long debated. This controversy is anchored in the **"double-crush theory" (9),** which states that two small subclinical injuries can result in a severe neuropathy that is more than additive. The double-crush theory has neither been confirmed nor been refuted definitively in humans.

   2. Several large studies **have associated the presence of severe spinal stenosis within the same area as the neuraxial intervention with epidural hematoma, epidural abscess, and CES (12).**

   3. **Other associations** exist for new or worsening neurologic deficits in those patients that have received neurotoxic chemotherapeutic drugs, that have open or repaired spinal dysraphisms, and/or that have severe diabetic polyneuropathy (17).

4. Postpolio syndrome, multiple sclerosis, amyotrophic lateral sclerosis, spina bifida, and mild-to-moderate spinal canal pathology do not appear to place patients at significant risk for new or worsening neurologic injury (17).

CLINICAL PEARL   Data neither confirm nor refute the relationship of preexisting neurologic injury to regional anesthetics. Practitioners are advised to always consider risk-to-benefit before determining their anesthetic plan.

III. Local anesthetic systemic toxicity

A. **LAST is a classic regional anesthetic complication, the characteristics of which have changed dramatically with the advent of UG as a tool of prevention and lipid emulsion therapy as an antidote for toxicity.**

B. **Pharmacokinetics**

1. LAST can occur immediately after an intravenous (IV) injection of local anesthetic or be delayed for up to 60 minutes in the case of prolonged soft tissue uptake into the systemic circulation.

2. Peak local anesthetic plasma concentration varies linearly with dose, that is, doubling the local anesthetic dose doubles peak plasma concentration.

3. Contrary to common belief, peak local anesthetic plasma concentration is not related to adult weight and/or body mass index (Fig. 14.6). Correlation improves in children or adults with small muscle mass. **The common practice of basing maximum local anesthetic dose on patient weight has no scientific foundation.**

4. The time to, and magnitude of, peak local anesthetic concentration is affected by block type (Fig. 14.7 and Table 14.1), which in turn is determined by local tissue vascularity and the surface area from which the drug is absorbed.

5. The free fraction of local anesthetic (non–protein-bound) is responsible for LAST. Because acidosis displaces local anesthetic from plasma protein–binding sites, the presence of metabolic or respiratory acidosis increases the risk of LAST and adversely affects its treatment.

6. Epinephrine-induced local vasoconstriction decreases peak local anesthetic plasma concentration by reducing drug clearance from the injection site.

7. Because of rapid hydrolysis, ester local anesthetics (2-chloroprocaine, procaine) are least likely to cause LAST. Levo-enantiomers are less cardiotoxic than the racemic mixtures. Ropivacaine and L-bupivacaine (no longer available in the United States) are levo-enantiomeric local anesthetics. Despite animal-based evidence that ropivacaine is less cardiotoxic than bupivacaine, this effect is not as pronounced in humans, in part because ropivacaine is less potent (18). Indeed, LAST with ropivacaine is reported frequently in the literature (5,19).

8. Importantly, **local anesthetic systemic toxicity is additive (LAST)**. Therefore, mixing two or more different local anesthetics does not reduce the risk of LAST.

CLINICAL PEARL   Although ropivacaine is less cardiotoxic than bupivacaine, it is so only by a matter of degree. Practitioners should not become less vigilant to LAST just because they are using ropivacaine.

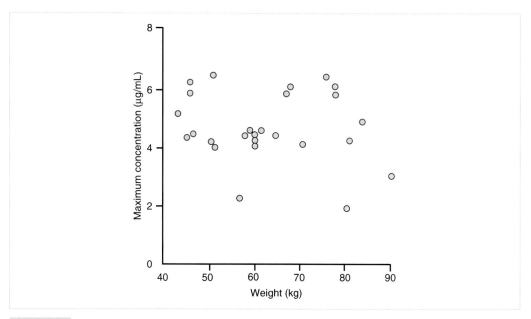

FIGURE 14.6 Lack of correlation between patient weight and peak plasma concentration after epidural administration of 400 mg of lidocaine. This same lack of a relationship between patient weight and peak plasma concentration has been demonstrated for multiple local anesthetics and different types of block. (Redrawn from Braid DP, Scott DB. Dosage of lignocaine in epidural block in relation to toxicity. *Br J Anaesth* 1966;38(8):596; by permission of Oxford University Press.)

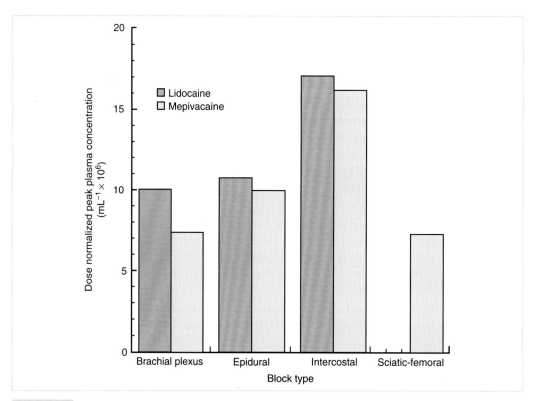

FIGURE 14.7 Dose-normalized peak plasma concentrations of lidocaine and mepivacaine following different types of nerve block. Highest concentrations occur following intercostal blocks.

TABLE 14.1 Typical C_{max} after regional anesthetics with commonly used local anesthetics

Local anesthetic	Technique	Dose (mg)	C_{max} (μg/mL)	T_{max} (min)	Toxic plasma concentration (μg/mL)
Bupivacaine	Brachial plexus	150	1.0	20	3
	Celiac plexus	100	1.50	17	
	Epidural	150	1.26	20	
	Intercostal	140	0.90	30	
	Sciatic/femoral	400	1.89	15	
Lidocaine	Brachial plexus	400	4.00	25	5
	Epidural	400	4.27	20	
	Intercostal	400	6.8	15	
Mepivacaine	Brachial plexus	500	3.68	24	5
	Epidural	500	4.95	16	
	Intercostal	500	8.06	9	
	Sciatic/femoral	500	3.59	31	
Ropivacaine	Brachial plexus	190	1.3	53	4
	Epidural	150	1.07	40	
	Intercostal	140	1.10	21	

C_{max}, peak plasma concentration; T_{max}, time until C_{max}.
Data from: Liu SS. Local anesthetics and analgesia. In: Ashburn MA, Rice LJ, eds. *The Management of Pain*. New York, NY: Churchill Livingstone; 1997:141–170; Berrisford RG, Sabanathan S, Mearns AJ, et al. Plasma concentrations of bupivacaine and its enantiomers during continuous extrapleural intercostal nerve block. *Br J Anaesth* 1993;70:201; Kopacz DJ, Helman JD, Nussbaum CE, et al. A comparison of epidural levo-bupivacaine 0.5% with or without epinephrine for lumbar spine surgery. *Anesth Analg* 2001;93:755; Crews JC, Weller RS, Moss J. Levo-bupivacaine for axillary brachial plexus block: a pharmacokinetic and clinical comparison in patients with normal renal function or renal disease. *Anesth Analg* 2002;95:219.

C. **Risk factors for LAST (18)**

  1. Some patient characteristics place them at greater risk for LAST. These factors include the following:

   a. **Small muscle mass** (muscles act as a depot for local anesthetic redistribution)

   b. History of **cardiac disease**, including conduction abnormalities

   c. **Extremes of age**

   d. **Impaired local anesthetic metabolism**, as might occur with congestive heart failure or hepatic disease

  2. Prolonged infusions of local anesthetic are generally safe, but can become problematic in patients with risk factors as listed earlier.

D. **Prevention of LAST (20)**

  1. Use the **smallest local anesthetic dose possible** (local anesthetic mass/dose = volume × concentration)

  2. Although not proven scientifically, frequent syringe **aspiration** to rule out IV needle or catheter placement is advised. False-negative aspiration occurs 1% to 2% of the time. **Incremental injection** of small aliquots (3 to 5 mL) of local anesthetic is also advised, ideally allowing a full circulation time (30 to 45 seconds) between injections.

  3. UG reduces the frequency of LAST throughout its continuum by approximately 65% (5).

  4. Consider an intravascular marker, especially when potentially toxic doses of potent local anesthetics such as ropivacaine and bupivacaine are used. There is evidence that the use of an IV test dose has substantially decreased the incidence of LAST associated with epidural anesthesia (20).

   a. **Epinephrine test dose**. A test dose containing 10 to 15 µg epinephrine facilitates detection of IV injection through the observance of a tachycardic response. The classic test dose (3 mL lidocaine 1.5% with 5 µg/mL epinephrine) is 100% sensitive and 100% specific for causing a 10- to-20-beat/minute heart-rate increase within 2 minutes of injection in a nonsedated, non–beta-blocked young adult (21).

   b. The expected tachycardic response to an epinephrine-containing IV test dose is tempered in patients older than 40 years, and especially in the elderly (Table 14.2). A similarly altered response is present in beta-blocked or anesthetized patients, or those with a thoracic epidural in place. In these patients, a 15-mm Hg increase in systolic blood pressure is more indicative of IV needle or catheter placement.

   c. **Mild sedation can mask patient awareness of the subjective signs of LAST**, for example, auditory changes, feeling of doom, circumoral numbness, or metallic taste. Therefore, epinephrine-containing IV test doses are recommended for all sedated or anesthetized patients receiving potentially toxic doses of local anesthetic.

   d. If epinephrine is contraindicated, fentanyl 100 µg is an alternative test dose regimen. When injected intravenously, nonsedated parturients exhibit signs of drowsiness or sedation.

5. **LAST presentation (19)**

   a. **The presentation of LAST can be quite variable** and changes with local anesthetic peak plasma concentrations. Classic LAST presentation involves progression from subjective central nervous system (CNS) symptoms (circumoral numbness, metallic taste, auditory changes, feelings of doom, and/or vocalization), to seizure and cardiovascular (CV) collapse. However, this classic presentation only occurs in about 40% of LAST episodes. Presentation typically begins with excitatory signs—for example, hypertension, cardiac dysrhythmias for CV, agitation, seizure, vocalization for CNS. Inhibitory signs and symptoms follow if not preempted by seizure or cardiac arrest. These signs include hypotension, bradycardia, or asystole for CV and drowsiness or confusion for CNS. The variability of presentation makes the diagnosis of LAST particularly challenging (Fig. 14.8).

TABLE 14.2 Hemodynamic responses to epinephrine test dose in different populations

Study population	Epinephrine dose (µg)	Maximal change in HR BPM (range)	Maximal change in SBP mm Hg (range)
Adult surgical patients (24)			
21–40 yr	15	39 (21–53)	28 (1–43)
41–60 yr	15	29 (20–45)	28 (20–53)
61–80 yr	15	31 (9–52)	33 (18–66)
Anesthetized adult patients (25)			
0.5 MAC	15	20 (12–35)	36 (16–54)
1.0 MAC	15	10 (1–18)	22 (6–44)
0.5 MAC	30	31 (18–42)	40 (25–60)
1.0 MAC	30	20 (5–50)	39 (15–66)
Acutely β-blocked adult volunteers (21)			
Control	15	37 (29–46)	26 (18–33)
β-blockade	15	−28 (−23–33)	35 (24–46)

BPM, beats per minute; HR, heart rate; MAC, minimum alveolar concentration; SBP, systolic blood pressure.

b. **About 10% of significant LAST episodes present with only cardiac signs and symptoms. The remaining patient presentations are divided equally between only CNS symptoms or a combination of CNS and CV symptoms**.

CLINICAL PEARL   Because systemic uptake of local anesthetic in amounts sufficient to induce LAST can be delayed 30 to 60 minutes, patients who receive potentially toxic doses of local anesthetic should be observed for at least 30 minutes after block placement.

6. **LAST treatment (18)**

   a. When LAST is suspected or in progress, **primacy of the airway** is paramount. Allowing the patient to become hypoxic, hypercarbic, or acidotic not only worsens LAST, but also impairs treatment effectiveness.

   b. If the patient experiences **seizures**, administer a benzodiazepine to stop cerebral hyperactivity. Many seizures abate quickly, but if not secure the patient's airway.

   c. When LAST occurs or is highly suspected, the administration of **lipid emulsion** acts as an antidote through lipid shuttling and cardiotonic mechanisms. Propofol is not a substitute for lipid emulsion because it contains relatively small amounts of lipid and worsens cardiac performance.

   d. Should cardiac arrest occur, it is of utmost importance to remember that **LAST-induced cardiac arrest is different from ischemic cardiac arrest**. Resuscitation drugs that reduce contractility or increase afterload are contraindicated. Thus, one should not administer more local anesthetic as an antiarrhythmic, use beta- or calcium-channel blockers, or administer vasopressin. If epinephrine is used, do so in small increments of 10 to 100 μg. Consider cardiopulmonary bypass early in recalcitrant episodes of LAST.

   e. Treatment of LAST is best managed through the use of a **checklist**, such as that produced as part of the frequently updated ASRA Practice Advisory on LAST (22) (Fig. 14.9).

IV. Cardiovascular complications

A. Intravascular pooling and local anesthetic blockade of the cardioaccelerator fibers of the thoracic spinal cord (T1–T4) contribute to the bradycardia that often accompanies neuraxial anesthesia. Heart rate can fall to 40 to 50 beats in 10% and to less than 40 beats in 1% of patients. Blockade of the lumbar sympathetic nerves contributes to hypotension, with decrements of 30% below baseline systolic pressure occurring in up to 10% of patients (Fig. 14.10). These hemodynamic changes can occur within 20 to 30 minutes of neuraxial block or be delayed up to an hour. When anesthesiologists are vigilant to these predictable changes in heart rate and blood pressure and treat them expeditiously with atropine (0.4 to 0.8 mg) and/or ephedrine (5 to 10 mg increments) or phenylephrine (80 to 100 μg increments), neuraxial anesthetic-induced cardiovascular side effects are seldom problematic. However, if left untreated or if they appear suddenly, these changes can lead quickly to cardiovascular collapse. When this occurs, rapid recognition and the use of epinephrine (10 to 100 μg) to restore contractility, vascular tone, and coronary perfusion pressure is paramount. The longer cardiovascular collapse persists, the more difficult it is to reverse. Although these patients experience lower-extremity venous pooling, they should not be placed in Trendelenburg position; doing so risks higher neuraxial block level and worsening hemodynamics. Associated risk factors for spinal hypotension and bradycardia are listed in Table 14.3.

B. **Hypotension and bradycardia have also been reported in sedated patients anesthetized with an interscalene block and placed in the beach chair position.** The combination of exogenous epinephrine and venous pooling are postulated to create the scenario of reflexive

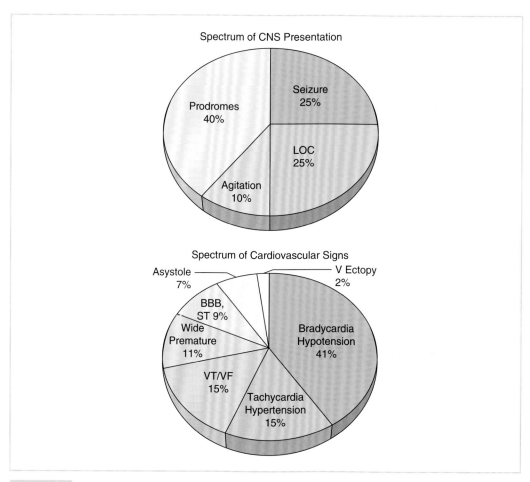

FIGURE 14.8 Spectrum of central nervous system and cardiovascular system signs reported in cases of local anesthetic systemic toxicity. BBB, ST, bundle branch block and ST-changes; LOC, loss of consciousness; V, ventricular; VT/VF, ventricular tachycardia and fibrillation. (Modified from Vasques F, Behr AU, Weinberg G, et al. A review of local anesthetic systemic toxicity cases since publication of the American Society of Regional Anesthesia recommendations. To whom it may concern. *Reg Anesth Pain Med* 2015;40(6):698–705, with permission.)

slowing of a relatively empty, but forcefully contracting, heart. Similar to spinal hypotension and bradycardia, presentation may be delayed for up to an hour after block placement. Treatment involves fluids, atropine, and/or vasopressors as appropriate.

V. Pulmonary complications

A. Hemidiaphragmatic paresis

1. Hemidiaphragmatic paresis (HDP) is a universal side effect of **percutaneous interscalene block techniques** that use 20 mL or more local anesthetic. The phrenic nerve is anesthetized from cephalad spread of local anesthetic to the 3rd and 4th cervical (C3–C4) nerve roots; an alternative pathway may involve unintended local anesthetic spread to the phrenic nerve as it crosses the anterior scalene muscle (Fig. 14.11).

2. **UG interscalene block** requires lower volumes of local anesthetic. Consequently, the incidence and intensity of HDP is reduced when only 5 to 10 mL of local anesthetic is

AMERICAN SOCIETY OF
REGIONAL ANESTHESIA AND PAIN MEDICINE

Checklist for Treatment
of Local Anesthetic Systemic Toxicity

The Pharmacologic Treatment of Local Anesthetic Systemic Toxicity (LAST) is Different from Other Cardiac Arrest Scenarios

- ❏ **Get Help**
- ❏ **Initial Focus**
    - ❏ **Airway management:** ventilate with 100% oxygen
    - ❏ **Seizure suppression:** benzodiazepines are preferred; **AVOID propofol** in patients having signs of cardiovascular instability
    - ❏ **Alert** the nearest facility having **cardiopulmonary bypass** capability
- ❏ **Management of Cardiac Arrhythmias**
    - ❏ **Basic and Advanced Cardiac Life Support (ACLS)** will require adjustment of medications and perhaps prolonged effort
    - ❏ **AVOID vasopressin, calcium channel blockers, beta blockers, or local anesthetic**
    - ❏ **REDUCE individual epinephrine doses to <1 mcg/kg**
- ❏ **Lipid Emulsion (20%) Therapy** (values in parenthesis are for 70kg patient)
    - ❏ **Bolus 1.5 mL/kg** (lean body mass) intravenously over 1 minute (~100mL)
    - ❏ **Continuous infusion 0.25 mL/kg/min** (~18 mL/min; adjust by roller clamp)
    - ❏ Repeat bolus once or twice for persistent cardiovascular collapse
    - ❏ Double the infusion rate to 0.5 mL/kg/min if blood pressure remains low
    - ❏ **Continue infusion** for at least10 minutes after attaining circulatory stability
    - ❏ Recommended upper limit: Approximately 10 mL/kg lipid emulsion over the first 30 minutes
- ❏ **Post LAST events at** www.lipidrescue.org and report use of lipid to www.lipidregistry.org

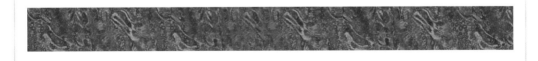

FIGURE 14.9   American Society of Regional Anesthesia and Pain Medicine (ASRA) checklist for treatment of local anesthetic systemic toxicity. (From Neal JM, Mulroy MF, Weinberg GL. American Society of Regional Anesthesia and Pain Medicine checklist for managing local anesthetic systemic toxicity: 2012 version. *Reg Anesth Pain Med* 2012;37(1):16–18, used with permission of ASRA.)

BE PREPARED
- We strongly advise that those using local anesthetics (LA) in doses sufficient to produce local anesthetic systemic toxicity (LAST) establish a plan for managing this complication. Making a *Local Anesthetic Toxicity Kit* and posting instructions for its use are encouraged.

RISK REDUCTION (*BE SENSIBLE*)
- Use the least dose of LA necessary to achieve the desired extent and duration of block.
- Local anesthetic blood levels are influenced by site of injection and dose. Factors that can increase the likelihood of LAST include: advanced age, heart failure, ischemic heart disease, conduction abnormalities, metabolic (e.g., mitochondrial) disease, liver disease, low plasma protein concentration, metabolic or respiratory acidosis, medications that inhibit sodium channels. Patients with severe cardiac dysfunction, particularly very low ejection fraction, are more sensitive to LAST and also more prone to 'stacked' injections (with resulting elevated LA tissue concentrations) due to slowed circulation time.
- Consider using a pharmacologic marker and/or test dose, e.g. epinephrine 5 mcg/mL of LA. Know the expected response, onset, duration, and limitations of "test dose" in identifying intravascular injection.
- Aspirate the syringe prior to *each* injection while observing for blood.
- Inject incrementally, while observing for signs and querying for symptoms of toxicity between each injection.

DETECTION (*BE VIGILANT*)
- Use standard American Society of Anesthesiologists (ASA) monitors.
- Monitor the patient during and after completing injection as clinical toxicity can be delayed up to 30 minutes.
- Communicate frequently with the patient to query for symptoms of toxicity.
- Consider LAST in any patient with altered mental status, neurological symptoms or cardiovascular instability after a regional anesthetic.
- Central nervous system signs (may be subtle or absent)
  - *Excitation* (agitation, confusion, muscle twitching, seizure)
  - *Depression* (drowsiness, obtundation, coma or apnea)
  - *Non-specific* (metallic taste, circumoral numbness, diplopia, tinnitus, dizziness)

- Cardiovascular signs (often the only manifestation of severe LAST)
  - *Initially may be hyperdynamic* (hypertension, tachycardia, ventricular arrhythmias), then
  - *Progressive hypotension*
  - *Conduction block, bradycardia or asystole*
  - *Ventricular arrhythmia* (ventricular tachycardia, Torsades de Pointes, ventricular fibrillation)
- Sedative hypnotic drugs reduce seizure risk but even light sedation may abolish the patient's ability to recognize or report symptoms of rising LA concentrations.

TREATMENT
- Timing of lipid infusion in LAST is controversial. The most conservative approach, waiting until after ACLS has proven unsuccessful, is unreasonable because early treatment can prevent cardiovascular collapse. Infusing lipid at the earliest sign of LAST can result in unnecessary treatment since only a fraction of patients will progress to severe toxicity. The most reasonable approach is to implement lipid therapy on the basis of clinical severity and rate of progression of LAST.
- There is laboratory evidence that epinephrine can impair resuscitation from LAST and reduce the efficacy of lipid rescue. Therefore it is recommended to avoid high doses of epinephrine and use smaller doses, e.g., <1mcg/kg, for treating hypotension.
- Propofol *should not be used* when there are signs of cardiovascular instability. Propofol is a cardiovascular depressant with lipid content too low to provide benefit. Its use is discouraged when there is a risk of progression to cardiovascular collapse.
- Prolonged monitoring (> 12 hours) is recommended after any signs of systemic LA toxicity, since cardiovascular depression due to local anesthetics can persist or recur after treatment.

The ASRA Practice Advisory on Local Anesthetic Toxicity is published in the society's official publication *Regional Anesthesia and Pain Medicine,* and can be downloaded from the journal Web site at www.rapm.org.

Neal JM, Bernards CM, Butterworth JF, Di Gregorio G, Drasner K, Hejtmanck MR, Mulroy MF, Rosenquist RW, Weinberg GL. ASRA practice advisory on local anesthetic systemic toxicity. *Reg Anesth Pain Med* 2010;35:152-161.

FIGURE 14.9   *(continued)*

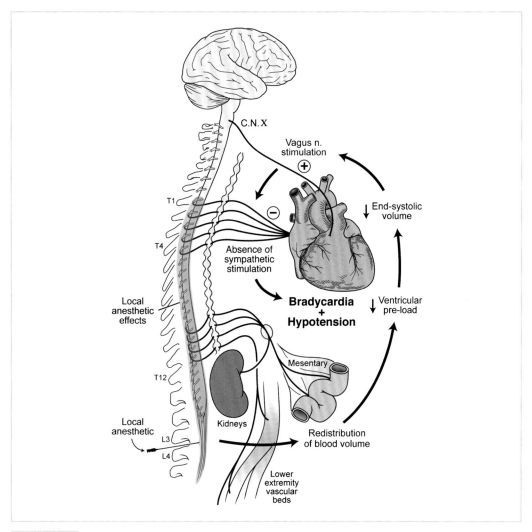

FIGURE 14.10 Factors that contribute to the development of hypotension and bradycardia associated with neuraxial local anesthetic blockade. (From Neal JM, Rathmell JP. *Complications of Regional Anesthesia and Pain Medicine.* 2nd ed. Philadelphia, PA: Lippincott Williams & Wilkins; 2013, used with permission.)

used, but importantly, HDP may still occur in an unpredictable manner. When using UG, the phrenic nerve resides fewer than 2 mm from the targeted C5 nerve root (Fig. 14.11).

3. Compared with the interscalene approach, HDP frequency is greatly reduced using the supraclavicular and lateral infraclavicular approaches, but still may happen unpredictably.

4. **HDP reduces spirometric measures of pulmonary function by upward of 30%**. Most patients not only tolerate this diminution of lung function, but also are unaware of it. However, some normal patients and especially those with severe pulmonary disease, for example, those on home oxygen therapy, experience significant pulmonary compromise and may require noninvasive respiratory support or intubation. Interscalene or supraclavicular blocks are relatively contraindicated in these patients because even low-volume UG techniques may adversely affect their pulmonary function.

TABLE 14.3 Spinal anesthesia–associated risk factors and odds ratios for hypotension and bradycardia

Risk factors	Odds ratio
Hypotension	
Peak sensory block height greater than T5	3.8
Chronic alcohol consumption	3.1
Urgency of surgery	2.9
Age >40 yr	2.5
Baseline systolic blood pressure <120 mm Hg	2.4
Chronic hypertension	2.2
Combined spinal-general anesthesia	1.9
Intrathecal injection at or above the L2–L3 IVS	1.8
Bradycardia	
Baseline heart rate <60 bpm	4.9–16.2
ASA physical status 1 (vs. 2 or 3)	3.5
Prolonged PR interval	3.2
β-Adrenergic blockade use	2.9
Peak block height above T5	1.7
Age <37 yr	1.4
Male gender	1.4
Case duration	2.0

BPM, beats per minute; IVS, intervertebral space.

5. HDP duration mirrors that of the local anesthetic. **Nearly all patients experience some degree of HDP when even dilute local anesthetic is infused around the brachial plexus for 24 hours**.

B. **Pneumothorax**

1. Pneumothorax is a complication of upper-extremity regional anesthetic techniques, especially with the **supraclavicular approach**. Pneumothorax occurs less frequently with the interscalene and medial infraclavicular approaches, as well as with paravertebral, intercostal, or suprascapular nerve blocks.

2. It is uncertain if UG has reduced the incidence of pneumothorax as compared with the percutaneous plumb-bob or subclavian perivascular techniques. Pneumothorax has been reported after UG supraclavicular and infraclavicular blocks. Even when ultrasound is used, **the risk of pneumothorax associated with supraclavicular block approaches 1/1,000 (upper limit of 95% confidence interval) (14).**

3. In the absence of positive pressure ventilation, the presentation of pneumothorax after a small-gauge needle injury to the pleura may be delayed 6 to 12 hours. Not all patients experience shortness of breath, but instead report ipsilateral pleuritic chest pain.

CLINICAL PEARL Although UG has reduced the incidence and intensity of HDP, and likely has reduced the incidence of pneumothorax, it has not completely eliminated these complications.

VI. **Local anesthetic–related complications and side effects**

A. **Total spinal anesthesia.** This term describes neuraxial blockade that ascends above the cervical region after local anesthetic administration anywhere along the neuraxis, including the lumbar

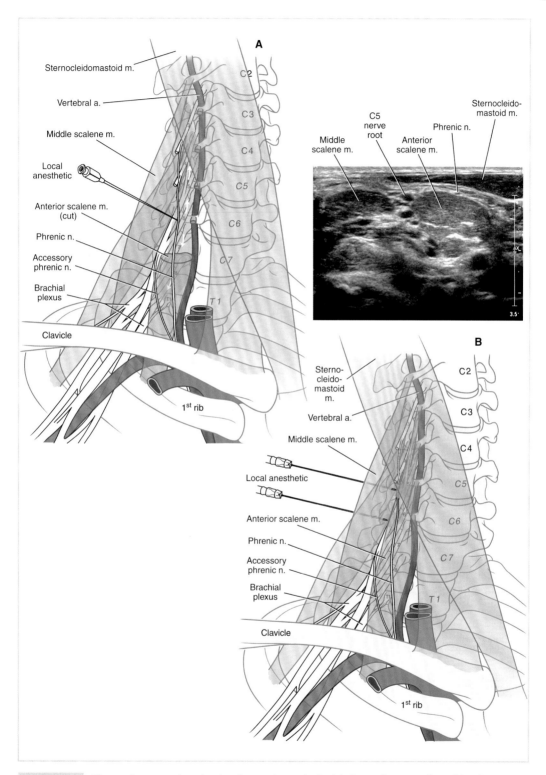

FIGURE 14.11   The panels compare how the phrenic nerve is anesthetized during performance of a traditional percutaneous interscalene block **(Panel A)** and an ultrasound-guided approach **(Panel B)**. (From Neal JM, Rathmell JP. *Complications of Regional Anesthesia and Pain Medicine.* 2nd ed. Philadelphia, PA: Lippincott Williams & Wilkins; 2013, used with permission.)

spine. Affected patients present with rapidly rising neuraxial block that is often accompanied by hypotension and bradycardia (up to complete cardiovascular collapse), respiratory distress, unconsciousness, and/or inability to phonate. Prompt recognition and treatment are essential to prevent further deterioration. Treatment includes rapid administration of volume, atropine to counteract blockade of the cardioaccelerator fibers, and vasopressors to ameliorate hypotension (including prompt use of **epinephrine to stimulate heart rate, increase systemic vascular resistance, and augment coronary perfusion pressure**). If the patient loses consciousness and/or stops breathing, airway support is indicated. Fortunately, the local anesthetic that reaches cephalad levels is rapidly diluted and therefore symptoms of low cerebral perfusion are often short lived.

7

B. **Neuraxial spread of local anesthetic.** A variant of total spinal anesthesia is the rare but potentially devastating complication of unintended spread of local anesthetic to the neuraxis. Local anesthetic access to the neuraxis during interscalene block occurs via long dural root sleeves, by intraneural injection with retrograde transport to the spinal cord, via tissue planes to the epidural space, or by direct epidural, subdural, or subarachnoid injection (Fig. 14.12).

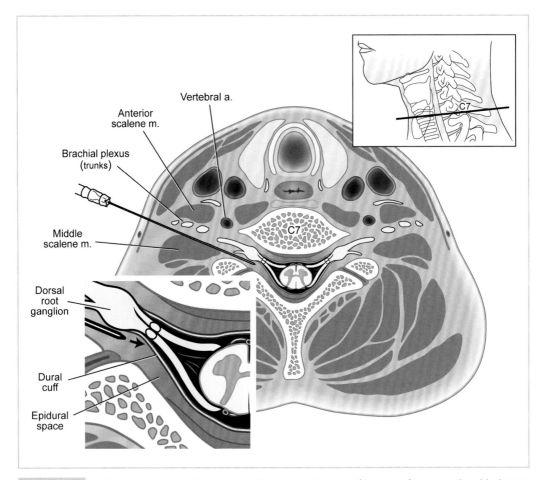

FIGURE 14.12 Pathways for local anesthetic to reach the neuraxis during performance of an interscalene block. Inset shows a needle near a long dural root sleeve. Local anesthetic may also spread retrograde to the neuraxis via intraneural injection, by translocation through tissue planes to the epidural space, or by direct epidural, subdural, or intrathecal injection. (From Neal JM, Rathmell JP. *Complications of Regional Anesthesia and Pain Medicine.* 2nd ed. Philadelphia, PA: Lippincott Williams & Wilkins; 2013, used with permission.)

The latter two mechanisms also apply to instances of neuraxial local anesthetic spread during paravertebral and psoas compartment blocks. Patients present with unexpected bilateral anesthesia, hypotension, bradycardia, and/or circulatory collapse. Prompt recognition of this complication is paramount. Failure to respond promptly to atropine and vasopressors mandates immediate administration of epinephrine to restore hemodynamic stability.

C. **Cervicosympathetic chain/stellate ganglion anesthesia.** The cervicosympathetic chain and stellate ganglion lie in close proximity to the brachial plexus (Fig. 14.13), especially when the supraclavicular approach is used. Local anesthetic blockade of these structures results in Horner syndrome (ipsilateral ptosis, miosis, and decreased sweating). The effect of low-volume UG techniques in reducing this side effect is unclear.

D. **Recurrent laryngeal nerve anesthesia.** The recurrent laryngeal nerve and vagus nerves reside close to the brachial plexus (Fig. 14.14) and are particularly vulnerable to unintended local anesthetic spread as a side effect of interscalene block. Symptoms dissipate with resolution of the local anesthetic effect.

E. **Urinary retention**

1. Neuraxial anesthetic blockade of parasympathetic neurons can be long lasting and result in inhibition of micturition with consequent urinary retention. This side effect can also happen after general anesthesia and/or administration of opioids. Timely return of bladder function is fostered by the use of shorter-acting intrathecal local anesthetic agents. When the patient has not voided before discharge, **measurement of bladder volume using an ultrasonographic device** aids in management. Bladder volumes of 400 mL or less can be safely discharged home, whereas volumes in excess of 600 to 700 mL require further observation and/or bladder catheterization.

2. Most **data suggest that thoracic epidural analgesia should not** *per se* **mandate an indwelling bladder catheter**. The occasional necessity to catheterize these patients postoperatively is offset by reduced bladder infection rates consequent to eliminating longer-term indwelling catheters.

F. **Local anesthetic allergy**

1. **True allergy to local anesthetic is rare**. Instead, most reported "allergies" are attributable to IV injection of adjuvant epinephrine (tachycardia, flushing), subjective symptoms from IV administration of local anesthetic (auditory changes, metallic taste, disinhibition, etc.), or vasovagal episodes.

2. **Ester local anesthetics**. Allergic reactions to esters are infrequent and typically involve reaction to the metabolite para-aminobenzoic acid (PABA). Patients with known PABA allergy (cosmetics, sunscreens) should not receive ester local anesthetics.

3. **Amide local anesthetics**. Allergic reactions to amides are extremely rare. There is probably no cross-reactivity between ester-allergic patients and amide local anesthetics.

4. Skin testing can be performed on patients suspected to be allergic to local anesthetic.

VII. **Transient neurologic symptoms**

A. TNS is a syndrome that **presents as low back pain and dysesthesia hours after resolution of a spinal anesthetic, with or without radiation to the buttocks and/or legs** (Fig. 14.15). The etiology of TNS is not fully understood, but most experts do not believe it to be a *forme fruste* of neurotoxicity (2).

B. **TNS is associated with spinal lidocaine to a much greater extent than with bupivacaine or 2-chloroprocaine.** Spinal mepivacaine is intermediate in risk. The syndrome has not been

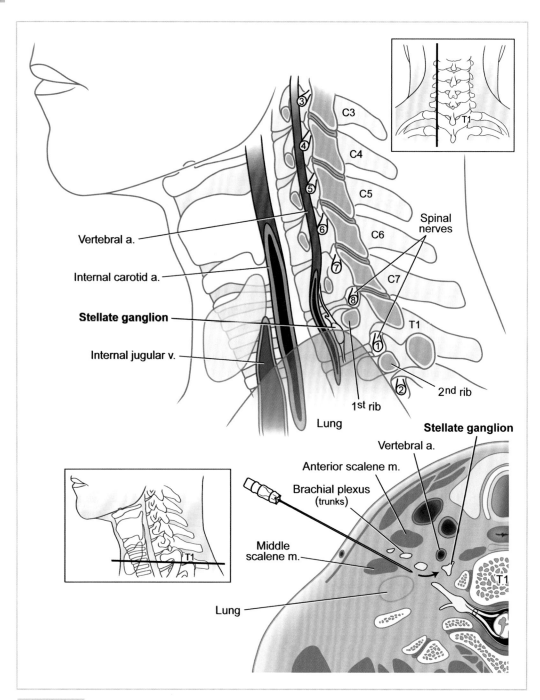

FIGURE 14.13 Pathways by which upper-extremity local anesthetic injection reaches the stellate ganglion and cervicosympathetic chain. Horner syndrome may result. (From Neal JM, Rathmell JP. *Complications of Regional Anesthesia and Pain Medicine.* 2nd ed. Philadelphia, PA: Lippincott Williams & Wilkins; 2013, used with permission.)

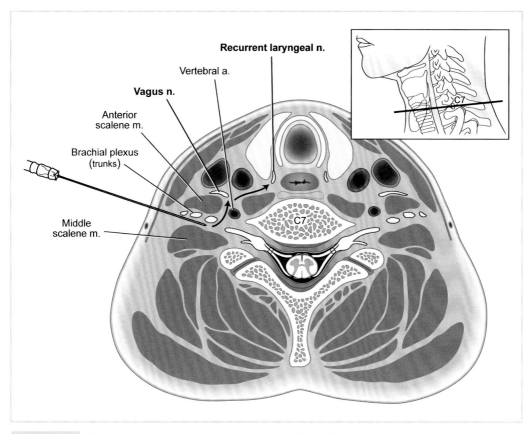

FIGURE 14.14   Pathways by which upper-extremity local anesthetic injection reaches the recurrent laryngeal and vagus nerves. Temporary hoarseness can result. (From Neal JM, Rathmell JP. *Complications of Regional Anesthesia and Pain Medicine.* 2nd ed. Philadelphia, PA: Lippincott Williams & Wilkins; 2013, used with permission.)

linked conclusively to early ambulation. Except perhaps at the lowest local anesthetic doses, TNS does not appear to be dose or concentration related, which is an argument for why it is thought not to be a neurotoxic phenomenon.

C. Besides the use of lidocaine, the most consistent predictors of TNS relate to patient position. The incidence of TNS using spinal lidocaine in patients positioned for **knee arthroscopy or in lithotomy** is reported between 16% and 31%.

D. TNS may last 3 to 7 days and is best treated with nonsteroidal anti-inflammatory drugs and rest. The presence of any neurologic deficit should prompt consideration of an alternative diagnosis.

VIII. Postdural puncture headache

A. Although firmly entrenched in the vernacular, postdural puncture headache (PDPH) is more properly thought of as postmeningeal puncture headache because it is the arachnoid, rather than the dura, that allows leakage of CSF.

B. PDPH was recognized the day after August Bier's first spinal anesthetic in 1898.

C. PDPH is believed to occur when a hole in the meninges permits leakage of CSF into the epidural space. Subsequently, buoyancy is lost and the brain sags when the patient assumes an upright

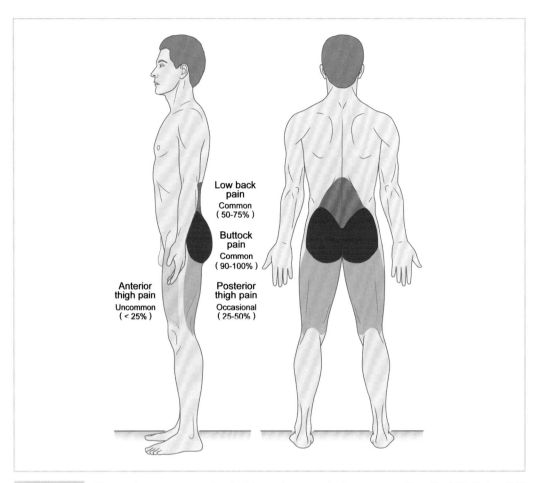

FIGURE 14.15 Signs and symptoms associated with transient neurologic symptoms. (From Neal JM, Rathmell JP. *Complications of Regional Anesthesia and Pain Medicine.* 2nd ed. Philadelphia, PA: Lippincott Williams & Wilkins; 2013, used with permission.)

position. **The pain is caused by stretching of innervated structures that bridge the brain to the cranium and is augmented by reflex cerebral vasodilation, which occurs in response to CSF volume loss.** Definitive treatment of PDPH is placement of an epidural blood patch (EBP), which seals the meningeal defect and allows reaccumulation of CSF. Temporary increased spinal pressure generated by the epidural injection of blood is responsible for the immediate headache relief that most patients experience.

D. **Risk factors for PDPH include the following:**

   1. **Younger age** (teenage through early 20s). The risk is less than 1% over age 40 years (Fig. 14.16).

   2. Females are often reported to be at higher risk for PDPH, but this relates to use of neuraxial blocks in young parturients.

   3. Epidural needles or **larger gauge** (22-gauge and lower) spinal needles with **cutting tips**, for example, Quincke needles.

   4. Conversely, atraumatic needle tip configurations reduce the risk, as is the case with Whitacre or Sprotte tips.

   5. Early ambulation does not increase the risk of PDPH.

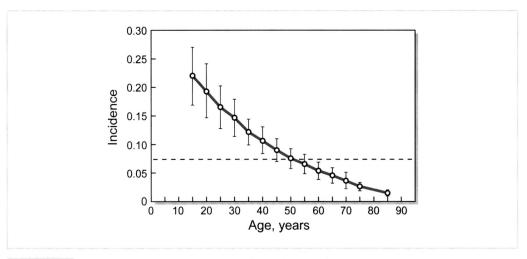

FIGURE 14.16   Incidence of postdural puncture headache as a function of age. (From Neal JM, Rathmell JP. *Complications of Regional Anesthesia and Pain Medicine.* 2nd ed. Philadelphia, PA: Lippincott Williams & Wilkins; 2013, used with permission.)

8

E. Signs and symptoms of PDPH

1. PDPH typically presents within 12 hours of meningeal puncture, but may occur immediately with large dural holes or be delayed if the CSF leak is slow.

2. **The cardinal feature of** PDPH is that it is positional—absent or much improved when supine, but worse with sitting or becoming erect. The headache itself is bilateral, dull, and throbbing. Importantly, PDPH is never associated with localizing neurologic findings, fever, or mental status changes. Presence of these signs and symptoms should prompt reconsideration of the diagnosis.

CLINICAL PEARL   If a patient with suspected PDPH exhibits localizing neurologic findings, is febrile, or shows signs of mental compromise, an alternate diagnosis should be considered along with neuroimaging.

F. Treatment of PDPH

1. Nearly all cases of PDPH resolve spontaneously within a week of onset. Cases associated with smaller-gauge needle punctures are likely to resolve sooner.

2. **Most conservative therapies for PDPH are ineffective**, including increased fluid intake, supplemental caffeine, abdominal binders, and the like.

3. When more immediate relief is desired, an **EBP is about 70% effective**. Repeat EBP 24 hours later is advisable, but progressively less effective.
    a. **The technique of EBP** involves aseptic acquisition of 20 mL of the patient's blood after his or her epidural space has been accessed. The blood is injected into the epidural space incrementally up to the full volume or until patient reports of back pain or radicular discomfort. The patient should remain flat for an hour and avoid lifting or straining for the next 24 hours.
    b. The safety of an autologous EBP in patients with cancer has not been established.

IX. Myotoxicity

A. All local anesthetics are myotoxic in animal models; however, it was generally accepted that clinically significant myotoxicity was not an issue in humans except as a complication of retrobulbar block.

B. Presumed local anesthetic-induced myotoxicity has now been reported after continuous adductor canal blocks in humans (23). These patients present with flaccid quadricep muscles 1 or 2 days after total knee arthroplasty. Because myoblasts are not affected, most but not all of the reported patients experienced near-total functional recovery weeks to months later.

C. The precise etiology is not understood. There are no known preventative measures or treatments.

ACKNOWLEDGMENTS

The author wishes to acknowledge Christopher M. Bernards, MD (d. 2012), who penned the 4th-edition version of this chapter. As Chris was fond of saying, "Never believe everything that you think."

REFERENCES

1. Phillips OC, Ebner H, Nelson AT, et al. Neurologic complications following spinal anesthesia with lidocaine: a prospective review of 10,440 cases. *Anesthesiology* 1969;30:284–289.
2. Pollock JE. Transient neurologic symptoms: etiology, risk factors, and management. *Reg Anesth Pain Med* 2002;27:581–586.
3. Moen V, Dahlgren N, Irestedt L. Severe neurological complications after central neuraxial blockades in Sweden 1990–1999. *Anesthesiology* 2004;101:950–959.
4. Neal JM, Barrington MJ, Brull R, et al. The second ASRA practice advisory on neurologic complications associated with regional anesthesia and pain medicine: Executive summary, 2015. *Reg Anesth Pain Med* 2015;40:401–430.
5. Barrington MJ, Kluger R. Ultrasound guidance reduces the risk of local anesthetic systemic toxicity following peripheral nerve blockade. *Reg Anesth Pain Med* 2013;38:289–297.
6. Jacob AK, Mantilla CB, Sviggum HP, et al. Perioperative nerve injury after total knee arthroplasty: regional anesthesia risk during a 20-year cohort study. *Anesthesiology* 2011;114:311–317.
7. Barrington MJ, Watts SA, Gledhill SR, et al. Preliminary results of the Australasian Regional Anaesthesia Collaboration. A prospective audit of over 7000 peripheral nerve and plexus blocks for neurological and other complications. *Reg Anesth Pain Med* 2009;34:534–541.
8. Welch MB, Brummett CM, Welch TD, et al. Perioperative peripheral nerve injuries. A retrospective study of 380,680 cases during a 10-year period at a single institution. *Anesthesiology* 2009;111:464–466.
9. Brull R, Hadzic A, Reina MA, et al. Pathophysiology and etiology of nerve injury following peripheral nerve blockade. *Reg Anesth Pain Med* 2015;40:479–490.
10. Horlocker TT, Wedel DJ, Rowlingson JC, et al. Regional anesthesia in the patient receiving antithrombotic or thrombolytic therapy: American Society of Regional Anesthesia and Pain Medicine Evidence-Based Guidelines (Third Edition). *Reg Anesth Pain Med* 2010;35:64–101.
11. Horlocker TT, Birnbach DJ, Connis RT, et al. Practice advisory for the prevention, diagnosis, and management of infectious complications associated with neuraxial techniques: a report by the American Society of Anesthesiologists Task Force on infectious complications associated with neuraxial techniques. *Anesthesiology* 2010;112:530–545.
12. Neal JM, Kopp SL, Lanier WL, et al. Anatomy and pathophysiology of spinal cord injury associated with regional anesthesia and pain medicine: 2015 update. *Reg Anesth Pain Med* 2015;40:506–525.
13. Hodgson PS, Neal JM, Pollock JE, Liu SS. The neurotoxicity of drugs given intrathecally (spinal). *Anesth Analg* 1999;88:797–809.
14. Neal JM, Brull R, Horn JL et al. The second ASRA evidence-based medicine assessment of ultrasound-guided regional anesthesia. Executive summary of 2015 update. *Reg Anesth Pain Med* 2016;41:181–194.

15. Neal JM. Effects of epinephrine in local anesthetics on the central and peripheral nervous systems: neurotoxicity and neural blood flow. *Reg Anesth Pain Med* 2003;28:124–134.

16. Staff NP, Engelstad J, Klein CJ, et al. Post-surgical inflammatory neuropathy. *Brain* 2010;133:2866–2880.

17. Kopp SL, Jacob AK, Hebl JR. Regional anesthesia in patients with pre-existing neurologic disease. *Reg Anesth Pain Med* 2015;40:467–478.

18. Neal JM, Bernards CM, Butterworth JF, et al. ASRA practice advisory on local anesthetic systemic toxicity. *Reg Anesth Pain Med* 2010;35:152–161.

19. Vasques F, Behr AU, Weinberg G, et al. A review of local anesthetic systemic toxicity cases since publication of the American Society of Regional Anesthesia recommendations. To whom it may concern. *Reg Anesth Pain Med* 2015;40:698–705.

20. Mulroy MF, Hejtmanek MR. Prevention of local anesthetic systemic toxicity. *Reg Anesth Pain Med* 2010;35:177–180.

21. Guinard JP, Mulroy MF, Carpenter RL, et al. Test doses: optimal epinephrine content with and without acute beta-adrenergic blockade. *Anesthesiology* 1990;73:386–392.

22. Neal JM, Mulroy MF, Weinberg GL. American Society of Regional Anesthesia and Pain Medicine checklist for managing local anesthetic systemic toxicity: 2012 version. *Reg Anesth Pain Med* 2012;37:16–18.

23. Neal JM, Salinas FV, Choi DS. Local anesthetic-induced myotoxicity after continuous adductor canal block. *Reg Anesth Pain Med* 2016;41:723–727.

24. Guinard JP, Mulroy MF, Carpenter RL. Aging reduces the reliability of epidural epinephrine test doses. *Reg Anesth* 1995;20:193–198.

25. Liu SS, Carpenter RL. Hemodynamic responses to intravascular injection of epinephrine-containing epidural test doses in adults during general anesthesia. *Anesthesiology* 1996;84:81–87.

15

Pediatric Regional Anesthesia

Kathleen L. McGinn

I. **Topical blocks**

II. **Neuraxial blocks**

  A. **Spinal anesthesia**

  B. **Epidural**

  C. **Caudal block**

III. **Peripheral nerve blocks**

  A. **Techniques**

  B. **Head and neck blocks**

C. **Rectus sheath block**

D. **Transversus abdominis plane block**

E. **Ilioinguinal and iliohypogastric nerve blocks**

F. **Penile block**

G. **Extremity blocks**

KEY POINTS

1. Performing regional blocks in children under general anesthesia has been shown to be safe and is regarded as the standard of care.

2. Pain is often undertreated in infants and children because of erroneous beliefs that it has no harmful long-term effect in this patient population.

3. There is an increased risk of local anesthetic systemic toxicity in infants cause by decreased plasma protein concentration, higher unbound fraction of local anesthetic, slower hepatic metabolism, slightly reduced plasma pseudocholinesterase activity, and decreased methemoglobin-reductase activity.

4. Topical anesthesia can decrease needle pain with intravenous placement or regional blocks, but it requires standard protocols for early placement to ensure adequate time for maximal effectiveness.

5. Caudal block is the most common pediatric regional technique for children up to school age.

6. Ultrasound-guidance for pediatric regional anesthesia facilitates the use of lower local anesthetic volume and greater block placement accuracy.

1 **THE USE OF REGIONAL BLOCKS** in pediatric anesthesia has increased dramatically with the advent of ultrasound guidance. However, nerve blocks still tend to be underutilized in children. This can be attributed to fear of neurologic complications, lack of experience, or lack of appropriate pediatric-sized equipment. In pediatric patients, it is standard to perform regional blocks under general anesthesia. The benefit of successful regional anesthesia lies in a more comfortable emergence. In turn, this reduces complications associated with parenteral opioids in vulnerable pediatric patients (neonates, ex-premature infants, and children with cystic fibrosis).

Although regional blocks confer similar advantages in children as in adults, the methods used for performing these techniques must be modified. Expectedly, the key to success lies in knowledge of anatomy, pharmacology, equipment, ultrasound, and preblock sedation or anesthesia. Because general anesthesia/sedation is often required, two individuals are helpful; one to perform the block and the other to monitor the child. All techniques, whether regional or general, carry risks, and the latter must be weighed against the potential benefits in anesthetized children. The current chapter focuses on how pediatric regional techniques differ from their adult counterparts. There exist excellent reviews of pediatric regional anesthetic techniques for readers who wish to pursue the latter in more detail (1–4).

I. Topical blocks

A. Topical local anesthesia can be used to **reduce needle pain** during intravenous (IV) catheter insertion or during regional techniques (5). Several products are available for use in pediatrics.

1. 2.5% lidocaine and 2.5% prilocaine (**eutectic mixture of local anesthetics [EMLA] cream**) is effective for anesthetizing the dermis to a depth of 5 mm. Lidocaine–prilocaine can cause the unwanted side effect of vasoconstriction. The benefit of decreasing a child's distress usually outweighs the disadvantage of vasoconstriction. It is recommended to apply lidocaine–prilocaine cream at least 45 minutes before needle insertion, but the longer it is on, the better the anesthesia. Because of this time constraint, lidocaine–prilocaine may be underutilized.

2. 4% liposomal lidocaine (**LMX4**) and 5% liposomal lidocaine (LMX5) are rapid-acting topical agents for intact skin that work by way of a liposomal delivery system. Studies demonstrate that a 30-minute application of LMX4 is as safe and as effective as a 60-minute application of the lidocaine–prilocaine cream. Additionally, LMX4 is reported to cause less blanching of the skin and less risk of methemoglobinemia as compared with lidocaine–prilocaine cream.

3. 4% tetracaine gel (Ametop or Amethocaine) is more lipophilic than lidocaine or prilocaine. Under an occlusive dressing, it anesthetizes the skin to the same depth as lidocaine–prilocaine cream in 30 minutes.

4. Lidocaine/tetracaine topical (Synera) is an adhesive patch containing lidocaine and tetracaine with an oxygen-activated heating element to help improve skin penetration of the local anesthetics. It can cover 10 cm^2 and penetrate to over 6 mm in 20 minutes. It is approved for children aged 3 years and older.

5. Iontophoretic drug delivery systems (e.g., **Numby stuff**) allow iontophoresis of 2% lidocaine and epinephrine through intact skin, thus providing topical anesthesia in approximately 20 minutes after application. This device employs a small electric current to provide the iontophoresis that some younger children find objectionable.

6. A popular alternative is a needleless injection system (**J-Tip**) that can be used for delivery of carbonated local anesthetic. Eighty-four percent of children reported no pain at the time of J-Tip lidocaine application compared to 61% in the EMLA group at the time of dressing removal (6). Children should be warned of the startling loud popping sound on injection.

7. Zingo is a newer needless delivery system. It contains 0.5 mg lidocaine powder that is propelled subcutaneously with compressed helium. It has the shortest time of onset (1 to 3 minutes) and duration (10 minutes). It is approved for children aged 3 years and older.

4 **CLINICAL PEARL** All topical local anesthetic preparations require application over the area to be anesthetized, and need variable amounts of time to become effective. Thus, standing protocols can improve the timing of application and efficacy of topical anesthetics.

B. Topical local anesthetics have also been employed successfully to provide surgical anesthesia for exposed **mucous membranes.**

1. Oral mucous membranes can be anesthetized to allow earlier placement of oral airways or laryngoscopy in infants and children with potentially difficult airways.

2. Topical lidocaine 1 to 2 mg/kg is often employed following induction of general anesthesia in infants who require diagnostic direct laryngoscopy in order for the otolaryngologist to view vocal cord movement.

3. Because it can penetrate the foreskin, EMLA has been used in addition to penile blocks for anesthesia for newborn **circumcisions** (7). Application must be done following amputation of the foreskin in order to expose the mucous membranes that will absorb these preparations. Because this is a topical technique, only enough local anesthetic is required to contact all of the "target" mucous membrane. If jelly or ointment is used, parents need to be reassured regarding the appearance of the wound, because the site of dried local anesthetic mixed with a tinge of blood may be unsettling.

II. Neuraxial blocks

A. Spinal anesthesia

This technique is rarely used outside the neonatal period, but has an important role in decreasing postoperative apnea in neonates after herniorrhaphy.

The techniques are the same as in adults, although with a short 22- or 25-gauge needle. In contrast to other pediatric regional techniques, spinal blockade is usually performed without sedation or general anesthesia.

CLINICAL PEARL   Spinal anesthesia is especially useful in the premature neonate who is at increased risk of periodic breathing, apnea, and bradycardia following general anesthesia.

B. Epidural

In the older and larger children, neuraxial blockade is usually performed under general anesthesia. Epidural anesthesia can be delivered by the thoracic, lumbar, or caudal route.

1. **Anatomy**. The depth of the epidural space varies with growth in children. A simple approximation from skin to space is 1 mm/kg between 10 and 50 kg. Shorter epidural needles are now available.

2. **Indications.** Continuous epidural infusions are frequently used in children for major lower extremity orthopedic surgery, abdominal procedures, and thoracotomies.

3. **Technique**. Because of the small child's increased resting heart rate and the variability of the general anesthesia technique when epidural test doses are being administered, local anesthetic test doses can be harder to interpret.

   a. The volume of a pediatric test dose is 0.1 mL/kg of a local anesthetic with 5 µg/mL of epinephrine. The cardiovascular systems response to epinephrine can vary with age. In younger children, an intravascular injection of test dose can increase T-wave amplitude within 20 to 40 seconds. In older children, T-wave inversion can occur. A few seconds later there may be a change in heart rate, most commonly an increase of more than 10 beats/min. However, there may be bradycardia, no change, or other dysrhythmias with an intravascular injection. Therefore, a negative test dose may be reassuring but does not rule out intravascular placement of the needle tip.

    b. Injection of local anesthetic should be slow with incremental aspiration every 0.1 to 0.2 mL/kg and close observation of the electrocardiography.

    c. In placing epidurals in children, air and/or saline are most commonly used for loss of resistance to confirm needle placement in the epidural space. There have been volume-related complications reported with the air-only technique such as pneumocephalus and venous air embolism, so the maximum volume of air recommended is 0.5 to 1 mL. The volume of saline for loss of resistance should also be minimized to avoid diluting the local anesthetic.

    d. Patient-controlled epidural analgesia has been used in patients as young as 5 years old.

  4. Complications. Most adverse events with pediatric epidurals are catheter related (dislodgement or kinking).

    a. Intraoperative. Intravascular injection, dural puncture (with possible postdural puncture headache requiring blood patch), and failed block have all been reported with pediatric epidurals.

    b. Postoperative. Infection, hematoma, unilateral block, and respiratory depression have also been reported with pediatric epidurals.

    c. To avoid masking compartment syndrome in children, less concentrated solutions such as 0.25% of bupivacaine should be used for single-shot nerve blocks and 0.1% used for continuous infusions (8).

C. Caudal block

As paresthesias cannot be detected in the anesthetized child, less experienced providers prefer approaching the epidural space caudally. The single-injection caudal block is one of the most popular and versatile pediatric regional anesthetic techniques. Placement of a catheter allows for redosing or continuous infusion of local anesthetic or local anesthetic and opioid mixture. A combination of caudal blockade supplemented with light general anesthesia allows for a quicker wake up because less inhalational anesthetic agent is required.

5

  1. Anatomy. Caudal blocks are **technically easier** to perform in children than in adults. The poorly developed gluteal musculature and limited amount of subcutaneous fat means that landmarks defining the sacral hiatus are not obscured. There is less bony fusion in the region of the sacral hiatus, and less distortion of bony landmarks in infants and children, who have not developed the gluteal fat pad commonly seen after puberty.

    a. The fifth sacral cornua are very prominent, lying well above the gluteal cleft.

    b. The sacrococcygeal ligament is not calcified in the infant or child; indeed, the distinct "pop" one encounters is quite similar to the tactile sensation experienced when entering a peripheral vein with an 18-gauge IV catheter in an adult.

    c. The **dural sac** ends between the second and third sacral vertebrae (Table 15.1), whereas the length of the sacrum is reduced in proportion to the overall size of the child. It is possible to pierce the fragile sacrum or perform a dural puncture in an infant. Most catastrophic complications of caudal blocks, such as cardiac arrest and seizure, have occurred in younger children (less than 11 months). Meticulous attention to technique is vital in these small patients.

  2. Indications

    a. A caudal block provides excellent perioperative **analgesia** for subumbilical surgery and most other surgeries below the diaphragm. This includes the commonly performed groin surgeries, such as **herniorrhaphy**, **orchidopexy**, and **hydrocele** repair. Children undergoing lower extremity **orthopedic** procedures (e.g., club foot) or **urologic** procedures also enjoy profound postoperative analgesia provided by a caudal block.

TABLE 15.1   Caudal anatomy in infants

	Dural sac ends at	Conus medullaris ends at
Infant	S2	L2
Adult	S1	L1

   b. Caudal blocks are usually performed following induction of general anesthesia and placement of an IV catheter. Only a very light plane of general anesthesia is required once the block has taken effect. The time spent placing the block before the beginning of surgery is recovered at the end because the child usually awakens faster.

3. Drugs. In children, most local anesthetics should be dosed in milliliter per kilogram to avoid toxicity associated with larger volumes used in adult blocks.

   a. Bupivacaine. A 0.25% concentration provides minimal motor blockade with adequate sensory blockade. An easy approximation of caudal dose is 1 mL/kg of 0.25% bupivacaine (Table 15.2). The total dose of bupivacaine should not exceed 3 mg/kg. In the epidural space, it lasts 4 to 6 hours.

   b. Other drugs and additives. 0.2% **ropivacaine** is also employed at 1 mL/kg. The most common additive is Clonidine (1 to 2 μg/kg can lengthen analgesia by 2 to 3 hours (9)).

CLINICAL PEARL   Neonates may have a **higher free drug level** and may be more susceptible to the toxic effects of local anesthetics. The bolus dose and infusion should be reduced by 30% for infants younger than 6 months to decrease the risk of toxicity.

4. Technique

   a. The patient is turned into the lateral position, and the hips and knees are flexed similar to that position appropriate for the performance of a lumbar puncture (Fig. 15.1).

   b. The cornua of the sacral hiatus are the most easily palpated as two bony ridges at the beginning crease of the buttocks. It can be useful to identify the **equilateral triangle** with the two posterior superior iliac spines as the base and the hiatus as the apex (see Fig. 15.1).

   c. After aseptic preparation of the area, it is started by breaking the skin with an 18-gauge needle to avoid tracking an epidermal plug into the epidural space. Then, 22-gauge IV catheter is inserted into the sacrococcygeal ligament at a 60-degree angle to the skin. If bone is encountered, the needle is withdrawn several millimeters and the angle with the skin is decreased before advancing again. A distinct "pop" will be felt as the needle punctures the sacrococcygeal ligament; the angle with the skin is decreased again into a plane parallel to the spinal axis, and the needle shaft is advanced an additional 2 mm to be certain that the entire bevel of the needle is in the caudal space. Then the IV cannula is advanced gently into the caudal space, taking care not to puncture the dural sac.

CLINICAL PEARL   The bevel should be maintained in the bevel ventral position to avoid puncture of the anterior wall of the caudal space (sacrum).

Desired block height	Volume (mL/kg)
Sacral	0.5
Lower thoracic	0.75
Upper thoracic	1.25

TABLE 15.2   Caudal block volumes

From Duflo F, Sautou-Miranda, V. Efficacy and plasma levels of ropivacaine for children: controlled regional analgesia following lower limb surgery. *Br J Anaesth* 2006;97(2):250 by permission of Oxford University Press.

d. **Test dose.** After negative aspiration for blood and cerebrospinal fluid, a test dose of the local anesthetic solution with epinephrine is injected (epinephrine 0.5 µg/kg) (10). Attention should be paid to the heart rate and electrocardiography tracing for 1 minute. An increase of >10 beats/min suggests intravascular injection. The sensitivity of the test dose is diminished in the anesthetized patient. A transient elevation of the T-waves, especially in V5, can also alert the provider to an intravascular injection of bupivacaine. The noninjecting hand can be placed superior to the injection site to detect any crepitus that occurs when the injection is subcutaneous rather than epidural.

e. Frequent **aspiration** and **incremental injection** of local anesthetic is the best safeguard against undetected intravascular injection because test doses can be unreliable in children. Intraosseous injections into the marrow have rapid uptake similar to intravascular injections.

f. **Caudal catheter.** A 22-gauge catheter can be threaded through the 18-gauge IV to allow repeated boluses of local anesthetics in longer cases or for postoperative infusions. Before placement, the catheter should be measured to determine the length from sacral hiatus to the desired dermatome. Catheter tip site can be confirmed with fluoroscopy or ultrasonography (11). A test dose should be done through the catheter before further dosing of local

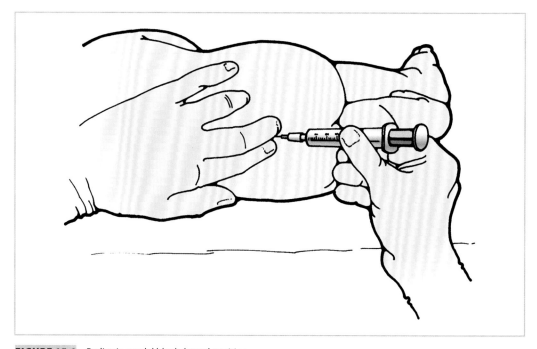

FIGURE 15.1   Pediatric caudal block, lateral position.

anesthetic. In patients younger than 5 years, the catheter can usually be easily advanced to the thoracic level. Care should be taken with the dressing to minimize fecal soiling.

5. **Complications**
   a. **Dural puncture** with resultant total spinal anesthesia is possible. Careful stabilization of the needle, careful advancement of the cannula, and frequent gentle aspiration will assist in avoiding this complication. A sacral dimple may be associated with spina bifida occulta, and the risk of neurologic complications is increased due to a tethered or low-lying spinal cord. Therefore, it is a relative contraindication to a caudal block.
   b. **Local anesthetics pose an increased risk of systemic toxicity in infants because of decreased plasma protein concentration, higher free fraction, slower hepatic metabolism, slightly reduced plasma pseudocholinesterase activity, and decreased methemoglobin-reductase activity.**
   c. Injection of local anesthetic **intravascularly** or **intraosseously** may lead to toxicity. Bupivacaine cardiac toxicity threshold in children may be increased by the concomitant use of volatile anesthetics. The central nervous system effect of the general anesthetic may obscure any signs of neurotoxicity until devastating cardiovascular effects are apparent. Dysrhythmias and cardiac arrest have occurred, usually in infants less than 10 kg. First-line treatment is 20% IV lipid emulsion (1.5 mL/kg over 1 minute, may repeat after 3 to 5 minutes) and doses more than 10 μg/kg of epinephrine may impair lipid resuscitation (12).
   d. Infection is possible but uncommon because most indwelling caudal catheters are removed within 2 to 3 days.

III. **Peripheral nerve blocks**
The use of peripheral nerve blocks in children has increased with progress in manufacturing pediatric-sized needles, catheters, and ultrasound transducers.

A. **Techniques**
   1. **Ultrasound**-guided nerve blocks have increased in popularity. Ultrasound can be very helpful for nerve localization as well as visualizing the spread of local anesthetic in the desired tissue plane. It is increasingly being studied in children (13), but the technology requires significant training to master. Smaller "hockey stick" probes are available that are more suited to the smaller anatomic relationships in children. Additional advantages of ultrasound-guided nerve blocks include the need for smaller local anesthetic volumes to achieve adequate block and reduced intravascular injection.

   2. **Nerve stimulator.** Like in adults, a nerve stimulator is a very helpful alternative for placing peripheral nerve blocks. It is crucial to remember to avoid muscle relaxants before placing a block with a nerve stimulator in the anesthetized child.

B. **Head and neck blocks.** The use of nerve blocks for head and neck procedures is increasing in pediatrics. Most are landmark-based field blocks of sensory nerves that can significantly improve postoperative pain management.
   1. **Supraorbital and supratrochlear** nerve blocks
      a. **Anatomy.** These are the end branches of the ophthalmic division (V1) of the trigeminal nerve. The supraorbital nerve exits the supraorbital foramen. The supratrochlear nerve exits 1 cm medial to the supraorbital nerve.
      b. **Indications.** This block can be useful in frontal craniotomies, ventriculoperitoneal shunt revisions, and scalp nevus excision.
      c. **Technique.** With the patient supine, palpate the supraorbital notch along the medial eyebrow in line with the midline pupil. After sterile preparation of the site, a 27-gauge

needle is inserted just superior to the notch so as to avoid the artery that travels through it. Aspirate before placing 1 mL of 0.25% bupivacaine. The needle is then withdrawn to skin level, redirected medially, and advanced several millimeters. Another 1 mL of bupivacaine is injected to block the supratrochlear nerve.

    d. Complications. The vascular periorbital tissue has the potential for hematomas. Pressure applied to the injection site can minimize this.

  2. Infraorbital nerve block. This simple block provides profound pain relief for 12 to 18 hours in children undergoing cleft lip repair or other surgery on the anterior hard palate, lower eyelid, side of nose, or upper lip (14). Local anesthetic injected directly into the surgical site by the surgeon has a shorter duration as compared with infraorbital nerve block.

    a. Anatomy. The infraorbital notch lies on a line connecting the supraorbital and mental foramina and the pupil of the eye (Fig. 13.9).

    b. Technique. There are two techniques for blocking this nerve: intraoral and extraoral. Both are field blocks and local anesthetic should not be injected in the notch or in the nerve.

      (1) Extraoral. First locate the infraorbital foramen with the index finger of the nondominant hand—approximately 0.5 cm from the midpoint of lower orbital margin. A 27-gauge needle is inserted at a 45-degree angle to the notch until touching bone. The needle is then withdrawn slightly so that the injection is not intraosseous, and 0.25 to 0.5 mL of local anesthetic is injected. A small skin wheal should be visible.

      (2) Intraoral. The second technique is transoral and will leave no mark on the face. Again the infraorbital foramen is palpated with the nondominant hand. The superior lip is elevated, and a 25-gauge needle of 1.5-in. is inserted parallel to the upper first premolar and guided toward the nondominant index finger palpating the notch. After aspiration, 0.5 to 1.5 mL of local anesthetic is injected. If this technique is planned, it should be performed before the surgery so that there is no risk of disruption of the surgery by the manipulation of the upper lip.

C. Rectus sheath block

  1. Indications. This block is used commonly in pediatrics, especially for surgeries around the umbilicus. Bilateral placement blocks the 10th intercostal nerves because they become the anterior cutaneous branch. The nerve passes between the transverse abdominis muscle and the internal oblique muscle and between the sheath and the posterior wall of the rectus abdominis muscle.

  2. Technique. The ultrasound probe is placed next to the umbilicus and the posterior rectus sheath is identified. A needle is inserted laterally to medially, and local anesthetic is injected into the potential space between the rectus abdominis and the posterior wall of the rectus sheath (15).

  3. Drug. After negative aspiration, 0.25% bupivacaine can be injected, 0.1 to 0.2 mL/kg on each side.

  4. Complications. Injection can be too superficial within the belly of the rectus abdominus muscle and not spread posteriorly to the nerve, resulting in a failed block. Intravascular injection is also possible in the muscle belly.

D. Transversus abdominis plane block

  1. Indications. This block is used commonly in pediatrics, especially for surgeries on the abdomen. The transversus abdominis plane is a potential space between the internal oblique and transversus abdominis muscles where the T8–L1 nerve roots pass.

2. **Technique.** The ultrasound transducer is placed in the mid-axillary line between the lower costal margin and the iliac crest, and the three muscle layers are identified. A needle is inserted laterally to medially, and local anesthetic is injected into the potential space between the internal oblique and the transversus abdominis muscles.

3. **Drug.** After negative aspiration, 0.25% bupivacaine can be injected, 0.3 mL/kg on each side, up to 20 mL, as a single injection or continuous infusion through a catheter.

4. **Complications.** Complications are rare but could include unintentional puncture of the peritoneum or abdominal organs (liver, spleen, and bowel) or vascular puncture (16).

E. **Ilioinguinal and iliohypogastric nerve blocks.** These blocks provide analgesia equivalent to that of caudal blockade for children undergoing **inguinal hernia, hydrocele, or orchidopexy repair.** If there is a contraindication to a caudal, such as a sacral dimple, or the child is old enough to be concerned about the loss of leg strength postoperatively, these blocks are advantageous.

1. **Technique.** Although using the landmark technique has been reliable historically, the use of ultrasound has increased the accuracy and consistency of this block (Fig. 15.2). The ultrasound probe is placed medial to the anterior superior iliac spine with the axis toward the umbilicus. The nerves are identified between the transversus abdominis and the internal oblique, and local anesthetic is injected under direct visualization (17).

2. **Dose.** Bupivacaine 0.25% or ropivacaine 0.2% are most often employed, in a dose of 0.1 to 0.4 mL/kg depending on patient size.

3. **Complications.** The use of ultrasound decreases the incidence of bowel puncture and intravascular injection with this block. Femoral nerve palsy is another possible adverse events (18).

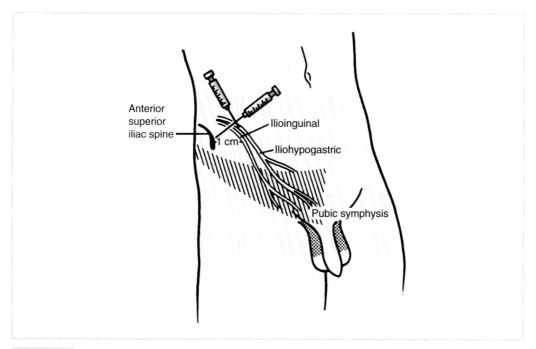

FIGURE 15.2   Ilioinguinal and iliohypogastric nerve blocks.

F. **Penile block.** This block is useful for perioperative analgesia for boys undergoing **circumcision or hypospadias repair.** The American Academy of Pediatrics does endorse the use of local anesthetics if the family desires a circumcision in the neonatal period. Both the topical application of LMX cream **and the ring block of the penis are simple and carry minimal risks for the newborn.**

1. **Technique.** Two approaches are commonly used.

   a. **Ring block.** The simplest way to block the dorsal penile nerves is to place a subcutaneous wheal of 0.25% to 0.5% bupivacaine **without** epinephrine around the base of the penis. This subcutaneous block places local anesthetic just superficial to the tough Buck fascia that surrounds the corpora, and the dorsal nerve, arteries, and veins of the penis. The local anesthetic is diffuse across this fascia to provide anesthesia.

   b. **Dorsal penile nerve block.** This well-established technique involves blockade of the dorsal penile nerves in the subpubic area (Fig. 15.3). Downward traction on the penis opens the subpubic space, and the injection of local anesthetic under Scarpa fascia (which is continuous with Buck fascia in the shaft of the penis). Two injections are made 0.5 to 1 cm lateral to the midline just caudal to the inferior ramus of the pubic bone. A 22-gauge needle is inserted slightly medial and caudad until the characteristic "pop" is felt as the needle traverses Scarpa fascia just below the pubis. One to two milliliters of local anesthetic is injected (if under 3 years) to a maximum 0.5 mL/kg of 0.25% bupivacaine. Ultrasound with a hockey stick probe may improve the failure rate ascribed to the landmark technique by 7.5% (19).

2. **Complications.** There have been no complications observed with the ring technique. Blockade of the dorsal penile nerve deep to Buck fascia in the shaft of the penis has been associated with decreased perfusion to the tip of the glans penis.

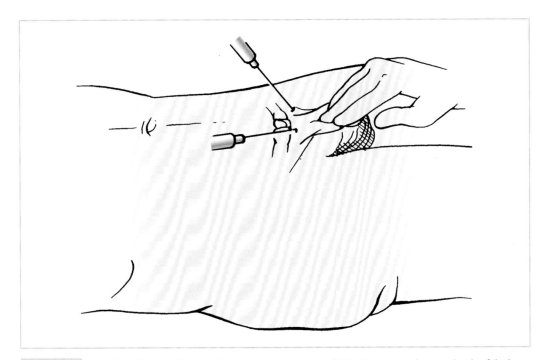

FIGURE 15.3 Dorsal penile block. The penis is retracted downward and injections are made on each side of the base, 0.5 to 1 cm lateral to the midline and below the symphysis pubis. The needle is inserted slightly medially and caudally to pierce Scarpa fascia.

G. Extremity blocks. The basic techniques for extremity blockade in infants and children are similar to those used in adults, with the exception that these blocks are usually carried out under general anesthesia. Ultrasound is important in the placement of extremity blocks in infants and children.

1. **Indications**
   a. **Upper extremity blocks** can provide muscle relaxation and anesthesia for the reduction of fractures as well as analgesia after an open procedure.
   b. A **femoral nerve block**, alone or in conjunction with a lateral femoral cutaneous nerve block, can provide anesthesia for muscle biopsy. Femoral nerve blockade also provides excellent analgesia and muscle relaxation for children with femur fractures, especially if the fracture is in the middle third of the femoral shaft.
   c. For older children having more extensive lower extremity surgery, both femoral and **sciatic nerve blockage** are often done. However, caudal blockade with its single injection is preferred for lower extremity surgery in children before they are school aged.

2. **Drugs.** The longer acting agents, bupivacaine and ropivacaine, provide effective anesthesia and analgesia for up to 12 hours. It must be remembered that toxicities are additive when compounding local anesthetics (Table 15.3). Ropivacaine has been widely studied in caudals and, less so, in extremity blocks for pediatric patients (20).

3. **Techniques**
   a. **Brachial plexus block**
      (1) According to the Pediatric Regional Anesthesia Network (PRAN) database, the most common approach to the brachial plexus in children is the supraclavicular approach (21). The safety of this approach in children has been improved with the use of ultrasound, thus decreasing the risk of pneumothorax and vascular puncture. The placement of supraclavicular block is the same as in adults (see Chapter 8). In children, ultrasound guidance with this block is more comfortable if placed awake and produces faster onset and longer duration of blockade (22).
      (2) For an **axillary block in children, ultrasound has resulted in lower volumes being used and less vascular puncture because the axillary artery and veins can be directly visualized.** Appropriate volumes of local anesthetics are noted in Table 15.3; these volumes usually include separate blockade of the musculocutaneous nerve.

CLINICAL PEARL   This block has been used in the neonatal intensive care unit for peripherally inserted central venous catheter placement and to treat limb ischemia after arterial catheterization (23).

      (3) The PRAN reviewed interscalene blocks in children under general anesthesia, because this was previously discouraged owing to a few case reports of adverse events in adults under anesthesia, and concluded that general anesthesia does not increase the risk of complications (24). However, these blocks should only be attempted by those most well trained to perform them.

TABLE 15.3   Drug volumes for pediatric regional techniques with 0.25% bupivacaine or 0.2% ropivacaine

Peripheral nerve block	Volume (mL/kg)
Brachial plexus	0.3
Femoral nerve block	0.3
Sciatic nerve	0.3
Transversus abdominus	0.3 per side

b. Lower extremity blocks

   (1) The **femoral nerve block** is described in Chapter 10; few modifications are required for pediatric patients. This is the most common lower extremity block in children and can be quite useful in femur fractures even in the emergency room (25) or for muscle biopsies. Ultrasound can be useful. A volume of 0.3 mL/kg is injected with epinephrine to detect intravascular placement. Adductor canal block is gaining popularity in providing pure sensory block with minimal effect on quadriceps strength.

   (2) The **sciatic nerve** is easily blocked more peripherally than in the classic description. Children often have a smaller gluteal fat pad and one can frequently palpate their sciatic groove. Place the child in the lateral (Sims) position; the ankle of the upper leg is placed on the knee of the lower leg. The child can also be supine with the leg elevated. Locate and mark the greater trochanter and the ischial tuberosity of the upper leg. The ultrasound probe can be placed transversely below the gluteal fold and the sciatic can be visualized below the gluteus maximus muscle. A total of 0.3 mL/kg to a maximum of 20 mL should be injected.

   (3) The **popliteal fossa** can be the ideal location for blocking the sciatic nerve. The sciatic nerve always bifurcates within the fossa in infants but cephalad of the fossa in adults. Children are usually anesthetized and supine, so the lateral approach would be advantageous. However, in small children, the leg can usually be lifted with ease to expose the popliteal fossa for the posterior approach. This block is described in Chapter 11. Bifurcation of the nerve can be identified with ultrasound guidance. In children, the volume of 0.25% bupivacaine injected should be 0.2 to 0.3 mL/kg.

   (4) Dosing. Because of the complex nerve supply from two plexuses, anesthetizing the leg requires larger doses of local anesthetic than upper extremity blocks. If multiple blocks are planned, remember that local anesthetic doses are additive with regard to LAST.

4. Continuous catheters

   a. There are many reports of improved postoperative pain management in children with continuous infusion of local anesthetics through a peripheral nerve catheter, both in the upper and lower extremities (20). Continuous infusions of local anesthetics are increasingly being used in children at home postoperatively allowing earlier discharge (26). Continuously infusing catheters serve to eliminate rebound pain that sometimes occurs the first night when the initial dose of local anesthetic wears off. Catheter sets are now available in pediatric sizes.

   b. Dose. For postoperative analgesia through a continuous catheter, the suggested starting dose of local anesthetic is 0.1 mL/kg/h of ropivacaine 0.2%, not to exceed 0.15 mL/kg/h.

   c. Clear postoperative instructions must be given to the parents about the block wearing off and the timing of oral analgesics. Regular dosing of acetaminophen and opioids can minimize a pain crisis or rebound when the block wears off. The parents should be explained about the importance of treating pain early and staying ahead of the pain with oral analgesics and of encouraging children to report sensations of discomfort early.

REFERENCES

1. Dalens BJ, Truchon R. Neural blockade for pediatric surgery. In: Cousins MJ, Bridenbaugh PO, eds. *Neural Blockade in Clinical Anesthesia and Management of Pain*, 3rd ed. Philadelphia, PA: Lippincott Williams & Wilkins; 2009.
2. Dadure C, Sola C, Dalens BJ, et al. Regional anesthesia in children. In: Miller RDM, ed. *Anesthesia*, 5th ed. Philadelphia, PA: Elsevier Saunders; 2015.

3. Ross, AK, Bryskin RB. Regional anesthesia. In: Motoyama E, Davis P, eds. *Smith's Anesthesia for Infants and Children*, 8th ed. Philadelphia, PA: Elsevier Saunders; 2011.

4. Sethna NF, Berde CB. Pediatric regional anesthesia. In: Gregory GA, ed. *Pediatric Anesthesia*, 5th ed. Hoboken, NJ: Wiley-Blackwell; 2011.

5. Young KD. Topical anaesthetics: what's new? *Arch Dis Child Educ Pract Ed* 2015;100(2):105–110.

6. Jimenez N. A comparison of a needle-free injection system for local anesthesia versus EMLA for intravenous catheter insertion in the pediatric patient. *Anesth Analg* 2006;102(2):411–414.

7. Paix BR, Peterson SE. Circumcision of neonates and children without appropriate anaesthesia is unacceptable practice. *Anaesth Intensive Care* 2012;40(3):511–516.

8. Ivani G, Suresh S, Ecoffey C, et al. The ESRA and ASRA Joint Committee Practice Advisory on Controversial Topics in Pediatric Regional Anesthesia. *Reg Anesth Pain Med* 2015;40:426–432.

9. Menzies F, Congreve K, Herodes V, et al. A survey of pediatric caudal extradural anesthesia practice. *Paediatr Anesth* 2009;19(9):829–836.

10. Tobias JD. Caudal epidural block: a review of test dosing and recognition of systemic injection in children. *Anesth Analg* 2001;93:1156–1161.

11. Long J, Joselyn AS, Bhalla T, et al. The use of neuraxial catheters for postoperative analgesia in neonates: a multicenter safety analysis from the Pediatric Regional Anesthesia Network. *Anesth Analg* 2016;122(6):1965–1970.

12. Presley JD, Chyka PA. Intravenous lipid emulsion to reverse acute drug toxicity in pediatric patients. *Ann Pharmacother* 2013;47(5):735–743.

13. Marhofer P, Willschke H, Kettner S. Imaging techniques for regional nerve blockade and vascular cannulation in children. *Curr Opin Anaesthesiol* 2006;19:293–300.

14. Simion C, Corcoran J, Iyer A. Postoperative pain control for primary cleft lip repair in infants: is there an advantage in performing peripheral nerve blocks? *Paediatr Anesth* 2008;18(11):1060–1065.

15. Hamill J, Rahiri J, Liley A, et al. Rectus sheath and transversus abdominis plane blocks in childrens: a systematic review and meta-analysis of randomized trials. *Pediatr Anesth* 2016;26(4):363–371.

16. Long JB, Birmingham PK, De Oliveira GS, et al. Transversus abdominis plane block in children: a multicenter safety analysis of 1994 cases from PRAN (Pediatric Regional Anesthesia Network) database. *Anesth Analg* 2014;119(2):395–399.

17. Willschke H, Bosenberg A, Marhofer P, et al. Ultrasonographic-guided ilioinguinal/iliohypogastric nerve block in pediatric anesthesia: what is the optimal volume? *Anesth Analg* 2006;102:1680–1684.

18. Bhalla T, Sawardekar A, Tobias J, et al. Ultrasound-guided truck and core blocks in infants and children. *J Anesth* 2013;27:109–123.

19. O'Sullivan M, Mislovic B, Alexander E. Dorsal penile block for male pediatric circumcision—randomized comparison of ultrasound-guided vs anatomical landmark technique. *Pediatr Anesth* 2011;21:1214–1218.

20. Visoiu M, Joy L, Chelly J. Effectiveness of ambulatory continuous peripheral nerve blocks for postoperative pain management in children and adolescents. *Pediatr Anesth* 2014;24(11):1141.

21. Polaner D, Taenzer A, Walker B, et al. Pediatric Regional Anesthesia Network (PRAN): a multi-institutional study of the use and incidence of complications of pediatric regional anesthesia. *Anesth Analg* 2012;115(6):1353–1364.

22. Amiri HR. Upper extremity surgery in younger children under ultrasound-guided supraclavicular brachial plexus block: a case series. *J Child Orthop* 2011;5:5.

23. Breschan C, Marhofer P. Axillary brachial plexus block for treatment of severe forearm ischemia after arterial cannulation in an extremely low birth-weight infant. *Paediatr Anaesth* 2004;14:681.

24. Taenzer A, Walker B, Bosenberg A, et al. Interscalene brachial plexus blocks under general anesthesia in children: is this safe practice? A report from the Pediatric Regional Anesthesia Network (PRAN). *Reg Anesth Pain Med* 2014;39:502.

25. Baker MD. Ultrasound-guided femoral nerve blocks. *Pediatr Emerg Care* 2015;31:864.

26. Duflo F. Efficacy and plasma levels of ropivacaine for children: controlled regional analgesia following lower limb surgery. *Br J Anaesth* 2006;97:250.

16

Acute Pain Medicine Service

Kevin E. Vorenkamp and Christine L. Oryhan

KEY POINTS

1. An organized acute pain medicine service (APMS) improves patient satisfaction and pain control.

2. A balanced multimodal approach can achieve optimal pain control while minimizing side effects for patients with pain.

3. Epidural analgesia provides superior analgesia as compared with systemic opioids. Vigilant assessment and treatment modification by the APMS serve to minimize epidural-related side effects.

4. Enhanced recovery after surgery (ERAS) protocols target early return to function using multimodal therapies aimed at minimizing effects of the surgical stress response.

5. Appropriate evaluation and vigilance are required to accurately diagnose and treat patients with painful conditions.

ESTABLISHING AN ORGANIZED REGIONAL ANESTHESIA-DRIVEN acute pain medicine service (APMS) is critical to provide essential postoperative pain medicine in both the hospital and ambulatory environments (1). Postoperative pain is the patient's greatest preoperative concern and remains undertreated. A **balanced multimodal approach** incorporating pharmacologic, nonpharmacologic, and regional anesthetic and analgesic interventions is essential. **Enhanced recovery after surgery** (ERAS) protocols are beneficial when incorporated into perioperative pain management treatment plans.

I. APMS structure

  A. Depending on the volume and demand of the service and the nature of the practice (academic vs. private practice), the APMS can be divided into an acute pain service (APS)/epidural service, a pain consult service, and a peripheral nerve catheter (PNC)/regional analgesia service. Alternatively, all the aspects can be combined into a comprehensive service.

  B. Roles for the APMS team should be defined and include:

    1. **Director** oversees direction of service, develops policies and protocols, directs educational and research initiatives, and collaborates with other services such as pharmacy and information technology.

    2. **APMS attending** daily rounds, supervises regional anesthesia/analgesia procedures, and pain consultations.

    3. **APMS resident/fellow** daily rounds, performs regional anesthesia/analgesia procedures and pain consultations, promptly responds to calls and questions regarding pain management and/or complications, and coordinates APMS recommendations with primary services.

    4. **APMS nurse specialist** provides continuity on service, daily rounds, educates ward nurses on policies/protocols, performs quality improvement, calls discharged patients with indwelling PNCs for follow-up, and coordinates APMS recommendations with primary services.

    5. Alternatively, and predominantly in nonacademic settings, a **physician assistant or nurse practitioner** can fill the role of APMS resident/fellow or nurse specialist, or this can also be done independently under the APS director's oversight.

  C. Challenges

    1. **Education** and frequent **communication** with nursing and physician staff regarding breadth and limitations of the services provided are essential.

    2. **Availability** of APMS on a 24-h/d and 7 d/wk basis is required to address unusual complications, technical malfunctions, and dose adjustments of neuraxial and PNCs. This requires commitment and support from the anesthesiology staff. Ideally, patients on the APMS should be evaluated twice daily, particularly those individuals with indwelling pain management catheters in place.

    3. The APMS should provide and communicate management recommendations to the primary service. There are times when the pain service will be the primary prescriber of analgesic medications. Typically, this will be the case when managing an epidural catheter or if the patient requires complex management beyond what the primary service is able to provide. There must be clear communication to avoid duplicate orders and to enable a smooth transition of care when the condition has stabilized.

D. APMS rounding

1. Key questions should include:
   a. Location of pain
   b. Pain score (0 to 10) at rest and with activity
   c. Any significant side effects, for example, nausea, sedation, itching, and weakness
   d. Baseline (preadmission) pain scores, locations, medications, and intolerances

2. Physical examination should include:
   a. General sensorium
   b. Lower extremity strength/sensation for epidural and lower extremity blocks and upper extremity strength/sensation for upper extremity blocks. For thoracic epidural catheters, assess the patient's strength with hip flexion because this movement requires use of the hip flexors (L1–L3) and quadriceps (L2–L4) which are more likely to be affected if there is local anesthetic in the upper lumbar spine. This is also a way to assess how pain is interfering with function.
   c. **Assessment of catheter insertion site.** Verify that the sterile occlusive dressing is intact without significant amounts of blood or leakage of infusate, that the catheter remains at an appropriate depth (compare with documentation on procedure note), and that the skin is without erythema, induration, or tenderness.

3. **For a sample APMS note template,** Figure 16.1.

II. Neuraxial analgesia

A. Epidural analgesia include continuous epidural infusion (CEI) and patient-controlled epidural analgesia (PCEA)

   3

   1. **Advantages**
      a. **Superior postoperative analgesia** (overall, at rest, and with activity) compared to intravenous patient-controlled analgesia (IV PCA) with opioids (2,3).
      b. **Improved respiratory function** (can prevent splinting), preventing postoperative atelectasis and pneumonia (3).
      c. **Decreased duration of ileus** versus systemic analgesia (3).

CLINICAL PEARL Epidural analgesia provides superior pain relief, improved respiratory function, and decreased duration of ileus compared to systemic opioids.

   2. Epidural placement level for select procedures (for specific considerations, see Chapter 7)
      a. The surgical incision site dictates the appropriate level for epidural placement. Mid-thoracic epidurals are ideal for thoracic surgery, low-thoracic epidurals are ideal for abdominal surgery, and lumbar epidurals are used for obstetric analgesia. Thoracic epidurals have a positive effect on respiratory function and splanchnic sympathetic block, which can help return of bowel function. Unlike thoracic epidurals, lumbar epidurals can impair ambulation, cause urinary retention, and lack the benefits of improved respiratory and bowel function (4).
      b. **Epidural spread** of infusate is preferentially cephalad rather than caudal in both the lower thoracic (2:1) and lumbar (3:1) spine following bolus injection (5); however, spread is typically equal in the mid-thoracic spine and preferentially caudad in the high-thoracic spine. Additionally, other factors such as spinal pathology, age, and bevel direction when threading the catheter may also influence the spread (4).

Anesthesia Pain Medicine Service Progress Note

Chief Complaint:

Plan:
Changes to current plan: ☐ None   other: _____
☐ Transition to oral analgesics at this time   ☐ Transition tomorrow AM early:
☐ Pain management catheter removed intact
Additional comments: _____
Continue to follow patient: ☐ YES   ☐ NO

Assessment:
Postoperative Day #: _____
Procedure: _____
Location of pain: _____
Subjective: _____
Pain score at rest: ☐
Pain score with activity: ☐
Current Diet: ☐ NPO   ☐ Clears   ☐ Full   Notes: _____

Significant other symptoms:
☐ Nausea
☐ Sedation
☐ Itching
☐ Leg weakness
☐ Other: _____

Physical Exam
Sensorium: ☐ Awake, clear speech, oriented   Other: _____
Lower Extremity Strength: ☐ normal   ☐ abnormal
Catheter site: ☐ intact, nontender   other: _____

Pain Therapy Details:
☐ PCEA (Patient Controlled Epidural Analgesia) 2 mL prn with lockout 10 minutes
☐ CEA (Continuous Epidural Infusion)
   Rate/Infusion: _____ mL/hr,
☐ PCA (Patient Controlled Intravenous Analgesia)
   Drug: ☐ hydromorphone
          ☐ morphine
   Bolus dose: ☐ mg   Lockout Interval: ☐ min   Continuous: ☐ mg/hr
24 hour shift total of IV narcotics: ☐ mg
☐ PNC (Perineural Catheter)
Type of catheter: ☐ femoral   ☐ interscalene   ☐ other: _____
Infusion: 0.2% ropivacaine   Rate _____ ml/hour
☐ Ketorolac   ☐ PRN   Scheduled ☐
Other Pain Medications: _____

FIGURE 16.1 Example of an acute pain medicine service (APMS) progress note template. (Modified with permission from *Acute Pain Service Template*. Seattle, WA: Department of Anesthesiology, Virginia Mason Medical Center. ©2017 Virginia Mason Medical Center.)

   c. Choice of epidural infusion rate and infusate (**for standard infusates,** Table 16.1)

   d. The options for medication delivery include **CEI**-only, bolus-only options, or **PCEA** including both a continuous and demand option. The continuous infusion rate can range from 0 to 14 mL/h (typical starting dose is 8 mL/h); standard demand dose is 2 mL every (q) 10 minutes.

   e. Special considerations

     (1) Changing the epidural infusate to local anesthetic alone (continuous only, no bolus) with the possible addition of an IV opioid PCA.

       (a) Consider in **opioid-tolerant patients** with chronic pain, especially patients taking greater than 30 oral morphine equivalents per day.

       (b) Consider if epidural **does not provide adequate analgesia** for the surgical incision(s) or if patient has baseline pain in an area not covered by the epidural.

       (c) Although this configuration may address inadequate analgesia in the situations mentioned, disadvantages related to higher doses of systemic opioids may occur (i.e., ileus, nausea, and confusion).

     (2) See below for adjustments based on prevalent side effects.

CLINICAL PEARL　Epidural flow is preferentially cephalad (2 of 3) rather than caudal in the lower thoracic spine, but equal in the mid-thoracic spine.

---

   3. Anticoagulation in the setting of epidural catheter

     a. For full anticoagulation guidelines for neuraxial and peripheral nerve blocks procedures, refer to **ASRA guidelines** (6).

     b. Concurrent epidural use is contraindicated with low-molecular weight heparin (e.g., enoxaparin) and clopidogrel

     c. Unfractionated **heparin** (IV or subcutaneous) should not be given 4 hours before or 1 hour after epidural catheter removal. Accidental removal of catheter or administration of heparin too close to manipulation warrants frequent (at least every 4 hours if asymptomatic) neurologic checks for 24 hours to assess for epidural hematoma.

     d. For perioperative management of neuraxial blocks in the setting of warfarin use (6), refer to ASRA guidelines.

   4. Risks/side effects (for details regarding neuraxial complications, see Chapter 14)

TABLE 16.1　Standard epidural infusates

Medication and concentration	Comments
Hydromorphone 0.005 mg/mL + bupivacaine 0.05%	Standard infusate
Hydromorphone 0.01 mg/mL + bupivacaine 0.05%	Higher concentration of opioid with standard local anesthetic concentration
Bupivacaine 0.05%	Lower concentration local anesthetic-only infusion for hypotensive patients who require systemic opioids or do not tolerate opioid side effects
Bupivacaine 0.1%	Ideal for hemodynamically stable patients who require systemic opioids or do not tolerate opioid side effects
Fentanyl 2–4 µg/mL + bupivacaine 0.05% or 0.1%	Alternative to hydromorphone
Morphine 0.04 mg/mL + bupivacaine 0.05% or 0.1%	Alternative to hydromorphone

    a. Hypotension, pruritus, urinary retention, and motor blockade are more common with PCEA/CEI than PCA. Nausea/vomiting and sedation can occur, but to a lesser degree than, with PCA administration (2).

    b. Epidural hematoma

        (1) The estimated incidence of neurologic dysfunction resulting from epidural hematoma when adhering to guidelines in patients undergoing epidural catheter placement is estimated between 1:50,000 and 1:150,000 (7,8). This has likely increased in the past few decades for several reasons, most notably the introduction of new anticoagulant and antiplatelet medications (9), as well as the aging population. See below for diagnosis and management.

    c. Epidural abscess and other neuraxial infections.

        (1) Serious infections such as meningitis and epidural abscess are rare, particularly in routine postsurgical patients. Risk factors for serious infection include patient factors (immunocompromised, serious illness, and preexisting infection of skin or spine), breaks in aseptic technique, and prolonged catheter in situ (10). Urgent (<12 hours) surgical intervention combined with broad-spectrum antibiotics is typically required when epidural abscess or discitis are present. See below for diagnosis and management.

CLINICAL PEARL Serious complications such as hematoma or abscess are exceedingly rare, but require urgent intervention when they occur.

    d. Nonfunctioning catheters are often the consequence of inappropriate placement or catheter migration. The overall failure rate may be as high as 21.6% (11), but the incidence of premature catheter dislodgement is closer to 5.7% (12).

5. Treatment of complications and side effects, postoperatively (for details on neuraxial complications, see Chapter 14).

    a. Parameters for abnormal vital signs and/or inadequate pain control should be included in standard order sets for ward nurses, in addition to periodic nursing education for what signs and symptoms to monitor in a patient with epidural analgesia.

    b. Respiratory depression (respiratory rate <10 breaths/min). Decrease rate or remove opioid from infusate. Use opioid antagonist if severe, increase monitoring vigilance. Administer **naloxone** 0.1 to 0.4 mg IV every 1 to 2 minutes for respiratory rate less than 8 breaths/min and/or the patient is unarousable.

    c. Sedation. Remove opioid from infusate, increase monitoring vigilance. Search for other physiologic (hypoxia, hypotension, and hypercarbia) and pharmacologic causes.

    d. Hypotension (blood pressure <20% of baseline or signs of decreased end-organ perfusion). Ensure adequate preload, contractility, afterload. If not improved with fluid administration and epidural suspected to be a contributing factor, consider decreasing rate or local anesthetic concentration. Contact surgery service if patient shows signs of persistent volume depletion or concern for postoperative bleeding.

    e. Pruritus. Most commonly treated with removal of opioid from infusate if intolerable. Although not believed to be histamine related, some patients do benefit from diphenhydramine 12.5 to 25 mg IV or 25 to 50 mg by mouth (PO) or nalbuphine 2.5 to 5 mg IV (13).

    f. Epidural hematoma. New neurologic deficits (urinary retention and motor blockade) as well as back or radicular pain. If suspected, immediate neurologic evaluation and diagnostic imaging. MRI is most sensitive, but may be contraindicated with the presence of some types of epidural catheters. Consider removing the epidural catheter if suspicion is high versus proceeding with CT imaging which is faster and does not require catheter removal. If confirmed, emergent surgical evacuation is most commonly warranted.

g. **Infection.** Local tenderness, erythema, fever, and leukocytosis noted with peripheral infection. Meningitis typically presents with fever, headache, photophobia, meningismus, and later altered mental status. Epidural abscess associated with back and/or radicular pain or signs of new neurologic deficits. Treat by removal of epidural catheter. If epidural abscess suspected and confirmed with diagnostic imaging, aggressive medical and/or surgical intervention may be necessary.

h. Postdural puncture headache (14) (for details, see Chapter 14).

i. **Inadequate analgesia** (Fig. 16.2, decision tree)

    (1) **Assess dermatomal level** if possible. Is the block one sided? Is there adequate dermatomal spread?

    (2) Consider **bolus** of local anesthetic (5 mL of either infusate solution or 1% lidocaine, depending on the initial blood pressure) or the performance of **epidurogram** if any uncertainty. Monitor for hypotension after local anesthetic bolus, particularly with higher concentration of local anesthetic. For epidurogram, under sterile conditions 5 mL of myelography contrast (i.e., Isovue-M300, Iopamidol injection 61%, Bracco Diagnostics Inc., Princeton, NJ, USA) should be injected through the

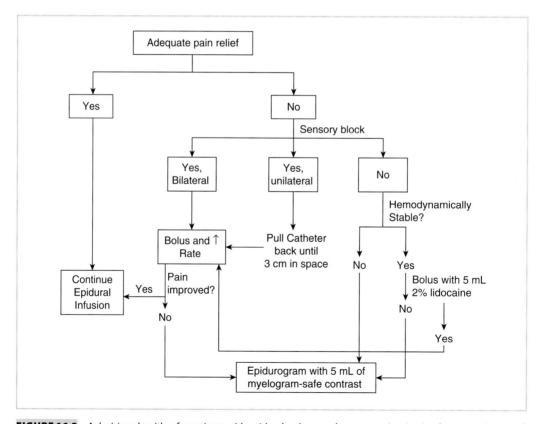

FIGURE 16.2 A decision algorithm for patients with epidural catheters who are experiencing inadequate pain control.

epidural catheter immediately prior to a plain film X-ray of the thoracic spine. Epidurograms can be performed in conjunction with the surgical closing film or in the recovery room or even on the wards. **The characteristic appearance of epidural contrast** demonstrates epidural spread within the confines of the pedicles, "fatty" appearance with characteristic lobules, and possible spread out of exiting neural foramen (for an example of an epidurogram and nonepidurogram, Fig. 16.3A and B, respectively).

(3) Also consider **epidural waveform analysis** (for details, see Chapter 7).

(4) Consider removing the epidural catheter and changing to PCA versus replacing the catheter.

6. **Transitioning from epidural to oral analgesic regimen**

   a. Once the patient tolerates a clear liquid diet, consider the addition of oral adjuncts such as acetaminophen and possibly gabapentin or nonsteroidal anti-inflammatory drugs (NSAIDs; see below).

   b. Once the patient is tolerating a full liquid diet, attempt to transition to oral opioids. In a patient who is not taking opioids prior to admission, oxycodone 5 to 10 mg or hydromorphone 2 to 4 mg every 4 hours is usually adequate.

   c. In patients taking chronic opioids prior to surgery (for >1 month), consider starting oral opioids anywhere from 50% to 100% greater than their dose prior to admission.

   d. For opioid intolerant patients, **tramadol** is a partial μ-agonist medication that is often better tolerated. Dosage is 50 to 100 mg orally every 6 to 8 hours as needed (maximum dose 400 mg/d). Alternatively, opioids can be used in smaller doses (oxycodone 2.5 mg or hydromorphone 1 mg) or avoided altogether.

   e. Place orders to pause the epidural infusate at the same time as giving a one-time dose of oral medication. Reassess the patient's pain control 2 hours later. After ensuring that administration of anticoagulants has been paused appropriately, and that the patient tolerated the transition, remove the epidural catheter and document that the catheter was removed with its tip intact.

   f. Remove epidural catheters after a maximum of **7 days** in most patients to reduce the risk of infection. If the patient is not yet tolerating a diet, consider transitioning to IV PCA. In very rare circumstances, epidural catheters may be kept longer than 7 days provided insertion site, white count, and temperature are monitored daily, and patient is made aware of increased risk of infection.

CLINICAL PEARL Once the patient is tolerating a clear liquid diet, consider the addition of oral adjuncts such as acetaminophen. Once the patient is tolerating a full liquid diet, attempt to transition to oral opioids.

B. **Intrathecal opioids (15–18)**

   1. Intrathecal morphine (hydrophilic) has slower plasma reuptake and remains in the cerebrospinal fluid longer than lipophilic opioids.

   2. Single injection intrathecal morphine can produce analgesia for up to 24 hours in doses ranging from 50 to 300 μg (lower dose if given with intrathecal local anesthetic).

   3. Pruritus and delayed respiratory depression (6 to 12 hours later) are the most significant side effects, and both are dose dependent.

   4. Hydrophilic opioids (i.e., fentanyl and sufentanil) have faster onset (10 to 15 minutes) but shorter duration of action (2 to 5 hours).

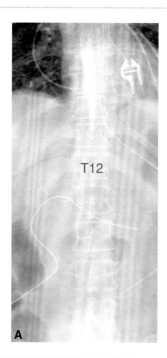 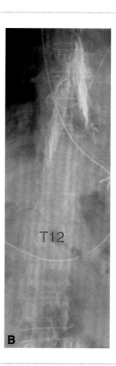

FIGURE 16.3 Epidurograms. **A:** Appropriate epidural contrast spread on thoracic radiogram after injection of 5 mL of contrast. Note the fluffy, bilateral appearance with fatty lobules present. Contrast (white) can be visualized from T11 to at least the top of the image (T6). **B:** *Non*epidural contrast spread on thoracic radiogram after injection of 5 mL of contrast. Although there is bilateral spread, the contrast exceeds the dimensions of the spinal canal and obliterates visualization of the pedicles on both sides.

III. Intravenous patient controlled analgesia

   A. Advantages/effectiveness

      1. **More effective analgesia** and **better patient satisfaction** as compared with nurse administered boluses (19).

      2. Effective administration of IV analgesia in a patient unable to take parenteral analgesics or with a contraindication to neuraxial analgesia.

      3. Once the patients can tolerate a full liquid diet, transition them back to oral opioids.

      4. See equianalgesic table (Table 16.2). Calculate the patients 24-hour total use of opioids via the PCA. Typically, start with a 50% dose reduction when converting.

CLINICAL PEARL When converting from IV hydromorphone to PO oxycodone, the calculated dose will be 10 times larger. For example, if the patient used 8 mg IV hydromorphone over 24 hours, then anticipate that the patient will need between 40 and 80 mg of oral oxycodone over 24 hours. Start with 10 mg PO q 3 to 4 hours as-needed (PRN) pain.

   B. Risks/side effects

      1. **Monitor** all patients with PCA for alertness and signs or symptoms of hypoxia or hypoventilation. Patients with obstructive sleep apnea are at particularly higher risk for both conditions. You may consider using smaller IV opioid doses in these patients.

TABLE 16.2   Equianalgesic dosing of opioids for pain management

Medication	Parenteral (IV) dosage (mg)	Oral (PO) dosage (mg)
Morphine	10	30
Hydrocodone	n/a	30
Hydromorphone	1.5–**2**	6–8
Oxycodone	10[a]	**20**
Oxymorphone	1	10
Fentanyl	0.1 (100 µg)	12.5 µg/h (transdermal)
Methadone	Variable[b]	Variable[b]
Tramadol	100[a]	120

[a]Not available in the United States.
[b]Methadone conversion tool available at http://www.agencymeddirectors.wa.gov/Calculator/DoseCalculator.htm.
IV, intravenous; PO, by mouth.

2. **Respiratory depression.** Ideally, all patients with PCA should have continuous respiratory rate and end-tidal CO_2 monitoring to assess for respiratory depression (20,21). At minimum, check respiratory rate and oxygen saturation every 4 hours and more frequently if sedation or respiratory depression is identified. Be aware that detecting hypoventilation with pulse oximetry can be delayed, particularly in patients receiving supplemental oxygen because the patient may have hypercarbia but not hypoxia.

3. **Sedation.** If sedation is noted, then the dose should be decreased. First, decrease the bolus dose and consider increasing the lockout interval. Educate the patient and family that only the patient should push the PCA button to minimize the risk of over sedation and respiratory depression. Certain patients may be at increased risk (e.g., those with sleep apnea or concomitant use of central nervous system depressants such as benzodiazepines).

4. Nausea and vomiting, pruritus, confusion, and opioid-induced constipation.

C. **Part of a multimodal approach to pain management**

D. **Typical IV opioids with dose and frequency** (Table 16.3)

IV. **Peripheral nerve catheters.** Peripheral nerve blocks and continuous catheters can provide excellent postoperative analgesia for both inpatients and outpatients and are opioid sparing.

A. For an in-depth discussion of catheter placement, see the peripheral nerve block chapters.

B. **Patient selection**

TABLE 16.3   Standard intravenous patient-controlled analgesia (PCA) medications

Medication and concentration	Typical starting rate with range	Comments
Hydromorphone (0.4 mg/mL)	0.2 mg every (q) 8 min, no continuous (0.1–0.5 mg q 8–15 min)	Standard PCA infusate/rate
Hydromorphone (1 or 5 mg/mL)	As above	Higher concentration for higher usage
Morphine (1 mg/mL)	1 mg q 8 min, no continuous (0.5–3 mg q 8–15 min)	Use for patient intolerant of hydromorphone
Morphine (5 mg/mL)	As above	Higher concentration for higher usage
Fentanyl (25 µg/mL)	10–25 µg q 6–10 min, no continuous	Alternative to hydromorphone and morphine

1. Inpatient PNCs are monitored and managed closely by ward nurses and the APMS team.

2. Ambulatory patients should be able to fully comprehend how to use the PNC delivery system (see below) and/or have a caregiver immediately available to assist them. Be sure that the patient can to be contacted and is able to call/page the APMS with any immediate questions or concerns.

3. If there is heightened concern for complications such as bleeding and infection, consider a single injection peripheral nerve block as an alternative to a continuous catheter.

C. **Delivery systems**

1. Pumps designed for epidural analgesia delivery can be used for inpatients (for details on these pumps, see Chapter 2).

2. Disposable battery-operated pumps can be used for both inpatient and outpatients (for details on disposable battery-operated pumps, see Chapter 2).
    a. Prior to discharge, use verbal and written instructions to inform the patient about pump function and possible malfunctions. Provide the patient with a 24-hour accessible contact phone or pager number.
    b. Daily phone calls should be made (by APMS nurse or resident) to assess the catheter and pain control while the catheter is still in place.

D. **Infusate.** Dilute local anesthetic solutions are ideally used, particularly long-acting amides, most commonly ropivacaine.

E. Complications and adverse effects are rare. Local inflammation and infection rates are less than 1% even when catheters remain in place for 4 to 7 days (22). Knotting of catheters around anatomic structures, including nerves, has been reported (23). If the patient has any difficulty removing the catheter (i.e., catheter not coming out easily or development of paresthesia), advise the patient to come in for assistance.

CLINICAL PEARL   Prior to discharge, inform the patient about pump function and possible malfunctions. Provide the patient with a 24-hour accessible contact phone or pager number. Daily phone calls should be made (by APMS nurse or physician) to assess the catheter and pain control while the catheter is still in place.

V. Transversus abdominis plane and rectus sheath blocks and catheters. These are typically performed under ultrasound guidance and can be done unilaterally or bilaterally for midline abdominal incisions (24–26). These are reasonable alternatives to epidural analgesia for abdominal surgery, particularly if a neuraxial procedure is contraindicated (see Chapter 12).

VI. **Adjunct IV analgesics**

A. **Ketamine infusion** may be considered for patients with baseline chronic pain and/or opioid resistance or intolerance.

1. NMDA receptor antagonist that provides analgesia at subanesthetic doses.

2. As part of a multimodal analgesia approach, low-dose intraoperative and perioperative ketamine bolus or infusion can reduce postoperative pain and decrease opioid consumption. Ketamine can attenuate central sensitization and hyperalgesia in opioid-tolerant patients (27).

3. Consider intraoperative bolus of 0.5 mg/kg followed by infusion of 0.05 to 0.2 mg/kg/h. Infusions can continue postoperatively, usually for 24 to 48 hours based on patient response.

4. When continued in the hospital, patients should have continuous respiratory monitoring (pulse oximetry or $EtCO_2$ monitoring) with mental status assessment.

CLINICAL PEARL   Hospital policy will vary regarding where to place patients on ketamine infusions. Although intensive care unit admission is not required in many hospitals, nursing education and care pathways for these patients are essential.

B. Dexmedetomidine infusion

1. $\alpha2$ Agonist that provides sedation, analgesia, anxiolysis, reduced anesthetic requirements, and preservation of respiratory function (28).

2. Consider intraoperative bolus of 1 µg/kg over 10 to 20 minutes, followed by infusion of 0.2 to 0.7 µg/kg/h. Infusion can be continued postoperatively, typically less than 24 hours. Dexmedetomidine can be given simultaneously with ketamine for opioid-tolerant patients.

C. Lidocaine infusion

1. As part of a multimodal analgesia approach, intraoperative lidocaine infusions can reduce postoperative pain and recovery of ileus in abdominal surgery patients versus placebo (3,29).

2. Limited by toxic plasma concentrations at higher doses. Patients at risk for local anesthetic systemic toxicity may require lower doses (see Chapter 14).

3. Consider intraoperative bolus of 1.5 mg/kg followed by 2 mg/kg/h intraoperatively.

D. Acetaminophen IV scheduled (**i.e.**, 1,000 mg IV q 6 hours × 48 hours). Use of IV acetaminophen should be limited to patient unable to take oral pills or solution. As soon as possible, transition from IV to PO acetaminophen. Rectal administration is also an option.

E. Ketorolac 15 to 30 mg IV q 6 hours (30,31)

VII. **Adjunct oral (PO) analgesics**. See also Chapter 4.

A. Acetaminophen PO scheduled (650 mg PO q 6 hours)

1. Less expensive than IV with similar benefit (32). Can start when the patient is tolerating a clear liquid diet.

B. NSAIDs PO (celecoxib 200 to 400 mg PO preoperatively, 100 mg PO BID starting POD#3, depending on the surgery). Celecoxib is preferred over other NSAIDs in the immediate postoperative period because as a cyclooxygenase-2 inhibitor, it does not affect platelet function.

C. Gabapentinoids

1. **Gabapentin** (600 to 900 mg PO preoperatively, 300 mg PO qhs or BID/TID postoperatively when the patient is tolerating a clear liquid diet)

2. **Pregabalin** (150 to 300 mg PO preoperatively, 50 to 75 mg PO BID postoperatively when the patient is tolerating a clear liquid diet)

    a. Pregabalin pharmacodynamics are more consistent as compared with gabapentin

D. Antidepressants

1. Tricyclic antidepressants may be beneficial for neuropathic pain. Use caution in patients at risk for cardiac toxicity and anticholinergic side effects (urinary retention, confusion, and constipation).

   a. Amitriptyline (25 to 50 mg PO qhs)

   b. Nortriptyline (10 to 25 mg PO qhs)

      (1) Nortriptyline can be less sedating than amitriptyline in some patients

2. Serotonin–norepinephrine reuptake inhibitors

   a. Duloxetine (30 to 60 mg PO q or BID)

      (1) The Food and Drug Administration approved for management of diabetic peripheral neuropathy, fibromyalgia, and chronic musculoskeletal pain. Most common adverse effect is nausea, may also see increased blood pressure, use cautiously in patients with hepatic failure.

E. Muscle relaxants

1. **Centrally acting.** Limit use for acute muscle spasms, useful for complex spine patients, and other orthopedic procedures. Not recommended for long-term use for pain, unless the patient has chronic spasticity caused by an underlying disorder (i.e., cerebral palsy, multiple sclerosis, spinal cord injury, etc.).

   a. Preferably use tizanidine 2 to 4 mg PO q 8 hours PRN or baclofen 5 to 10 mg PO q 8 hours PRN (cyclobenzaprine and methocarbamol can be more sedating).

   b. Tizanidine is also an $\alpha2$ agonist and may have additional analgesic benefit.

   c. Avoid abrupt cessation of baclofen can precipitate withdrawal (spasticity, nausea, hypotension, fevers, and altered mental status).

VIII. Enhanced recovery after surgery

A. ERAS is an evidence-based multidisciplinary approach to the care of the surgical patient.

4. B. The goals of ERAS are to **enhance the patient's surgical recovery and reduce complications.** In order to achieve this, protocols are instituted that focus on minimizing surgical stress and improving the patient's response to stress (33).

C. Implementing an ERAS protocol requires **close coordination** with the surgical team, anesthesiology team, nursing, dieticians, and physical therapists.

D. **Evidence-based guidelines** for different types of surgery should be continuously updated and address goals for the preadmission, preoperative, intraoperative, and postoperative phases of care.

IX. Nonsurgical acute pain. The APMS provides consultative service for assistance with management of nonsurgical acute pain (e.g., sickle cell crisis, pancreatitis, and rib fractures) or patients with acute exacerbations of chronic or cancer-related pain. As outlined above, the first step is a thorough evaluation to determine the etiology of the pain, prior pain treatments and future goals with care. One should query state prescription monitoring programs to verify opioid dosing and evaluate for multiple prescribing sources. Also, utilize adjunct medications and regional anesthesia procedures when appropriate.

X. Special considerations

A. **Opioid-tolerant patients.** Patients with preexisting chronic pain on chronic opioid therapy require additional consideration. Despite requiring higher doses of opioids to achieve adequate analgesia, they are still at risk for the same opioid-related side effects. These patients are mostly likely to benefit from the addition of nonopioid analgesics and regional anesthesia procedures. These options are discussed earlier in this chapter.

B. Patients taking buprenorphine for pain or substance use disorder.

1. Buprenorphine is a partial opioid agonist at the μ-receptor and an antagonist at the κ-receptor. At high doses (up to 32 mg PO once daily); it is effective for treatment of opioid use disorder. At lower doses, usually in divided doses twice or three times daily (BID or TID), buprenorphine may be beneficial for treatment of chronic pain. Given the high affinity for the μ-receptor (1,000× higher than morphine), acute and perioperative pain are difficult to treat in patients taking buprenorphine because the μ-opioid receptors are already saturated (34).

2. Several options are available for the perioperative management of patients receiving buprenorphine. The most important first step is to arrange a preoperative visit with a preanesthesia clinic or pain management physician to develop a plan. All patients on buprenorphine must be educated on multimodal pain control, with a focus on nonopioid adjunct analgesics and regional anesthesia if appropriate.

    a. For minor surgical procedures, an ideal option is to continue the current dose of buprenorphine through the perioperative procedure and supplement with additional buprenorphine or opioid if necessary.

    b. For intermediate and major surgical procedures, the best option is to **stop the buprenorphine for 5 days** prior to surgery (given the variable half-life, particularly at higher doses). Coordinate with the prescribing physician and convert the patient to a full agonist opioid preoperatively if needed, with the eventual resumption of buprenorphine postoperatively once the pain has returned to manageable levels. If opioids are to be avoided completely (sometimes per the patient's request), holding for 3 days may be adequate. Regardless, these patients may still require higher doses of opioids intra- and postoperatively given opioid tolerance (34,35).

    c. For emergent surgery or if holding buprenorphine is not an option, supplement pain control with larger doses of full agonist opioids, in addition to multimodal analgesia.

CLINICAL PEARL   For elective intermediate and major surgical procedures, patients should **stop the buprenorphine for 5 days** prior to surgery.

ACKNOWLEDGMENTS

The authors wish to acknowledge Susan B. McDonald, MD, who wrote the fourth edition version of this chapter.

REFERENCES

1. Schwenk ES, Baratta JL, Gandhi K, et al. Setting up an acute pain management service. *Anesthesiol Clin* 2014;32(4):893–910.
2. Wu CL, Cohen SR, Richman JM, et al. Efficacy of postoperative patient-controlled and continuous infusion epidural analgesia versus intravenous patient-controlled analgesia with opioids: a meta-analysis. *Anesthesiology* 2005;103(5):1079–1088; quiz 1109–1110.
3. Chou R, Gordon DB, de Leon-Casasola OA, et al. Management of postoperative pain: A Clinical Practice Guideline From the American Pain Society, the American Society of Regional Anesthesia and Pain

Medicine, and the American Society of Anesthesiologists' Committee on Regional Anesthesia, Executive Committee, and Administrative Council. *J Pain* 2016;17(2):131–157.

4. Visser WA, Lee RA, Gielen MJ. Factors affecting the distribution of neural blockade by local anesthetics in epidural anesthesia and a comparison of lumbar versus thoracic epidural anesthesia. *Anesth Analg* 2008;107(2):708–721.

5. Yokoyama M, Hanazaki M, Fujii H, et al. Correlation between the distribution of contrast medium and the extent of blockade during epidural anesthesia. *Anesthesiology* 2004;100(6):1504–1010.

6. Horlocker TT, Wedel DJ, Rowlingson JC, et al. Regional anesthesia in the patient receiving antithrombotic or thrombolytic therapy: American Society of Regional Anesthesia and Pain Medicine Evidence-Based Guidelines (Third Edition). *Reg Anesth Pain Med* 2010;35(1):64–101.

7. Moen V, Dahlgren N, Irestedt L. Severe neurological complications after central neuraxial blockades in Sweden 1990–1999. *Anesthesiology* 2004;101(4):950–959.

8. Tryba M. [Epidural regional anesthesia and low molecular heparin: Pro]. *Anasthesiol Intensivmed Notfallmed Schmerzther* 1993;28(3):179–181.

9. Horlocker TT, Wedel DJ. Bleeding complications. In: Neal JM, ed. *Complications in Regional Anesthesia adn Pain Medicine*. Philadelphia, PA: Lippincott Williams & Williams; 2013:29–43.

10. Niesen AD, Wedel DJ, Horlocker TT. Infectious complications. In: Neal JM, ed. *Complications in Regional Anesthesia and Pain Medicine*. Philadelphia, PA: Lippincott Williams & Williams; 2013:44–58.

11. Auyong DB, Hostetter L, Yuan SC, et al. Evaluation of ultrasound-assisted thoracic epidural placement in patients undergoing upper abdominal and thoracic surgery: a randomized, double-blind study. *Reg Anesth Pain Med* 2017;42(2):204–209.

12. Wu CL, Ouanes J. Complications associated with continuous epidural analgesia. In: Neal JM, ed. *Complications in Regional Anesthesia and Pain Medicine*. Philadelphia, PA: Lippincott Williams & Williams; 2013:219–234.

13. Jannuzzi RG. Nalbuphine for treatment of opioid-induced pruritus: a systematic review of literature. *Clin J Pain* 2016;32(1):87–93.

14. Harrington BE. Postdural puncture headache and the development of the epidural blood patch. *Reg Anesth Pain Med* 2004;29(2):136–163; discussion 135.

15. Mugabure Bujedo B. A clinical approach to neuraxial morphine for the treatment of postoperative pain. *Pain Res Treat* 2012;2012:612145.

16. Hamber EA, Viscomi CM. Intrathecal lipophilic opioids as adjuncts to surgical spinal anesthesia. *Reg Anesth Pain Med* 1999;24(3):255–263.

17. Rathmell JP, Lair TR, Nauman B. The role of intrathecal drugs in the treatment of acute pain. *Anesth Analg* 2005;101(Suppl 5):S30–S43.

18. Giovannelli M, Bedforth N, Aitkenhead A. Survey of intrathecal opioid usage in the UK. *Eur J Anaesthesiol* 2008;25(2):118–122.

19. Hudcova J, McNicol E, Quah C, et al. Patient controlled opioid analgesia versus conventional opioid analgesia for postoperative pain. *Cochrane Database Syst Rev* 2006;(4):CD003348.

20. Vorenkamp KE, Durieux ME. Patient-controlled analgesia. *J Neurosurg* 2009;111(2):340–342; discussion 341–342.

21. Weinger M. *Danger of Postoperative Opioids*. Anesthesia Patient Safety Foundation Newsletter, 2006.

22. Wiegel M, Gottschaldt U, Hennebach R, et al. Complications and adverse effects associated with continuous peripheral nerve blocks in orthopedic patients. *Anesth Analg* 2007;104(6):1578–1582; table of contents.

23. Offerdahl MR, Lennon RL, Horlocker TT. Successful removal of a knotted fascia iliaca catheter: principles of patient positioning for peripheral nerve catheter extraction. *Anesth Analg* 2004;99(5):1550–1552; table of contents.

24. Wada M, Kitayama M, Hashimoto H, et al. Brief reports: plasma ropivacaine concentrations after ultrasound-guided rectus sheath block in patients undergoing lower abdominal surgery. *Anesth Analg* 2012;114(1):230–232.

25. Petersen PL, Hilsted KL, Dahl JB, et al. Bilateral transversus abdominis plane (TAP) block with 24 hours ropivacaine infusion via TAP catheters: a randomized trial in healthy volunteers. *BMC Anesthesiol* 2013;13(1):30.

26. Sviggum HP, Niesen AD, Sites BD, et al. Trunk blocks 101: transversus abdominis plane, ilioinguinal-iliohypogastric, and rectus sheath blocks. *Int Anesthesiol Clin* 2012;50(1):74–92.

27. Nielsen RV, Fomsgaard JS, Siegel H, et al. Intraoperative ketamine reduces immediate postoperative opioid consumption after spinal fusion surgery in chronic pain patients with opioid dependency: a randomized, blinded trial. *Pain* 2017;158(3):463–470.

28. Naaz S, Ozair E. Dexmedetomidine in current anaesthesia practice—a review. *J Clin Diagn Res* 2014;8(10):GE01–GE04.

29. Vigneault L, Turgeon AF, Côté D, et al. Perioperative intravenous lidocaine infusion for postoperative pain control: a meta-analysis of randomized controlled trials. *Can J Anaesth* 2011;58(1):22–37.

30. Bergese SD, Candiotti K, Ayad SS, et al. The shortened infusion time of intravenous ibuprofen part 1: a multicenter, open-label, surveillance trial to evaluate safety and efficacy. *Clin Ther* 2015;37(2):360–367.

31. Gan TJ, Candiotti K, Turan A, et al. The shortened infusion time of intravenous ibuprofen, part 2: a multicenter, open-label, surgical surveillance trial to evaluate safety. *Clin Ther* 2015;37(2):368–375.

32. Jibril F, Sharaby S, Mohamed A, et al. Intravenous versus oral acetaminophen for pain: systematic review of current evidence to support clinical decision-making. *Can J Hosp Pharm* 2015;68(3):238–247.

33. Ljungqvist O, Scott M, Fearon KC. Enhanced recovery after surgery: a review. *JAMA Surg* 2017;152(3):292–298.

34. Bryson EO, Lipson S, Gevirtz C. Anesthesia for patients on buprenorphine. *Anesthesiol Clin* 2010;28(4):611–617.

35. Chern SY, Isserman R, Chen L, et al. Perioperative pain management for patients on chronic buprenorphine: a case report. *J Anesth Clin Res* 2013;3(250):1000250.

INDEX

Page numbers followed by f or t indicate material in figures or tables, respectively.